THE BIG PICTURE

PATHOLOGY

THE BIG PICTURE

PATHOLOGY

Walter L. Kemp, MD

Deputy State Medical Examiner
Forensic Science Division, Montana State Department of Justice
Missoula, Montana
and
Clinical Assistant Professor
The University of Texas Southwestern Medical Center at Dallas
Dallas, Texas

Dennis K. Burns, MD

Professor of Pathology
Distinguished Teaching Professor
The University of Texas Southwestern Medical Center at Dallas
Dallas, Texas

Travis G. Brown, MD

Resident, Department of Family Medicine
John Peter Smith Hospital
Forth Worth, Texas

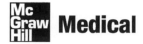

New York   Chicago   San Francisco   Lisbon   London   Madrid   Mexico City
New Delhi   San Juan   Seoul   Singapore   Sydney   Toronto

The *McGraw·Hill* Companies

Pathology: The Big Picture

1 2 3 4 5 6 7 8 9 0 CTP/CTP 0 9 8 7

ISBN: 978-0-07-147748-2
MHID: 0-07-147748-9

This book was set in Minion by Aptara.
The editors were Jason Mally, Susan Kelly, and Karen W. Davis.
The production supervisor was Phil Galea.
Project management was provided by Aptara.
The text designer was Alan Barnett.
The cover designers were Alan Barnett and Elizabeth Pisacreta.
Cover image caption: Detail of color-enhanced scanning electron micrograph (SEM) of metastasis, the spread of cancer cells.
Credit: Science Source/Photo Researchers, Inc.
China Translation & Printing Service, Ltd., was printer and binder.

This book is printed on acid-free paper.

Library of Congress Cataloging-in-Publication Data
Kemp, Walter L.
   Pathology : the big picture / by Walter L. Kemp, Dennis K. Burns, and Travis G. Brown.
      p. ; cm.
   ISBN-13: 978-0-07-147748-2 (pbk. : alk. paper)
   ISBN-10: 0-07-147748-9
   1. Pathology—Examinations, questions, etc. I. Burns, Dennis K.
II. Brown, Travis G. III. Title.
   [DNLM: 1. Pathology—Examination Questions. QZ 18.2 K32p
2007]
   RB119.K46 2007
   616.07076—dc22
                                                    2007024855

International Edition:
ISBN: 978-0-07-128729-6
MHID: 0-07-128729-9

DEDICATION

To my mom, dad, and sister, for your love, support, and encouragement.

To Julie Ann, for making me finally realize that spare time
should be treasured and used wisely and not wasted.

To Kris, for sharing Montana with me.

To my good friend, Brian Kieffer, for showing me how an individual can persevere
in the face of real and not imagined hardship, and that all the "rigors" of becoming a doctor
are truly an imagined hardship when compared to the challenges others face.

—*Walter L. Kemp*

My small contribution to this work is dedicated with love and gratitude to my wife, Carol,
and to my children, Kelly and Evan, my greatest sources of encouragement and inspiration.

—*Dennis K. Burns*

Dedicated to the memory of Earnest Franklin Brown (December 19, 1929–March 6, 2004)
and to my friend and classmate Kelly Dianne Werlinger, MD (March 19, 1974–July 10, 2006).

—*Travis G. Brown*

CONTENTS

About the Authors viii

Acknowledgments ix

How to Use This Book x

CHAPTER 1   Cellular Pathology 1

CHAPTER 2   Inflammation and Repair 13

CHAPTER 3   Pathology of the Immune System . . . 23

CHAPTER 4   Neoplasia 35

CHAPTER 5   Environmental and Nutritional Pathology 47

CHAPTER 6   Genetic Disorders 55

CHAPTER 7   Pediatric Pathology 71

CHAPTER 8   Hemodynamics 81

CHAPTER 9   Vascular Pathology 93

CHAPTER 10   Cardiac Pathology 109

CHAPTER 11   Neuropathology 133

CHAPTER 12   Hematopathology 173

CHAPTER 13   Pulmonary Pathology 209

CHAPTER 14   Gastrointestinal Pathology 231

CHAPTER 15   Pathology of the Liver, Gallbladder, and Pancreas 261

CHAPTER 16   Pathology of the Kidney and Bladder 283

CHAPTER 17   Pathology of the Male and Female Reproductive Tract and Breast 309

CHAPTER 18   Endocrine Pathology 337

CHAPTER 19   Pathology of the Bones and Joints 361

CHAPTER 20   Dermatopathology 379

CHAPTER 21   Practice Examination 391
                      Answers 413

Index 423

ABOUT THE AUTHORS

Walter L. Kemp, MD, completed his residency in Anatomic and Clinical Pathology and fellowship in Forensic Pathology at The University of Texas Southwestern Medical Center in Dallas, Texas. After completing his forensic fellowship, he was appointed Assistant Professor at UT Southwestern, where he taught for two years. In each of his two years as a faculty member, he received one of the Outstanding Teacher awards given by the second-year medical students. He is currently the Deputy State Medical Examiner in his home state of Montana, and continues to teach a two-week pathology course in the summer at UT Southwestern.

Dennis K. Burns, MD, is a full-time faculty member at The University of Texas Southwestern Medical Center, where he currently serves as Associate Director of the Division of Neuropathology, co-director of the first year medical neuroscience course, and director of the second year pathology course. In 2006, Dr. Burns was elected to the University of Texas Southwestern Academy of Teaching and to the University of Texas Academy of Health Science Education, and he received the title of Distinguished Teaching Professor. For his efforts, Dr. Burns has been awarded fourteen teaching awards by medical students and pathology residents at The University of Texas Southwestern Medical Center.

Travis G. Brown, MD, is a graduate of The University of Texas Southwestern Medical School in Dallas, Texas, and is currently a resident in the Department of Family Medicine at John Peter Smith Hospital in Fort Worth, Texas. He has served as a teaching assistant for the second-year pathology course, a course instructor for the USMLE examinations, and continues to teach the pathology section of the **spring** USMLE preparation course at UT Southwestern.

ACKNOWLEDGMENTS

To me, success in life is the result of many people's contributions, and this book is the result of the contributions of many people who have knowingly or unknowingly helped in this pursuit. Having the chance to write this book is one pinnacle of my career, and I would like to acknowledge and thank everyone who helped me reach this point.

To all of my grade school, junior high, and high school teachers for giving me an excellent background for college. To my high school English teacher Rose Goyen for proofreading my draft manuscript. To my college professors, most notably Father Joseph Harrington and Dr. John Addis, for giving me the best preparation possible for medical school.

To Dr. Tom Nicholas for calling me in to watch an autopsy, an experience that I had not signed up for but one that instantly decided my career path. To Drs. Kenneth Sims, William "Bill" Hunter, and Gary Dale for guiding my initial steps into pathology as a career. To Drs. Jeffrey Barnard, Joe Prahlow, Dave Dolinak, Joseph Guileyardo, and Steve Cohle for their willingness to do more than was required of them to further my education in autopsy and forensic pathology. To all of the pathologists at University of Texas Southwestern (UTSW) for giving me a broad and firm knowledge base in pathology. To Dr. Reade Quinton for pulling me out of the dark ages and teaching me that digital photography is a useful tool.

To Drs. Al Hesser and Ramiah Subramanian for supporting and encouraging my initial teaching efforts. To Dr. Swapan Nath for having faith in my teaching efforts and recommending me to Jason Malley as an author for this book.

To Jason Malley and McGraw-Hill for accepting my book proposal, and for guiding my efforts in the publication of this book. To Susan Kelly for her editorial expertise and constructive comments. And, to everyone at McGraw-Hill who turned the finished manuscript and images into the final product.

To Bill Unger, Dr. Gary Dale, and the Montana State Department of Justice for bringing me back to my home state of Montana. Lolo Peak, Mt. Sentinel, and the Bitterroot Mountains provided wonderful scenic inspiration for me while I wrote this book.

Although I created the majority of the images used in this text, I thank colleagues Drs. Janis Townsend-Parchman, Sheila Spotswood, Jill Urban, Gary Dale, Steve Cohle, Dominick Cavuoti, and Sean Hussey for contributing images that were not in my own collection. To Hamo Muergerditchian, Erin Duddleston, J.B. Watts, Sidney Eakin, Pamela Steger, and the other Dallas County Medical Examiner autopsy technicians for helping me take pictures, and to Beth McHenry, for taking some of the pictures used in the book. To Beverly Shackelford and Dr. Ramiah Subramanian for providing me the medical student glass slide study set to photograph. To Drs. Brad Barker, Jeffrey Barnard, Dave Dolinak, Buddy Fuda, Brian Levenson, Joni McClain, Keith Pinckard, Reade Quinton, Steven Kroft, Joseph Zhou, and Lynn Salzberger for allowing me to photograph their cases.

To Jesse Yanes, UTSW medical student, for reading a draft and offering helpful suggestions to improve the manuscript.

To Dr. Travis Brown, for his contributions and knowledge of clinical medicine, for sharing his recent test-taking expertise, for his strong continuing interest in pathology, and for his willingness to join this project at a late stage, coordinating his efforts with the demands of his busy residency program.

To Dr. Dennis Burns for being an outstanding mentor, colleague, and friend to a young pathologist and for his work on Chapters 1, 2, 4, 6, 8, 9, 10, 11, and 18.

Finally, to all the medical students I have had the privilege to work with for encouraging and promoting my enthusiasm for pathology and for teaching. And, to all the patients, who, through their deaths, have educated me, and who will continue to help teach future physicians. Thank you.

—*Walter L. Kemp*

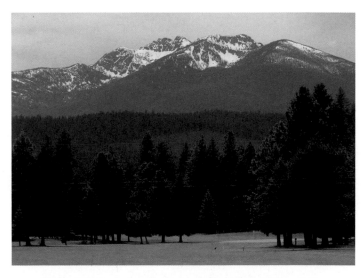

Libby, Montana, at the base of the Cabinet Mountains

HOW TO USE THIS BOOK

This pathology text offers medical students a concise and organized (i.e., "Big Picture") approach to the presentation of information needed for second-year medical school pathology courses and for study for the USMLE Step 1 licensing examination. In addition, pathology residents as well as other residents and physicians who want to brush up on their pathology may find the text useful.

Pathology: The Big Picture includes several features to facilitate learning and comprehension of the material.

■ Outline format discussion of pathologic conditions, with each condition's features divided by subheadings to promote access of information through an organized approach to each topic.

■ About 435 four-color images depicting important gross and microscopic pathologic conditions, complete with a detailed figure legend that explains the pathologic features and clinical presentation of the condition.

■ Integration of pathology and clinical information in support of the ongoing trends in medical education.

■ About 60 succinct tables highlighting key points (i.e., often those requiring memorization), as well as key comparison and contrast tables.

■ Practice examination of 130 questions, with clinical scenarios, and answers explained in relevant detail. In addition, 20 questions utilize images of common pathologic conditions with classic features.

Although the text is extensive, it primarily highlights common and uncommon conditions and common and uncommon causes of those conditions. Remember that the text is not an exhaustive source for material, and should be used as a review book or as a supplemental source to a general pathology textbook.

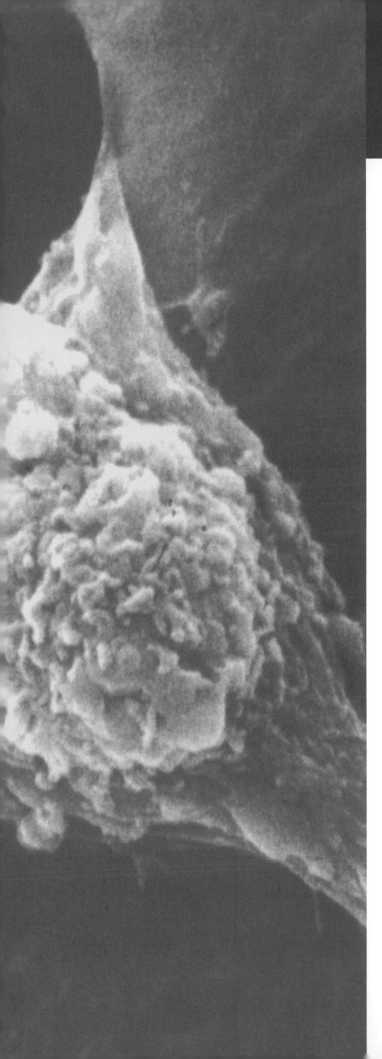

CHAPTER 1

CELLULAR PATHOLOGY

OVERVIEW

Pathology, in the broadest terms, is the **study of disease.** Disease occurs for many reasons. Some diseases represent spontaneous alterations in the ability of a cell to proliferate and function normally, and in other cases, disease results when external stimuli produce changes in the cell's environment that make it impossible for the cell to maintain homeostasis. In such situations, cells must adapt to the new environment. These adaptations include **hyperplasia, hypertrophy, atrophy,** and **metaplasia,** and can be physiologic or pathologic, depending upon whether the stimulus is normal or abnormal. A cell can adapt to a certain point, but if the stimulus continues beyond that point, failure of the cell, and hence the organ, can result. If cells cannot adapt to the pathologic stimulus, they can die. This chapter will discuss cellular adaptation, cell injury, cellular accumulations, and cellular aging.

CELLULAR ADAPTATION

Overview: The four basic types of cellular adaptation to be discussed in this section are hyperplasia, hypertrophy, atrophy, and metaplasia.

HYPERPLASIA

Basic description: Increase in the number of cells.

Types of hyperplasia

■ **Physiologic hyperplasia:** Occurs due to a normal stressor. For example, increase in the size of the breasts during pregnancy, increase in thickness of endometrium during menstrual cycle, and liver growth after partial resection.

■ **Pathologic hyperplasia:** Occurs due to an abnormal stressor. For example, growth of adrenal glands due to production of adrenocorticotropic hormone (ACTH) by a pituitary adenoma, and proliferation of endometrium due to prolonged estrogen stimulus.

Important point regarding hyperplasia: Only cells that can divide will undergo hyperplasia; therefore, hyperplasia of the myocytes in the heart and neurons in the brain does *not* occur.

HYPERTROPHY

Basic description: Increase in the size of the cell.

Types of hypertrophy

▪ **Physiologic hypertrophy:** Occurs due to a normal stressor. For example, enlargement of skeletal muscle with exercise.

▪ **Pathologic hypertrophy:** Occurs due to an abnormal stressor. For example, increase in the size of the heart due to aortic stenosis. Aortic stenosis is due to a change in the aortic valve, which obstructs the orifice, resulting in the left ventricle working harder to pump blood into the aorta.

Morphology of hyperplasia and hypertrophy: Both hyperplasia and hypertrophy result in an increase in organ size; therefore, both cannot always be distinguished grossly, and microscopic examination is required to distinguish the two (Figure 1-1).

Mechanisms by which hyperplasia and hypertrophy can occur: Up regulation or down regulation of receptors and induction of new protein synthesis. The two processes can occur together. For example, up regulation of receptors results in the induction of new protein synthesis; or up and down regulation of receptors and induction of new protein synthesis can occur as independent processes. The types of new proteins induced include transcription factors (e.g., c-Jun, c-Fos), contractile proteins (e.g., myosin light chain), and embryonic proteins (e.g., β-myosin heavy chain).

ATROPHY

Basic description: Decrease in the size of a cell that has at one time been of normal size.

Types of atrophy

▪ **Physiologic atrophy:** Occurs due to a normal stressor. For example, decrease in the size of the uterus after pregnancy.

▪ **Pathologic atrophy:** Occurs due to an abnormal stressor. In general, atrophy is due to the loss of stimulus to the organ. Specific types of loss of stimulus include loss of blood supply or innervation, loss of endocrine stimulus, disuse, mechanical compression, decreased workload, or aging.

Gross morphology of atrophy (Figure 1-2): The organ is smaller than usual. Atrophy occurs in a once normally developed organ. If the organ was never a normal size (i.e., because it did not develop normally), the condition is called **hypoplasia**.

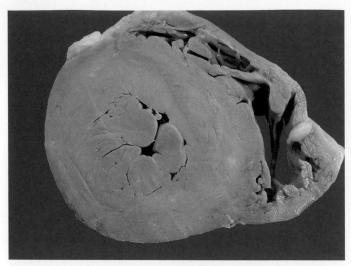

Figure 1-1. Cross-section of the heart of a patient with systemic hypertension. The patient had high blood pressure, which increased the workload of the left ventricle and resulted in concentric hypertrophy of the left ventricular myocardium. In response to the increasing pressure load, the cardiac myocytes increased their content of contractile proteins, resulting in enlargement of individual myocytes.

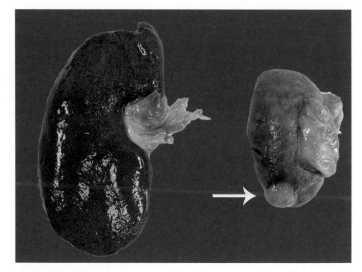

Figure 1-2. Kidneys from two different patients. The kidney on the left is normal in size, whereas the kidney on the right is atrophic. The kidney on the right was from a patient who had severe atherosclerosis of the renal artery, which led to ischemia (i.e., decreased perfusion) of the organ. Due to an insufficient supply of oxygen and nutrients, the cells of the kidney decreased in size to adapt. An incidental renal cell carcinoma is visible near the pole of the atrophic kidney (*arrow*).

METAPLASIA

Basic description: Change of epithelium at a site, or location, from one type of epithelium to another type. In metaplasia, the epithelium is normal in appearance but in an abnormal location.

Mechanism of metaplasia: The epithelium normally present at a site cannot handle the new environment so it converts to a type of epithelium that can adapt.

Examples: Barrett esophagus is due to reflux of gastric contents into the esophagus, which causes the epithelium type to convert from squamous to glandular (Figure 1-3 A and B). Squamous metaplasia in the lungs is due to exposure of respiratory epithelium to toxins in cigarette smoke.

CELL INJURY

Overview: Cell injury occurs when the cells cannot adapt to their new environment.

Causes of cell injury: Hypoxia (decreased oxygen), **ischemia** (decreased blood flow), physical and chemical agents, trauma, infectious agents, radiation and toxins, metabolic abnormalities (genetic or acquired), immune dysfunction (hypersensitivity reactions and autoimmune disease), aging, and nutritional imbalances.

Important points regarding cell injury

- Hypoxia and ischemia are two common sources of cellular injury. Of the two, ischemia is much more damaging because it involves hypoxia plus a lack of other nutrients and an accumulation of toxic cellular metabolites.

- When does injury occur? This varies from cell to cell. It depends upon the type, duration, and severity of injury, and the type, adaptability, and makeup of the affected cell.

- Cellular injury may or may not result in the death of the cell. Four cellular systems are especially vulnerable to cellular injury, and include:

  1. DNA
  2. Cell membranes
  3. Protein generation
  4. Adenosine triphosphate (ATP) production

- Although some of the causes of cellular injury have specific mechanisms, the mechanism of cellular injury due to many substances is not understood.

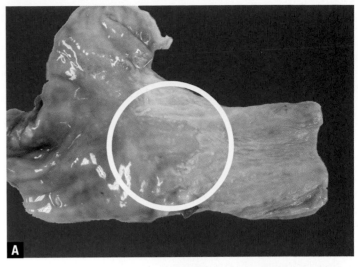

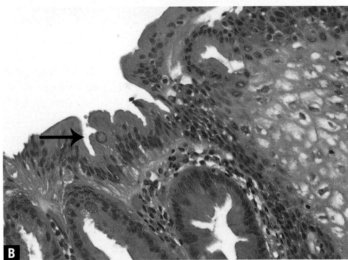

Figure 1-3. Barrett esophagus (glandular metaplasia). **A**, This specimen is taken from the region of the gastroesophageal junction and includes a segment of proximal stomach (on the left side) in continuity with the distal esophagus (on the right side). A small patch of mucosa with an appearance similar to the gastric mucosa extends proximally (*circle*), above the gastroesophageal junction. In this area, the normal stratified squamous epithelium of the esophagus has been replaced by glandular epithelium. Glandular metaplasia of the esophagus occurs in response to gastric acid reflux. **B**, The right side of the image shows stratified squamous epithelium, and the left side shows glandular epithelium, with goblet cells present (*arrow*). Transformation of one type of tissue to another type of tissue is termed metaplasia; in this case, stratified squamous epithelium was transformed to intestinal-type epithelium. Hematoxylin and eosin, 200×.

Mechanisms of cellular injury

1. **Hypoxia:** In general, decreased oxygen results in decreased production of ATP. ATP is normally required by the Na/K^+ pump and Ca^{2+} pump. When ATP levels decrease, these pumps fail and sodium (along with water, which follows sodium) enters the cell, causing swelling. Also, calcium enters the cell, which activates endonucleases, proteases, phospholipases, and DNAses, which damage the cell. Cells switch to anaerobic respiration to produce ATP, which results in accumulation of lactic acid. The accumulation of lactic acid decreases the cellular pH. Decreased pH causes disaggregation of ribosomes from endoplasmic reticulum.

2. **Generation of oxygen-derived free radicals by a stressing agent**

Basic description of free radical: A free radical is a molecule with an unpaired electron in the outer orbit. Another term for oxygen-derived free radicals is **reactive oxygen species.**

How free radicals are generated: Free radicals are generated by normal physiologic reduction-oxidation reactions, ultraviolet light, x-rays and ionizing radiation, and transitive metals. Also, metabolism of exogenous chemicals, such as carbon tetrachloride, induces formation of reactive oxygen species.

Damage by free radicals: Lipid peroxidation (damages cell membranes), DNA fragmentation, and protein cross-linking (e.g., sulfhydryl groups), which results in increased degradation and decreased activity.

Methods to prevent formation of reactive oxygen species

- **Catalase,** which degrades hydrogen peroxide.
- **Superoxide dismutase,** which converts superoxide to hydrogen peroxide.
- **Glutathione,** which catalyzes breakdown of hydroxyl radicals.
- **Vitamins A, C, and E,** which have an antioxidant effect.

3. **Chemical injury:** Some chemicals are directly toxic to the cells, and others require conversion to a toxic metabolite. For example, ethylene glycol (antifreeze) is not toxic, but its metabolite, oxalic acid, is. In contrast, cyanide directly inactivates cytochrome oxidase, which impairs the formation of ATP.

4. **Increased mitochondrial cytosolic calcium:** Increased mitochondrial cytosolic calcium leads to lipid peroxidation and formation of mitochondrial permeability transition (a nonselective pore that dissipates the proton gradient). Also, increased mitochondrial cytosolic calcium causes release of cytochrome c, which in turn activates apoptosis.

Two types of cellular injury

- **Reversible cellular injury:** As described above in the discussion of mechanisms of cellular injury, the decreased production of ATP causes sodium to enter the cell, bringing water and causing cellular and organelle swelling. The conversion from aerobic to anaerobic respiration decreases the pH of the cell. These changes are all reversible. If ATP is once again produced by the cell, the Na/K^+ ratio and pH will be corrected.

- **Irreversible cellular injury:** This type of injury occurs with damage to plasma or lysosomal membranes, loss of DNA, or loss of mitochondria. In these cases, the damage cannot be reversed. The two most important factors determining irreversible damage are membrane disturbances and the inability to reverse mitochondrial dysfunction.

Light microscope morphologic changes of cellular injury
- **Reversible injury:** Cellular swelling and fatty change.
- **Irreversible injury: Nuclear karyolysis** (loss of basophilia), **pyknosis** (shrinkage of nucleus), and **karyorrhexis** (fragmentation of nucleus).

Electron microscope morphologic changes of cellular injury
- **Reversible injury:** Cellular blebs and small mitochondrial densities.
- **Irreversible injury:** Ruptured lysosomes, myelin figures (which indicate phospholipid precipitation), lysis of endoplasmic reticulum, and large calcium rich mitochondrial densities.

CELL DEATH

Overview: There are two forms of cell death, **apoptosis** and **necrosis.** Apoptosis is controlled (programmed) breakdown of cells occurring in response to damage to DNA or as part of normal growth and development. Necrosis is uncontrolled break down of cells in response to injurious stimuli.

APOPTOSIS

Basic description: Programmed cell death.

Patterns of occurrence of apoptosis
- During growth and development, some cells serve a function in the growth phase but need to be removed after their purpose is fulfilled. In neonates, a rapid cell growth rate is necessary; in adults, however, unrestrained cell growth can lead to cancer.
- When DNA sustains irreparable damage (e.g., after low-dose radiation exposure), the cell must be destroyed so mutations that have developed will not be propagated. In this manner, apoptosis serves as a safety step by removing damaged cells from the body.

Phases of apoptosis
- **Initiation** is the phase in which **caspases** (*c*ysteine *asp*artic acid prote*ases*) become catalytically active.
- **Execution** is the phase in which the action of caspases causes death of cell.

Mechanism of apoptosis: There are multiple pathways by which apoptosis is initiated, including the extracellular and intracellular pathways. Both pathways share similar endpoints, culminating with the use of caspases and prevention of inflammatory reaction.
- **Initiation of extracellular pathway:** In Fas-Fas ligand binding, the Fas ligand binds to a member of the tumor necrosis

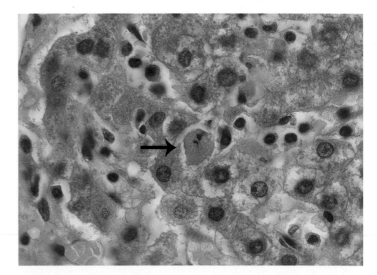

Figure 1-4. Acidophil body in the liver. The acidophil body (*arrow*) represents apoptosis, or programmed cell death. The nucleus is condensed and fragmented, and no inflammatory reaction has been elicited. Hematoxylin and eosin, 1000×.

factor family known as the Fas receptor. The activated Fas receptor in turn activates FADD (*Fas-associated death domain*), which in turn activates caspases.

- **Initiation of intracellular pathway:** The mitochondria release cytochrome c, which combines with Apaf-1 (*apoptosis activating factor-1*) to activate caspases.

- Caspases, which cleave DNA, are activated. DNA is cleaved in a coordinated manner so the fragments, if analyzed on a gel, will form a ladder. In contrast, in necrosis (an uncoordinated breakdown of DNA), the gel will be a smear.

- Apoptosis does not generate an inflammatory reaction as necrosis does. Fragments of cells express phosphatidyl serine, which is recognized by macrophages; therefore, fragments can be engulfed without generating an inflammatory reaction.

Morphology of apoptosis: The key feature microscopically is chromatin condensation and fragmentation (Figure 1-4).

NECROSIS

Basic description: Necrosis is a term used to describe uncontrolled death of cells due to one of the various causes of cellular injury.

Gross morphology of necrosis: Necrosis is typically manifested by softening and discoloration of the organ. Other processes can have a similar appearance, so the gross appearance of necrosis is not specific.

Microscopic morphology of necrosis: The two main types of necrosis are coagulative necrosis and liquefactive necrosis; however, there are several other variants.

- **Coagulative necrosis**

  Basic description: Coagulative necrosis is the type of necrosis in which protein denaturation is more prominent than enzymatic breakdown.

  Microscopic morphology of coagulative necrosis (Figure 1-5): There is increased eosinophilia of the cytoplasm and decreased basophilia of the nucleus; both are associated with preservation of the general cellular architecture (the organ type is identifiable).

  Organs affected by coagulative necrosis: Coagulative necrosis may occur in any organ. In organs with a high fat content, such as the brain, coagulative necrosis is followed rapidly by liquefactive necrosis.

- **Liquefactive necrosis**

  Basic description: Liquefactive necrosis occurs in situations in which enzymatic breakdown is more prominent than protein denaturation or in organs that lack a substantial protein-rich matrix (e.g., lipid-rich organs such as the brain).

  Microscopic morphology of liquefactive necrosis (Figure 1-6): There is loss of organ cellular architecture. In liquefactive necrosis of the brain, there are sheets of lipid-laden macrophages that replace the dead tissue.

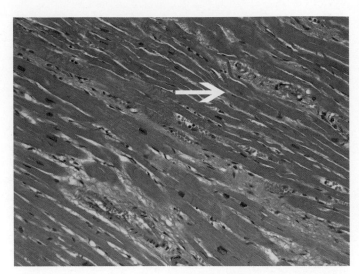

Figure 1-5. Coagulative necrosis of the myocardium. In the right upper half of the image (*arrow*), the cellular architecture is preserved; however, the cells are necrotic. The cytoplasm is eosinophilic from loss of protein, which imparts basophilia, and karyolysis of the nuclei has occurred (few cardiac myocyte nuclei are visible). Compare these features to the cells in the left lower half of the figure, which represent non-necrotic cardiac myocytes. Hematoxylin and eosin, 200×.

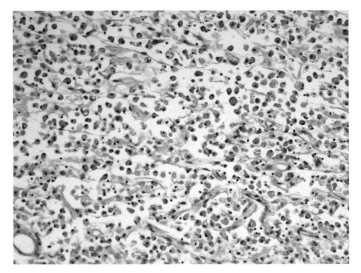

Figure 1-6. Liquefactive necrosis of the brain. The field contains sheets of foamy macrophages. In contrast to coagulative necrosis, the native tissue architecture has been lost. The foamy macrophages contain engulfed lipid-rich myelin and cellular debris. Liquefactive necrosis is common in tissues with relatively low protein content (e.g., the brain) or in situations where there is a high local concentration of proteolytic enzymes (e.g., abscesses; necrosis of pancreatic tissue). Hematoxylin and eosin, 200×.

Organs affected by liquefactive necrosis: Liquefactive necrosis is most commonly associated with organs that have a high fat and low protein content (e.g., the brain), or those with a high enzymatic content (e.g., the pancreas).

▨ **Fat necrosis:** Fat necrosis is a term applied to a change in adipose tissue due to trauma or the release of enzymes from adjacent organs (e.g., the pancreas). The trauma or enzymatic action causes a breakdown of lipid and a release of fatty acids, which combine with calcium to form chalky deposits.

▨ **Caseous necrosis** (Figure 1-7 *A* and *B*): Caseous necrosis is a "cheesy-looking" necrosis associated with tuberculosis infections and other granulomatous disease processes. Granulomas are a form of chronic inflammation due to some infections (e.g., mycobacterial), foreign bodies, and other chronic stimuli.

Important points regarding necrosis

▨ The terms coagulative and liquefactive necrosis are not mutually exclusive. For example, the death of heart muscle begins as coagulative necrosis, but once neutrophils enter the tissue as part of an inflammatory reaction and release enzymes, cellular architecture is lost (more consistent with liquefactive necrosis).

▨ Cell death involves the release of intracellular enzymes into blood. These enzymes in the blood can be measured and used clinically to detect disease.

▨ Cell death affects morphology (the shape of the cell) and function. Morphologic changes (both gross and microscopic) can develop over a period of time, while loss of function may occur almost immediately. Because of this immediate loss of function, the clinical manifestations of cellular injury may be present before the morphologic changes occur.

CELLULAR ACCUMULATIONS

Overview: Substances can accumulate in cells as a result of damage to the cell, or they can accumulate in the cells as the result of an intrinsic abnormality in metabolic function (e.g., genetic disease). The accumulation of substances in a cell may or may not cause damage to the cell. Substances that commonly accumulate are **lipofuscin** (also referred to as wear-and-tear pigment), calcium, protein, iron, fat, cholesterol, glycogen, and pigments.

General mechanisms of cellular accumulations: Include acquired or hereditary enzymatic defects, deposition of exogenous substances, and decreased metabolism of substances, which then accumulate.

LIPOFUSCIN

Basic description: Wear-and-tear pigment.

Mechanism of formation: Lipofuscin is a product of lipid peroxidation, which accumulates in lysosomes as the cell ages. The cell cannot rid itself of these lipofuscin-laden lysosomes.

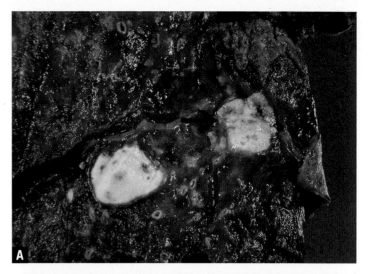

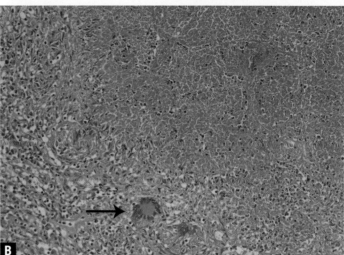

Figure 1-7. Caseous necrosis of the lung due to pulmonary tuberculosis. **A**, Gross section. The soft, cheese-like nature of the process is apparent (*arrows*). **B**, Microscopic section. The right side of the section shows central necrosis, and the left side shows large, activated ("epithelioid") histiocytes and a multinucleated giant cell (*arrow*). As in the case of liquefactive necrosis, tissue architecture is completely obliterated in foci of caseous necrosis. Hematoxylin and eosin, 200×.

Organs with lipofuscin accumulation: The most common organs where lipofuscin accumulates are the heart and liver.

Gross morphology of lipofuscin accumulation: Lipofuscin accumulation can impart brown discoloration to organ. Such organs may also be atrophic, giving rise to the term "**brown atrophy**."

Microscopic morphology of lipofuscin accumulation (Figure 1-8): Finely granular, yellow-brown pigment, which often surrounds the nucleus.

CALCIUM ACCUMULATION

Two forms of calcium deposition: Metastatic and dystrophic

Mechanism of metastatic calcification: Patients who have hypercalcemia have deposition of the calcium within normal or abnormal tissue. Some causes of hypercalcemia include increased parathyroid hormone (PTH) by a parathyroid adenoma or parathyroid gland hyperplasia; destruction of bone by tumors, vitamin D intoxication, or renal failure; and **sarcoidosis,** where macrophages activate vitamin D precursor.

Mechanism of dystrophic calcification: Patients who have normal levels of calcium have deposition of the calcium only within abnormal tissue, such as necrotic tissue.

Organs most commonly affected by calcium accumulation: Vasculature, kidneys, and lungs.

Gross morphology of calcium accumulation (Figure 1-9): Hard yellow nodules.

Microscopic morphology of calcium accumulation: Chunky, smooth, purple granules.

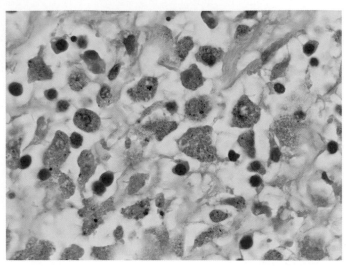

Figure 1-8. Lipofuscin pigment in macrophages in the liver. Almost all the cells in the photomicrograph contain finely granular, yellow-brown pigment, which is lipofuscin. Lipofuscin is the product of lipid peroxidation and free radical injury (wear-and-tear pigment) and, therefore, accumulates as the cell ages. This patient had centrilobular necrosis of the liver (normal hepatocytes are *not* visible in this section). Centrilobular hepatocytes normally contain lipofuscin, and the death of the hepatocytes releases the pigment for engulfment by macrophages. Hematoxylin and eosin, 400×.

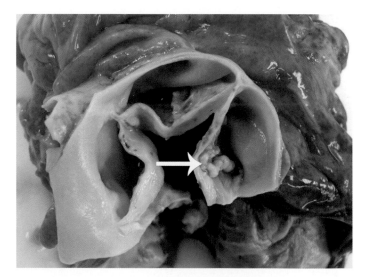

Figure 1-9. Dystrophic calcification of a tricuspid aortic valve. Dystrophic calcification involves damaged tissue such as would occur in an abnormal aortic valve (e.g., a bicuspid aortic valve, necrotic tissue, or normal age-related wear and tear, such as the aortic valve in elderly patients). The cusp on the right side of the photograph has prominent nodules of calcium on the sinus side of the valve leaflets (*arrow*).

PROTEIN ACCUMULATION

There are many different causes of protein accumulation. Accumulations often involve intermediate filaments; for example, **Mallory hyaline** in the liver (Figure 1-10) and neurofibrillary tangles seen in **Alzheimer disease.**

IRON ACCUMULATION

Two forms of iron accumulation: Hemosiderosis and hemochromatosis

Hemosiderosis: Accumulation of iron in organs without resultant side effects. The iron pigment is frequently within macrophages. Hemosiderin is a term used for aggregates of ferritin micelles (it stains positive with a Prussian blue stain).

Hemochromatosis

Basic description: Accumulation of iron in parenchymal cells resulting in side effects, including **congestive heart failure, diabetes mellitus** (from damage to the pancreas), and **cirrhosis.** Hemochromatosis can be acquired or hereditary.

Organs affected by hemochromatosis: Most common organs affected are the liver, skin, pancreas, and heart.

Microscopic morphology of iron accumulation (Figure 1-11): Chunky, yellow-brown granules.

FAT ACCUMULATION (STEATOSIS)

Organs affected: Most common organs affected are the liver, kidney, heart, and skeletal muscle.

Gross morphology of steatosis: Yellow discoloration of an organ.

Microscopic morphology of steatosis (see Figure 1-10): One or several clear vacuoles within the cell.

Important point regarding steatosis: Steatosis can indicate reversible damage or may be the sign of an intrinsic abnormality in fat metabolism.

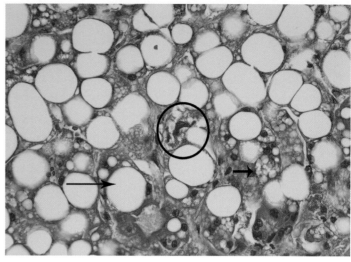

Figure 1-10. Fatty liver with Mallory hyaline. The hepatocytes in this photomicrograph show macrovesicular steatosis (one vacuole per cell) (*long arrow*) and microvesicular steatosis (many vacuoles per cell) (*short arrow*). The liver, along with the kidney and heart, are most commonly affected by fatty accumulations. In the center of the image is Mallory hyaline, the ropy, eosinophilic condensation within the cleared-out hepatocyte (*circle*). Mallory hyaline is a protein accumulation that is most commonly associated with alcohol use, and is composed of intermediate filaments. Hematoxylin and eosin, 200×.

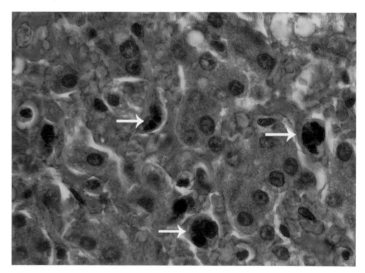

Figure 1-11. Hemosiderin within Kupffer cells in the liver. The hemosiderosis in this patient resulted from extravascular hemolysis. The hemosiderin represents iron accumulation from the breakdown of red blood cells. It has a characteristic chunky, yellow-brown appearance (*arrows*). Hematoxylin and eosin, 400×.

CHOLESTEROL ACCUMULATION

Organs affected: Blood vessels (by the process of atherosclerosis) or at sites of hemorrhage. Cholesterol accumulates within phagocytic cells.

GLYCOGEN ACCUMULATION

Organs affected: Glycogen accumulates as part of glycogen storage disorders (genetic diseases with a defect in enzymatic pathway of glycogen, such as **McArdle syndrome**). The most common organs affected are liver and skeletal muscle.

PIGMENTS

- **Exogenous pigments:** Tattoos and anthracotic pigment, which is carbonaceous debris from urban dwelling or cigarette smoking (Figure 1-12 *A* and *B*).
- **Endogenous pigments:** Melanin; bilirubin (Figure 1-13 *A* and *B*).

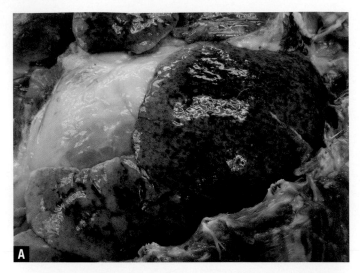

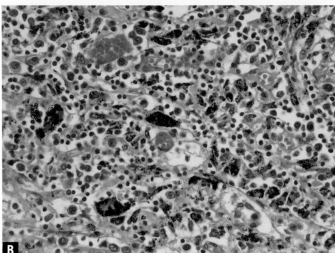

Figure 1-12. Anthracosis of the lung. Anthracotic pigment is carbonaceous material that accumulates in the lungs of smokers, coal miners, and persons living in a polluted environment such as a large city. The black anthracotic pigment typically accumulates in the pleural lymphatics (**A**), and microscopically has a finely stippled black appearance, found in interstitial and alveolar macrophages (**B**). Hematoxylin and eosin, 200×.

CELLULAR AGING

Basic description: Tissue cells have a fixed number of divisions, which they are capable of undergoing. Telomeres, or TTAGGG repeats, protect the ends of the chromosome, and they shorten with cell divisions. When the telomere is too short, the DNA is interpreted as broken.

Immortal cells: Telomerase (present in germ cells and stem cells) adds telomeres to the end of the chromosome, allowing the cell's lifespan to continue indefinitely.

WERNER SYNDROME

Manifestation: Premature aging.

Mutation: Defective DNA helicase.

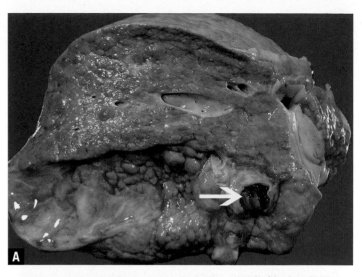

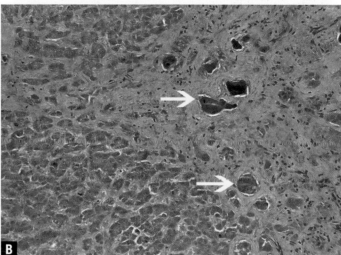

Figure 1-13. Cholestasis within a cirrhotic liver. Cholestasis is the accumulation of bile, an endogenous pigment produced by the liver. Its accumulation can result from many processes, including obstruction of the bile ducts. **A,** Grossly, cholestasis will result in a green discoloration of the liver. The arrow indicates a portal vein thrombus. **B,** Microscopically, bile is globular and yellow-green (right side of the slide, within the dilated bile ductules). The arrows indicate the accumulations of bile. Hematoxylin and eosin, 200×.

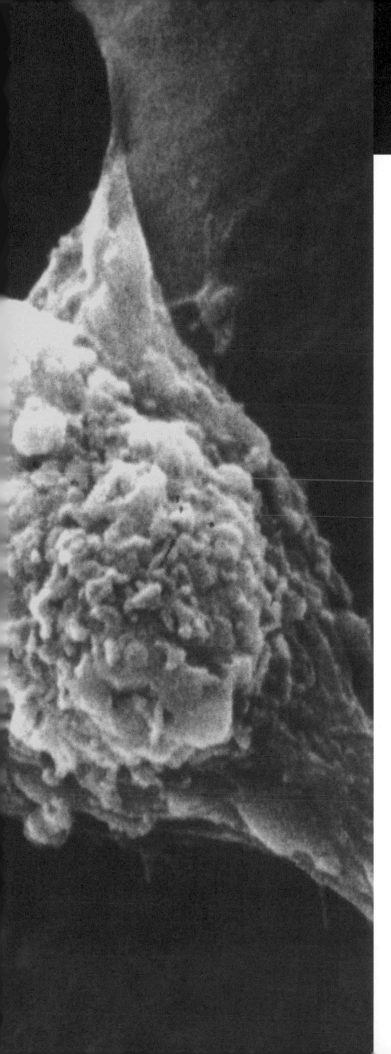

CHAPTER 2

INFLAMMATION AND REPAIR

OVERVIEW

Inflammation is the body's mechanism for coping with agents that could damage it. In other words, inflammation is a protective response to rid the body of the cause of cell injury and the resultant necrotic cells that cell injury produces. Although the processes of acute and chronic inflammation are an important protective mechanism used by the body to deal with potentially damaging agents, they are potentially damaging to the body and must be closely regulated. The basic steps in acute inflammation allow white blood cells to move from the blood to the tissue location where they are required. Acute inflammation can resolve completely if the inciting agent is removed, or it can have one of several other sequelae, including chronic inflammation. This chapter will discuss general concepts of acute and chronic inflammation, specific features of acute inflammation (including cardinal signs, causes, steps, and morphology and outcomes), specific features of chronic inflammation, and repair.

GENERAL CONCEPTS OF ACUTE AND CHRONIC INFLAMMATION

Overview: The body must undergo changes locally through vasodilation and increased vascular permeability in the area of the agent inciting the inflammatory reaction to allow white blood cells to accumulate. The white blood cells must then leave the blood vessel, cross the basement membrane, and be drawn to the area where they are needed. The process by which white blood cells are drawn to the area where they are needed is referred to as **chemotaxis.** Acute inflammation has a rapid onset, lasts for minutes to days, and is characterized by exudation of fluid and protein from vessels and emigration of neutrophils. Acute inflammation is a protective process that is designed to rid the body of the inciting agent and set up the process of repair. Chronic inflammation has a longer time course (days to years) and involves different cell types than does acute inflammation (lymphocytes and macrophages versus neutrophils). Also, *in chronic inflammation, tissue repair coexists with tissue destruction.*

ACUTE INFLAMMATION

Cardinal signs of acute inflammation: Rubor (red discoloration), calor (heat), dolor (pain), tumor (mass effect), and loss of function.

Causes of acute inflammation: Infection, trauma, physical and chemical agents, necrosis, foreign bodies, and immune reactions.

Stages of acute inflammation (Table 2-1)

1. **Vasodilation** (after a transient vasoconstriction)
   - **How:** Vasodilation occurs through release of mediators from cells. These mediators include histamine, prostacyclin (PGI_2), and nitric oxide (NO).
   - **Why:** Vasodilation increases the hydrostatic pressure by causing slowing (sludging) of blood flow. Sludging of blood also causes margination of leukocytes along the wall of the blood vessel.

2. **Increased vascular permeability** (increased leakiness of vessels)
   - **How:** Increased vascular permeability occurs through release of mediators from cells. These mediators include histamine and leukotrienes C_4, D_4, and E_4.
   - **Why:** Increased vascular permeability allows fluid to cross into the interstitial tissue, which increases protein levels in the interstitial tissue, thereby decreasing osmotic pressure in the blood and increasing osmotic pressure in the interstitial tissue. These changes cause fluid to flow out of the vessel, leading to edema of the interstitial tissue.
   - **Mechanisms of increased vascular permeability:** Several mechanisms increase vascular permeability, some of which are physiologic and some of which are pathologic.

TABLE 2-1. Mediators of Acute Inflammation

Effect Produced	Mediator Responsible
Vasodilation	Histamine, PGI_2, NO
Increased vascular permeability	Histamine, bradykinin, TNF, IL-1 Leukotrienes C_4, D_4, and E_4
Rolling of white blood cells	Sialyl-Lewis-X on white blood cells E-selectin on endothelium
Pavementing of white blood cells	LFA-1 and Mac-1 on white blood cells ICAM-1 and VCAM-1 on endothelium
Transmigration	CD31 (PECAM) on white blood cells and endothelium
Chemotaxis–endogenous mediators	C5a, LTB_4, IL-8
Opsonins	IgG, C3b, Collectins

PGI_2, prostacyclin; NO, nitric oxide; TNF, tumor necrosis factor; IL, interleukin; LFA-1, leukocyte function-associated antigen-1; ICAM, intercellular adhesion molecule; VCAM, vascular cell adhesion molecule; PECAM, platelet endothelial cell adhesion molecule; LTB_4, leukotriene B_4.

Endothelial contraction and retraction are physiologic mechanisms and are due to mediators. Direct endothelial injury is a pathologic mechanism due to damaging agents not under the body's control.

- **Endothelial contraction** (referred to as immediate-transient response)
  - **Mediators:** Histamine, bradykinin, and leukotrienes.
  - **Vessels affected:** Postcapillary venules.
  - **Time course:** Immediate; short lived (up to 30 minutes).
- **Endothelial cell retraction**
  - **Mediators:** Tumor necrosis factor (TNF) and interleukins (e.g., IL-1).
  - **How:** Structural rearrangement of cytoskeleton.
  - **Time course:** 4–6 hours (referred to as delayed response); long lived.
- **Direct endothelial injury**
  - **Mediators:** Bacterial enzymes.
  - **Vessels affected:** All.
  - **How:** Endothelial cell necrosis.
  - **Time course:** Immediate (referred to as immediate-sustained response).
- **Delayed prolonged response**
  - Due to ultraviolet light, x-ray, and mild thermal injury.
  - Uncertain mechanism.
- **Leukocyte-mediated damage**

3. **Movement of white blood cells from blood vessels into soft tissue at the site of inflammation:** The steps required are **rolling, pavementing,** and **transmigration. Chemotaxis** is the process by which white blood cells are drawn to the site of acute inflammation.

Rolling

- **Basic description:** Loose, intermittent contact of white blood cells with endothelium, partially due to margination of white blood cells from stasis of blood.
- **Mediators:** Sialyl-Lewis X molecules on white blood cells bind with E-selectins on endothelial cells.

Pavementing

- **Basic description:** Tight, constant contact of white blood cells with endothelium.
- **Mediators:** Leukocyte function-associated antigen-1 (LFA-1) and Mac-1 on white blood cells bind with intercellular adhesion molecule 1 (ICAM-1) and vascular cell adhesion molecule 1 (VCAM-1) on endothelial cells.

Transmigration

- **Basic description:** White blood cells crossing through the endothelial layer.
- **Mediators:** CD31 or platelet endothelial cell adhesion molecule (PECAM) on both white blood cells and endothelial cells.

CHEMOTAXIS

Basic description: Process by which white blood cells are drawn to the site of inflammation.

Mediators

▪ **Exogenous mediators:** Bacterial polysaccharides.

▪ **Endogenous mediators:** C5a, leukotriene B_4 (LTB_4), and IL-8. The endogenous mediators act through various mechanisms. With most, however, the activation of G-protein receptors ultimately results in activation of GTPases, which cause polymerization of actin.

The role of leukocytes (see Table 2-1)

▪ White blood cells recognize foreign particles through mannose and scavenger receptors. Opsonins are particles that bind to foreign material and signal leukocytes to remove it. **Types of opsonins** include:

1. IgG (recognized by Fc receptor on white blood cells).

2. C3b (recognized by CR 1, 2, and 3 on leukocytes).

3. Collectins (recognized by C1q on leukocytes).

▪ White blood cells engulf the foreign particles (most often bacteria) using the above-mentioned receptors.

▪ Killing and/or degradation of foreign substances occurs by one of several methods:

○ **Reduced nicotinamide adenine dinucleotide phosphate (NADPH) oxidase** (has membrane and cytoplasmic component). It uses two oxygen molecules to produce a superoxide radical ($O_2^{\cdot-}$), and the superoxide radical converts to hydrogen peroxide.

○ **Myeloperoxidase:** Converts hydrogen peroxide and halogen (Cl^-) to $HOCl^{\cdot}$, which causes halogenation or lipid or protein peroxidation.

○ Other methods of bacterial killing include bactericidal permeability increasing protein, lysozyme, and major basic protein.

DISEASES ASSOCIATED WITH IMPAIRED INFLAMMATORY RESPONSE

CHRONIC GRANULOMATOUS DISEASE

Basic description: Loss of NADPH oxidase results in chronic granulomatous disease. NADPH oxidase has two components—membrane and cytoplasmic; both components must be brought together for the enzyme to function.

Inheritance: The mutation for the autosomal recessive form of chronic granulomatous disease results in a defective cytoplasmic component, and the mutation for the X-linked form of chronic granulomatous disease results in a defective membrane component.

Effect of mutation: Inability to form hydrogen peroxide.

Important point regarding chronic granulomatous disease: Many bacterial organisms produce hydrogen peroxide. The hydrogen peroxide produced by bacteria can be utilized by myeloperoxidase, thus bypassing the need for NADPH oxidase. However, many organisms produce catalase, which degrades the hydrogen peroxide they produce.

CHÉDIAK-HIGASHI SYNDROME

Inheritance of Chédiak-Higashi syndrome: Autosomal recessive.

Mutation: A mutation occurs in a cytosolic protein, which plays a role in vesicle traffic.

Effects of mutation: Decreased cellular killing of bacteria because of reduced transfer of lysosomal enzymes to phagocytic vesicles. Other effects of mutation include albinism, nerve defects, and platelet disorders.

MORPHOLOGY OF ACUTE INFLAMMATION

Overview: Types of acute inflammation include serous, fibrinous, and purulent; however, mixed forms with features of one or more of these types may be seen.

- **Serous inflammation**
  - **Appearance:** Relatively clear, watery fluid.
  - **Contents of fluid:** Few cells; most of the inflammation is fluid (i.e., a transudate; a protein-poor fluid with a specific gravity < 1.012).
  - **Seen in:** Viral infections and burns.
- **Fibrinous inflammation**
  - **Appearance:** Finely particulate, thick fluid.
  - **Contents of fluid:** Much more protein and cells than serous inflammation (i.e., an exudate; a protein-rich fluid with a specific gravity > 1.020).
  - **Seen in:** Uremic and postmyocardial infarct pericarditis.
- **Purulent inflammation** (Figure 2-1 *A, B,* and *C*)
  - **Appearance:** Pus (thick, white-yellow fluid).
  - **Contents of fluid:** Neutrophils, protein, and necrotic cells (i.e., an exudate).
  - **Seen in:** Bacterial and fungal infections.

OUTCOMES OF ACUTE INFLAMMATION

Overview: Outcomes of acute inflammation include resolution, abscess formation, ulcers, fistula formation, chronic inflammation, and scar formation.

- **Resolution**
  - **Basic description:** The inciting agent is removed, and all damage done by the inciting agent and inflammatory cells is repaired.
  - **Requirements for resolution:** The organ affected must be capable of regeneration, and the body must be capable of completely dealing with the inciting agent.

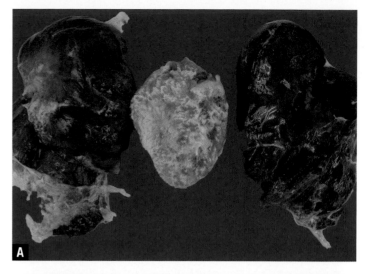

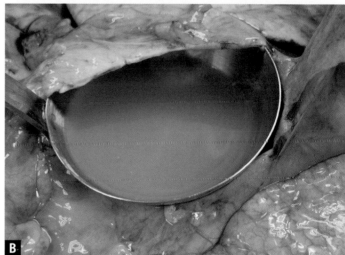

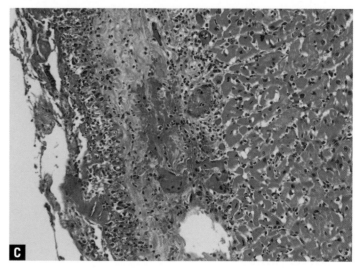

Figure 2-1. Purulent pericarditis and purulent pleuritis. **A,** In the center of the photograph is a heart, with the respective lungs to the right and left side of it. Covering most of the epicardial surface of the heart and a patchy distribution of the visceral pleurae of the lungs is a thick, yellow-white fluid, which is pus. Pus (i.e., purulent fluid) is composed predominantly of neutrophils admixed with plasma proteins and cellular debris. The source of most purulent infections is often bacterial organisms. **B,** Pus within the pericardial sac. **C,** A photomicrograph of the epicardial surface of the heart. Note the thick layer of inflammatory cells, predominantly neutrophils on the left side of the image. Hematoxylin and eosin, 200×.

- **Important point:** For epithelium to regenerate, the basement membrane must be intact because it serves as the guide upon which new cells are laid down. If the basement membrane is destroyed, the new cells can be laid down, but they are unorganized. For organs to regenerate, the framework (i.e., the connective tissue scaffold) of the organ must be intact.

- **Abscess** (Figure 2-2 *A* and *B*)
  - **Basic description:** Walled off collection of pus (neutrophils and necrotic debris).
  - **Requirements for abscess formation:** The body cannot rid itself of the inciting agent, or the process of repair and scarring is occurring more rapidly in the tissue around the site of the abscess.
  - **Location:** Any organ in the body.
  - **Complications of an abscess:** Pain, fever, rupture, and swelling.

- **Ulcer** (Figure 2-3)
  - **Basic description:** Loss of the mucosa and deeper tissues. If only the mucosa is lost, the correct term is an **erosion.**
  - **Requirements for ulcer formation:** The body cannot rid itself of the inciting agent.
  - **Microscopic morphology of an ulcer:** The ulcer has four layers, which recapitulate steps from acute inflammation to repair. The layers, from superficial to deep, are fibrin, neutrophils, granulation tissue, and fibrosis.
  - **Location:** Most commonly seen in the gastrointestinal tract.
  - **Complications of an ulcer:** Pain; hemorrhage, if the ulcer involves a vessel; and perforation, resulting in hemorrhage within a cavity or the lumen of the gastrointestinal tract, or seeding of the peritoneal cavity with the contents of the gastrointestinal tract, causing peritonitis.

- **Fistula** (Figure 2-4 *A*, *B*, and *C*)
  - **Basic description:** Anomalous patent connection between two organs; most commonly organs with a lumen.
  - **Requirement for fistula formation:** Inflammatory process involving full thickness of the wall of an organ, duct, or blood vessel. The wall adheres to an adjacent wall, which is subsequently involved by the inflammatory process, allowing communication between the lumens.
  - **Example:** Enterocutaneous fistula (skin to colon, occurring in colon cancer or inflammatory bowel disease).
  - **Complications:** Depends upon the nature of the two organs involved. For example, the fistula can serve as a conduit by which infection can enter other organs or as a conduit between a vessel and an organ, resulting in massive hemorrhage.

- **Chronic inflammation**

- **Scar formation**
  - **Basic description:** Replacement of lost parenchyma with disorganized connective tissue (e.g., collagen).
  - **Requirements for scar formation:** Loss of tissue in an organ not capable of regeneration or loss of basement membrane or other framework required for successful regeneration.
  - **Complications:** Loss of function.

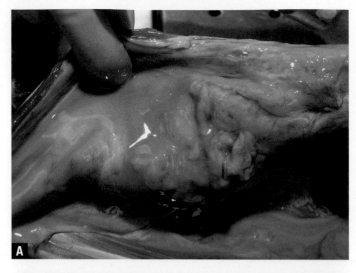

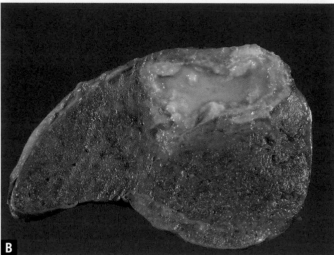

Figure 2-2. Abdominal wall and splenic abscesses. An abscess is a walled-off collection of pus. **A**, The abscess is in the right side of the abdominal wall. **B**, The abscess is in the spleen. Abscesses can rupture and release their contents (including bacteria) into body cavities and hollow organs, such as the gastrointestinal tract.

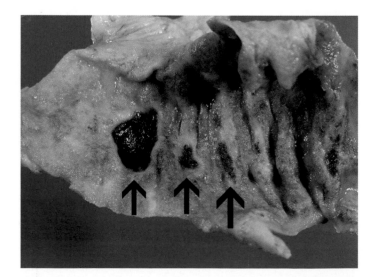

Figure 2-3. Duodenal ulcers. The arrows indicate superficial ulcers in the duodenum. Peptic ulcer disease is a chronic condition, often due to infection with *Helicobacter pylori*. Stress ulcers, as shown in the photograph, develop acutely, often due to burns, head injuries, or other forms of physical stress.

CHRONIC INFLAMMATION

Overview: Prolonged inflammation consisting of active inflammation and tissue destruction and repair, all occurring simultaneously. Chronic inflammation can follow acute inflammation, but it can also occur as a low-grade, asymptomatic, prolonged response to an inciting agent.

Causes of chronic inflammation: Viral, persistent microbial infection, prolonged exposure to toxin, and autoimmune dysfunction.

Cells involved in chronic inflammation: Macrophages and lymphocytes (Figure 2-5).

■ **Activated macrophages produce**

  ○ Proteases, IL-1, TNF, arachidonic acid metabolites, NO (IL-1 and TNF activate lymphocytes).

  ○ Angiogenesis and growth factors, such as platelet-derived growth factor (PDGF) or fibroblast growth factor (FGF).

■ **Activated lymphocytes produce**

  ○ FGF stimulates fibroblasts to produce collagen, which results in scarring.

  ○ PDGF and transforming growth factor-β (TGF-β).

  ○ Interferon-γ (activates macrophages).

Important type of chronic inflammation: Granulomatous inflammation

■ **Basic description of granuloma:** Collection of epithelioid histiocytes.

■ **Morphology of granuloma:** Collection of activated macrophages (i.e., epithelioid histiocytes); can have multinucleated giant cells (Figure 2-6).

■ **Causes:** Mycobacteria, fungi, foreign material, sarcoidosis, and silica.

REPAIR

Overview: The process of repair begins very early. Repair involves regeneration of the parenchyma or replacement of damaged tissue with a scar if regeneration is not possible. The process of complete regeneration (i.e., resolution of acute inflammation) requires an organ that is composed of cells that can divide and an intact basement membrane and connective tissue scaffolding.

Definitions: Healing versus regeneration

■ **Regeneration** is complete replacement of damaged cells, with no scar formation.

  ○ Can occur in renewing tissues (e.g., gastrointestinal tract and skin).

  ○ Can occur in stable tissues (e.g., compensatory growth in the liver and kidney).

  ○ Regeneration requires an intact connective tissue scaffold.

■ **Healing** is regeneration of cells combined with scarring and fibrosis.

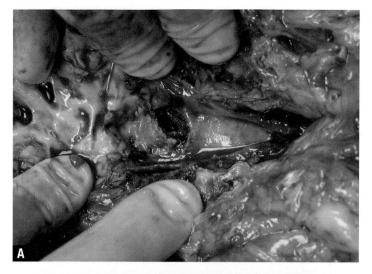

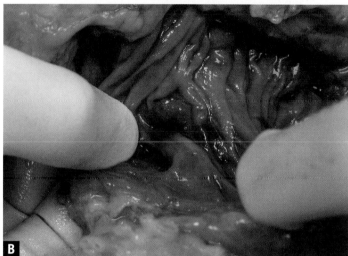

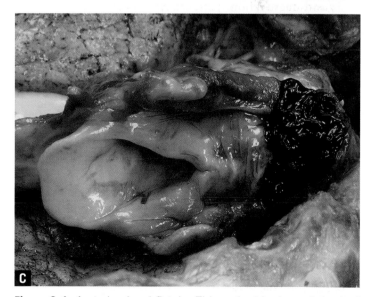

Figure 2-4. Aortoduodenal fistula. This patient had an abdominal aortic aneurysm, which was repaired with a graft. The graft became infected and was surgically replaced with a neointimal saphenous vein graft, which also became infected. A tract developed between the neointimal graft and the duodenum. There is a defect in the neointimal aortic graft (**A**) (center of the photograph), which communicated with the duodenum (**B**) through a fistula, resulting in a massive amount of blood entering the gastrointestinal tract, which is visible in the esophagus of the patient (**C**).

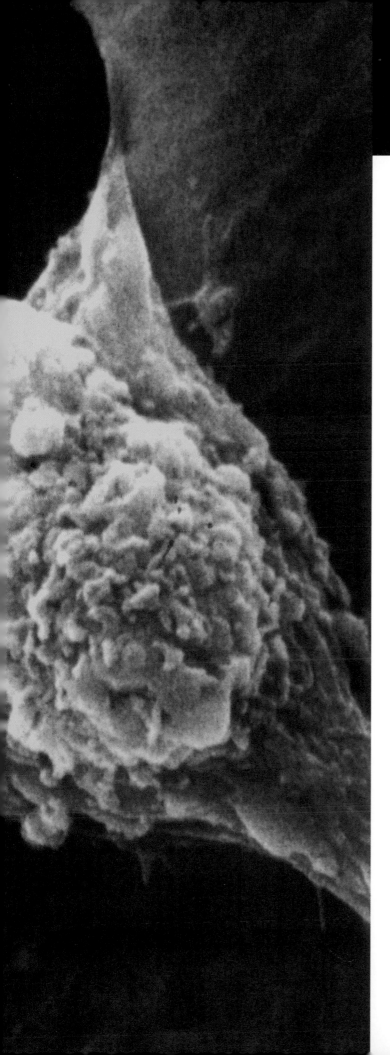

CHAPTER 3

PATHOLOGY OF THE IMMUNE SYSTEM

OVERVIEW

Diseases of the immune system take many forms, including **hypersensitivity reactions, autoimmune disorders,** and **immunodeficiency states.** Hypersensitivity reactions occur as one of four types (types I–IV). Autoimmune diseases are the result of a failure in the immune system to recognize self-antigens, resulting in production of antibodies that react against normal components of cells. Most of the autoimmune diseases are associated with one or more specific antibodies, which can be identified by laboratory tests to aid in diagnosis. Immunodeficiency states can be hereditary or acquired. A major cause of acquired immunodeficiency is human immunodeficiency virus (HIV) infection. The concepts of immunity are also important in regard to transplantation efforts. This chapter will discuss hypersensitivity reactions, transplantation pathology, autoimmune diseases, amyloidosis, and both hereditary and acquired immunodeficiency.

HYPERSENSITIVITY REACTIONS

Overview: There are four types of hypersensitivity reactions, each of which has a different mechanism. These four types of hypersensitivity reactions will be discussed below.

TYPE I HYPERSENSITIVITY REACTION

Mechanism: Exposure to an antigen results in the formation of IgE. The antigen reacts with $CD4^+$ cells, which differentiate to T_H2 cells. T_H2 cells release interleukin-3 (IL-3), IL-4, and IL-5. IL-5 stimulates eosinophils, and IL-4 activates IgE-producing B cells. The IgE binds to mast cells. Subsequent exposure to the same antigen results in binding of the antigen to IgE bound to mast cells, with the consequence of degranulation of the mast cells and release of mediators (e.g., histamine). The release of mediators causes increased vascular permeability, leading to edema and increased smooth muscle contraction and eventually to bronchoconstriction.

Sequence of events in type I hypersensitivity reaction

1. **Early phase** (occurs within 5–30 minutes of exposure to antigen): Characterized by vasodilation, increased vascular

permeability, and increased smooth muscle contraction. The early phase is due to binding of antigen to IgE bound to mast cells, with subsequent degranulation of the mast cells and release of mediators.

2. **Late phase** (occurs after 2–24 hours and lasts for days): Characterized by infiltration by neutrophils, eosinophils, basophils, and monocytes, and results in mucosal damage due to release of mediators by these recruited inflammatory cells.

Forms of type I hypersensitivity reactions

- **Systemic anaphylaxis:** Due to parenteral administration of antigen; for example, a bee sting or a reaction to penicillin.

- **Local reaction:** Urticaria (hives).

Causes: Penicillin, angiotensin-converting enzyme (ACE) inhibitors, intravenous (IV) contrast and other drugs, proteins (e.g., insect venoms), and food.

Clinical presentation of type I hypersensitivity reaction: Symptoms and signs include abrupt onset (within 30 minutes of exposure to antigen) of rash, nausea and vomiting and facial swelling, wheezing and stridor, and hypotension and tachycardia. Serum tryptase is a marker of anaphylaxis.

Complications of systemic anaphylaxis: Death due to airway compromise from laryngeal edema.

TYPE II HYPERSENSITIVITY REACTION

Overview of general mechanism: Antibodies directed against target antigens on cells or in extracellular matrix. The target antigens may be endogenous or absorbed exogenous antigens.

Specific mechanisms: There are three specific mechanisms by which type II hypersensitivity reactions occur. The three mechanisms are complement-dependent reactions, antibody-dependent cell-mediated cytotoxicity, and antibody-mediated cellular dysfunction.

- **Complement-dependent reactions**
  - **Mechanism:** Antibody bound to antigen can fix complement and cause direct lysis of the cell through production of the membrane attack complex (MAC), or the complement can coat cells with C3b (an opsonin) and promote phagocytosis of the antigen.
  - **Example:** Glomerulonephritis.
- **Antibody-dependent cell-mediated cytotoxicity**
  - **Mechanism:** Cell types that bear receptors for the Fc portion of IgG, such as neutrophils, eosinophils, macrophages, and natural-killer (NK) cells, mediate removal of antigen.
  - **Examples:** Transfusion reactions, **erythroblastosis fetalis,** and autoimmune hemolytic anemia.
- **Antibody-mediated cellular dysfunction**
  - **Mechanism:** Antibodies themselves affect function of the antigen.
  - **Examples: Graves disease** is due to an antibody that activates the thyroid-stimulating hormone (TSH) receptor,

resulting in hyperthyroidism. **Myasthenia gravis** is due to antibodies against the acetylcholine (ACh) receptor, impairing neuromuscular transmission.

TYPE III HYPERSENSITIVITY REACTION

Mechanism: Antibodies bind to the antigen, forming an immune complex. The antigens can be exogenous (e.g., viral proteins) or endogenous (e.g., DNA). These immune complexes can form in situ, or they can form in the vasculature and subsequently be deposited in organs, where they cause damage. The immune complex causes activation of the complement cascade. Note that immune complexes are commonly formed for various reasons, but only under certain circumstances do they elicit an immune reaction.

Examples: Immune–complex-mediated vasculitis and forms of glomerulonephritis.

TYPE IV HYPERSENSITIVITY REACTION

General mechanism: Mediated by sensitized T cells rather than by antibodies.

Specific mechanisms

- **Delayed form of type IV hypersensitivity reaction:** $CD4^+$ helper T cells (T_H1 type) sensitized from previous exposure to an antigen secrete interferon-γ, which activates macrophages. Activated macrophages secrete IL-12, which causes differentiation of T_H1 cells.
  - **Microscopic morphology:** Stimulation of macrophages results in granulomas (i.e., collections of epithelioid histiocytes).
  - **Inciting agents:** Mycobacteria, fungi, and parasites.
  - **Examples:** Tuberculin reaction and contact dermatitis.
- **Cell-mediated cytotoxicity:** Sensitized $CD8^+$ cells kill antigen-bearing cells. The antigens are presented by class I major histocompatibility complex (MHC) molecules. There are two mechanisms by which this occurs: the perforin-granzyme system and the FAS-FAS ligand system.
  - **Perforin-granzyme system:** Perforin produces holes in the plasma membrane of cells, allowing granzyme to enter the cells. Granzyme then activates apoptosis through stimulation of caspase activity.
  - **FAS-FAS ligand system:** The sensitized T lymphocytes have FAS ligand, which binds to FAS on target cells, leading to apoptosis.

TRANSPLANTATION PATHOLOGY

Overview: Rejection of transplanted organs may be cellular or humoral, with cellular rejection mediated by T cells, and humoral rejection mediated by antibodies. In addition, rejection may be classified based upon its timing following the transplant procedure. The rejection can be hyperacute, acute, or chronic.

CELLULAR REJECTION

Mechanism: Cellular rejection is due to hypersensitivity of the recipient's CD4$^+$ cells, which results in killing of graft cells by CD8$^+$ cells that have matured into cytotoxic T lymphocytes. The cytotoxic T lymphocytes kill graft cells through the perforin-granzyme pathway or the FAS-FAS ligand pathway.

Forms of cellular rejection

■ **Direct:** The body recognizes MHC molecules on the surface of the antigen-presenting cells in the graft.

■ **Indirect:** Antigens of the graft are presented by the recipient's cells.

HUMORAL REJECTION

Overview: Humoral rejection is due to preformed antibodies or formation of antibodies against graft vasculature.

CLASSIFICATION OF FORMS OF REJECTION BASED UPON TIMING OF REJECTION AFTER TRANSPLANTATION

Hyperacute rejection

■ **Mechanism:** Humoral reaction due to preformed antibodies to graft endothelium.

■ **Time course:** Minutes following transplantation.

■ **Morphology:** Grossly, there is cyanosis of the organ and a mottled parenchyma; microscopically, there is endothelial injury, neutrophils in arterioles, and infarcts of parenchyma.

Acute rejection

■ **Mechanism:** Cellular or humoral reaction.

■ **Time course:** Days to months to years following transplantation.

■ **Microscopic morphology of acute cellular rejection** (Figure 3-1): Interstitial mononuclear infiltrate, edema, interstitial hemorrhage, and endothelialitis (i.e., swollen endothelial cells).

■ **Microscopic morphology of acute humoral rejection:** Necrotizing vasculitis, neutrophilic infiltrate, and infarcts of parenchyma.

■ **Important point:** An acute cellular rejection will respond to cyclosporine.

Chronic rejection

■ **Mechanism:** Possibly, the indirect form of cellular rejection plays an important role.

■ **Time course:** 4–6 months to years following the graft.

■ **Microscopic morphology:** Vascular changes, interstitial fibrosis, interstitial mononuclear infiltrate, and ischemia with subsequent tissue loss.

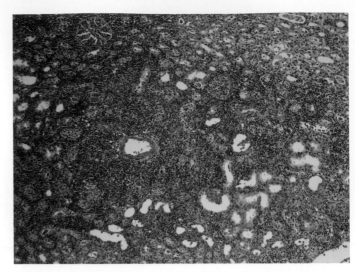

Figure 3-1. Acute cellular rejection in the kidney. In this low-power view of a renal transplant, note the infiltrate of lymphocytes among the glomeruli and renal tubules. Hematoxylin and eosin, 100×.

HEMATOPOIETIC TRANSPLANTATIONS

GRAFT VERSUS HOST DISEASE (GVHD)

Basic description: Immune competent cells in the graft recognize antigens in the host.

Occurrence: In bone marrow transplants; in solid organ transplants when the organ is rich in lymphocytes (e.g., liver); and in non-irradiated blood.

Forms of GVHD

- **Acute GVHD**
  - **Time course:** Days to weeks.
  - **Organs affected (and complications):** Skin (rash), bile ducts (jaundice), and gastrointestinal mucosa (bloody diarrhea).
  - **Associated findings:** Acute GVHD results in immunodeficiency and thus patients can have secondary infections, including cytomegalovirus (CMV) pneumonia.
- **Chronic GVHD**
  - **Organs affected (and complications):** Dermis and skin appendages (fibrosis), bile ducts (cholestatic jaundice), and esophagus (strictures).
  - **Associated findings:** Chronic GVHD results in immunodeficiency; thus patients can have secondary infections, including CMV pneumonia.

AUTOIMMUNE DISEASES

Overview: Autoimmune disease results from a failure of self-tolerance. In self-tolerance, the body inactivates its immune response against antigens, which are present on and in its own cells. Autoimmune diseases can be organ specific or systemic, and are often associated with a specific antibody (Table 3-1).

General mechanism: Loss of self-tolerance. Contributing factors include susceptibility genes (e.g., certain HLA types such as *B27* in **ankylosing spondylitis**) and infections. Infections may upregulate expression of costimulatory proteins on antigen-presenting cells, or microbes can have antigens that are similar in structure to self-antigens. Antibodies against these foreign antigens then cross-react with self-antigens.

TABLE 3-1. Autoimmune Diseases and Their Associated Antibodies

Disease	Associated Antibodies
Systemic lupus erythematosus	Anti-dsDNA, anti-Smith
Drug-induced lupus	Antihistone
Rheumatoid arthritis	IgM versus Fc portion of Ig
Sjögren syndrome	Anti-SSA and anti-SSB
CREST syndrome	Anti-centromere
Diffuse scleroderma	Anti-scl70

CREST, calcinosis, Raynaud phenomenon, esophageal dysfunction, sclerodactyly, telangiectasis.

ankylosis). **Rheumatoid nodules** have a central fibrinoid necrosis surrounded by palisading macrophages, with an outer rim of lymphocytes and plasma cells (Figure 3-3 A and B).

3. Sjögren syndrome

Epidemiology: Usually occurs in women between the ages of 50 and 60 years.

Clinical presentation of Sjögren syndrome: Triad of dry mouth, dry eyes, and an autoimmune disorder (usually rheumatoid arthritis).

Associated antibodies

- Anti-SSA (anti-ribonucleoprotein); patients with a high titer of anti-SSA are more likely to have systemic manifestations.
- Anti-SSB (anti-ribonucleoprotein).

Microscopic morphology: Lymphocytic and plasmacytic infiltrate of salivary and lacrimal glands, which is associated with ductal damage (Figure 3-4).

Complications of Sjögren syndrome: MALToma (neoplasm of mucosa-associated lymphoid tissue); patients can also have extraglandular involvement producing synovitis, pulmonary fibrosis, and neuropathy.

4. Systemic sclerosis (scleroderma)

Basic description: Autoimmune condition associated with fibrosis of organs involved.

Epidemiology: Usually occurs in individuals 50 to 60 years of age and older; the ratio of occurrence is 3:1 female to male.

Clinical presentation

- **Limited scleroderma** (also called **CREST syndrome**): **C**alcinosis, **R**aynaud phenomenon, **E**sophageal dysfunction, **S**clerodactyly, and **T**elangiectasia.
- **Diffuse scleroderma:** Widespread skin and visceral involvement, including pulmonary fibrosis resulting in hypertension and renal involvement resulting in oliguric renal crises.

Associated antibodies

- CREST syndrome: Anticentromere.
- Diffuse scleroderma: Anti-Scl70 (against DNA topoisomerase I).

Microscopic morphology of systemic sclerosis: Fibrosis involving dermis, muscularis of gastrointestinal tract, and alveolar septae in the lung and interlobular arteries in the kidney and heart.

5. Mixed connective tissue disorder

Clinical presentation: Findings suggestive of SLE, polymyositis, rheumatoid arthritis, and systemic sclerosis.

Associated antibodies: To ribonucleoprotein (RNP) particle containing U1.

Important points: Patients have little or no renal disease and respond well to treatment with corticosteroids.

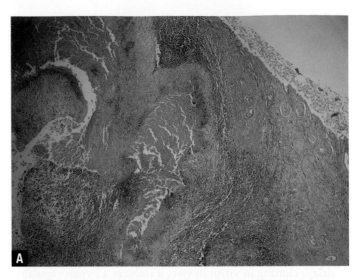

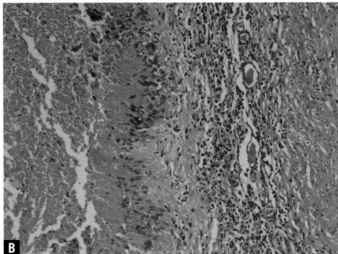

Figure 3-3. A, A low-power view of a rheumatoid nodule. **B,** A closer view showing the central necrosis on the left side of the photomicrograph, with successive layers of palisading macrophages and lymphocytes (to the right of the necrosis). Hematoxylin and eosin, A, 40×; B, 400×.

AMYLOIDOSIS

Overview: Amyloidosis is due to abnormal production and deposition of protein. Within tissues of the body, there are several types of amyloid, each of which is composed of a different protein and is associated with certain diseases (Table 3-2).

Microscopic morphology of amyloidosis

▪ **Light microscope:** Amorphous, hyaline deposition that has apple-green birefringence upon polarization after Congo red staining (Figure 3-5).

▪ **Electron microscope:** Most forms of amyloid are 7.5 to 10-nanometer fibrils in a β-pleated sheet configuration.

Some organs affected by amyloidosis: Kidney, spleen, liver, and heart.

Clinical presentation: Diastolic heart failure, macroglossia, carpal tunnel syndrome, and chronic renal disease. Amyloidosis is one of four causes of chronic renal disease associated with enlarged kidneys; the other three causes are diabetes mellitus, polycystic kidney disease, and HIV nephropathy.

HEREDITARY IMMUNODEFICIENCY STATES

Overview: There are many hereditary causes of immunodeficiency. Major points regarding six of the more common forms (X-linked agammaglobulinemia of Bruton, common variable immunodeficiency, isolated IgA deficiency, hyper-IgM syndrome, severe combined immunodeficiency disease [SCID], and Wiskott-Aldrich syndrome) are discussed below.

X-LINKED AGAMMAGLOBULINEMIA OF BRUTON

Inheritance pattern: X-linked recessive.

Mutated gene: Gene for B cell tyrosine kinase.

Mechanism: Failure of maturation of B cells. The B cells undergo heavy chain rearrangement and then stop maturing.

Epidemiology: Manifest by the age of 6 months. The delay in manifestations is because of the presence of maternal IgG.

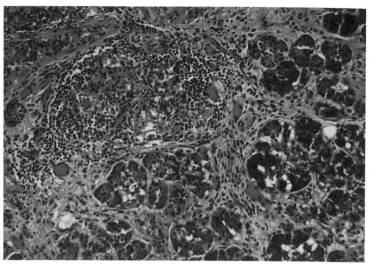

Figure 3-4. Salivary gland in a patient with Sjögren syndrome. This section of submandibular salivary gland has a lymphocytic infiltrate (in the left upper corner of the photomicrograph), associated with some disruption of the glandular parenchyma. With such destruction of salivary gland tissue, the inability to produce saliva is impaired; hence, the dry mouth associated with Sjögren syndrome. Hematoxylin and eosin, 200×.

TABLE 3-2. Amyloidosis: Types, Constituent Protein, and Associated Diseases

Forms of Amyloidosis	Type of Amyloid	Protein	Associated Disease
Systemic amyloidosis	AL	Ig light chain	Multiple myeloma
	AA	Serum amyloid-associated protein	Chronic inflammatory conditions; hereditary amyloidosis
	ATTR	Transthyretin	Systemic senile amyloidosis
Localized amyloidosis	Aβ	Amyloid precursor protein	Alzheimer disease
	A Cal	Calcitonin	Medullary thyroid carcinoma

GALACTOSEMIA

Mutation: Gene for galactose-1-phosphate uridyltransferase (GALT), which is required to convert galactose to glucose.

Manifestations of galactosemia

- Cirrhosis.
- Opacification of the lens (cataracts)—due to accumulation of galactitol, the lens absorbs water and swells.
- Mental retardation.
- Aminoaciduria due to accumulation of galactose in the kidney, which impairs amino acid transport.

Diagnosis: Positive urinary-reducing substance.

HEREDITARY HEMOCHROMATOSIS

Mutation: *HFE* gene on chromosome 6p21.3.

Epidemiology: 1 in 250 individuals of European descent are homozygous; incidence is higher in males than in females.

Mechanism: Increased intestinal absorption of iron leads to iron buildup in organs.

Manifestations of hereditary hemochromatosis

- Bronze skin discoloration due to iron deposition.
- Diabetes mellitus due to pancreatic fibrosis.
- Cirrhosis of the liver.
- Dilated or restrictive cardiomyopathy.

Clinical presentation: The classic triad of symptoms is arthralgia or arthritis, impotence, and fatigue.

Laboratory studies: Elevated transferrin saturation and ferritin concentration; the definitive test is a liver biopsy or DNA testing.

Treatment: Regular removal of blood (phlebotomy).

PHENYLKETONURIA (PKU)

Mutation: Gene for phenylalanine hydroxylase.

Mechanism: Changes are the result of hyperphenylalaninemia, due to inability to breakdown phenylalanine.

Manifestations of PKU

- Impairment of brain development due to high levels of phenylalanine and relatively low tyrosine levels with resultant microcephaly, severe mental retardation, and seizures. Patients may develop motor abnormalities later in life.
- Affected infants have fair hair and skin, blue eyes, and a "mousy odor."

Treatment: Phenylalanine-free diet, especially during infancy and childhood because of vital neurologic development occurring at that time. Because this disease has significant morbidity and is easily treated by dietary restrictions, most neonates are tested.

Important point regarding PKU: Adults can follow a less restrictive diet; however pregnant patients must return to a phenylalanine-free diet as phenylalanine will cross the placenta and affect the fetus.

WILSON DISEASE (HEPATOLENTICULAR DEGENERATION)

Mutation: Adenosine triphosphate (ATP)-dependent copper transporter gene on chromosome 13, which is expressed at highest levels in the liver and brain.

Mechanism: Failure to export copper from cells normally, with resultant increased copper accumulation in the liver and brain. Defective copper export in turn is associated with decreased excretion of copper into bile, which is the primary route for copper excretion.

Laboratory studies: Decreased serum ceruloplasmin, increased hepatic copper content (determined by liver biopsy), and increased urinary excretion of copper.

Manifestations of Wilson disease

- Liver damage (e.g., fatty change, acute hepatitis, chronic hepatitis, and cirrhosis).
- Neurologic abnormalities appearing after adolescence include tremor, speech abnormalities (dysarthria), painful muscle spasms, and dementia. Examination of the brain will reveal atrophy, hyperpigmentation, and cavitation of the putamen. Other basal ganglia nuclei (i.e., caudate and globus pallidus) and the thalamus and brainstem may also be affected.
- **Kayser-Fleischer rings** (i.e., green copper deposits in Descemet membrane at the limbus of the cornea).

ALKAPTONURIA

Mutation: Gene for homogentisic oxidase (3q21).

Mechanism: Inadequate breakdown of homogentisic acid.

Manifestations: Homogentisic acid accumulates in connective tissue, tendons, and cartilage, causing blue-black pigmentation (i.e., **ochronosis**) and making cartilage lose its resilience and become brittle, resulting in degenerative arthropathy. Classically, the urine turns black if allowed to sit, secondary to oxidation.

MAPLE SYRUP URINE DISEASE

Mutation: Gene for branched-chain ketoacid dehydrogenase.

Incidence: 1 in 180,000 births.

Mechanism: Accumulation of the branched-chain amino acids, leucine, valine, and isoleucine, causes neurologic symptoms and "maple syrup" odor of urine.

Manifestations: Alternating hypotonia and hypertonia, hypoglycemia, acidosis, and convulsions.

MYOPATHIC FORMS OF GLYCOGEN STORAGE DISEASE

Characteristic condition: McArdle disease (due to deficiency of muscle phosphorylase).

Manifestations: Cramps with exercise; no exercise-induced increase in lactate.

MISCELLANEOUS FORMS OF GLYCOGEN STORAGE DISEASE

Overview: Some forms of glycogen storage disease may have less conspicuous liver involvement, although skeletal muscle abnormalities are often present, along with cardiac involvement.

Characteristic condition: Pompe disease is due to a deficiency of acid maltase; all organs have increased glycogen accumulation associated with increased lysosomal activity. Cardiac involvement is the most prominent feature of infantile onset cases. Skeletal muscle weakness is conspicuous in adult-onset cases, with increased lysosomal glycogen accumulation (Figure 6-5).

GENETIC CONDITIONS WITH X-LINKED INHERITANCE PATTERN

DUCHENNE MUSCULAR DYSTROPHY

Epidemiology: 1 in 3000 infants; profound male predominance; female carriers of the disease are often asymptomatic.

Mutations: Dystrophin gene at Xp21.

Mechanism: Dystrophin is believed to help transfer the force of muscular contraction to connective tissue. In dystrophin deficiency, the cell membrane of the muscle fiber is damaged when the muscle contracts. Dystrophin is also expressed in organs other than skeletal muscle, including the brain and myocardium. Therefore, dystrophin abnormalities may also be associated with cardiac and neurologic defects.

Clinical presentation of Duchenne muscular dystrophy

- **Clinical course:** Disease manifests by the age of 5 years. The associated muscular weakness leads to immobility by the early teens and usually death by the early twenties. Cardiomyopathy and nonprogressive cognitive abnormalities are also fairly common.

- **Signs and symptoms:** Weakness of pelvis first, with delayed ability to walk; **pseudohypertrophy** (i.e., enlargement of calf muscles due to replacement with fat). Patients use their hands to rise to a standing position (Gower maneuver). Muscle atrophy and weakness progress relentlessly, with most patients becoming wheelchair-bound by the second decade. In most cases, death occurs by the end of the second decade, usually due to some combination of respiratory insufficiency and cardiac failure.

Microscopic morphology of Duchenne muscular dystrophy: By immunohistochemical staining, most fibers show an absence of dystrophin, although a few dystrophin-positive fibers (so-called "revertant fibers") are usually present. In symptomatic cases, there is marked variation in muscle fiber size, accompanied

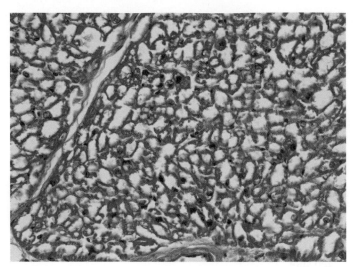

Figure 6-5. Pompe disease. Pompe disease is one of the glycogen storage disorders that affects heart and skeletal muscle. The myocardial cells have a central, fairly well-defined, cleared-out region representing sites of abnormal glycogen accumulation. Hematoxylin and eosin, 200×.

by muscle fiber degeneration, regeneration, and increased amounts of connective tissue. In advanced cases, the muscle is mostly replaced by adipose and connective tissue.

BECKER MUSCULAR DYSTROPHY

Mutation: Dystrophin gene on Xp21. Patients have decreased levels of dystrophin compared to normal individuals, or they may produce a mutant, defective form of dystrophin.

Clinical presentation of Becker muscular dystrophy: Variable. Some patients may follow a course indistinguishable from Duchenne muscular dystrophy, but most affected individuals present roughly a decade later than patients with Duchenne muscular dystrophy and remain ambulatory for several decades. In very mild cases, patients can have a nearly normal life span. Cardiac abnormalities may predominate in some cases.

GENETIC CONDITIONS WITH MIXED INHERITANCE PATTERNS

EHLERS-DANLOS SYNDROME

Mutation: Ehlers-Danlos syndrome occurs as one of many types. In each type, one of the multiple genes involved in collagen synthesis is affected. Depending upon which gene is involved, the inheritance pattern can be autosomal dominant, autosomal recessive, or X-linked recessive.

Types of Ehlers-Danlos syndrome

1. **Kyphoscoliosis type**

Mutated gene: Lysyl hydroxylase.

Manifestations: Hypotonia, joint laxity, and scoliosis.

2. **Vascular type**

Mutated gene: *COL3A1* gene of type III collagen.

Features: Thin skin; arterial rupture.

Manifestations: Hyperelasticity of the skin with hypermobile joints.

ADDITIONAL GENETIC ABNORMALITIES

Overview: Genome mutations (trisomies 21, 18 and 13) and chromosomal mutations (22q11.2 deletion and Cri-du-chat) are discussed below.

TRISOMY 21 (DOWN SYNDROME)

Epidemiology: 1 in 700 live births (1 in 1550 if the mother is younger than 20 years of age, and 1 in 25 if the mother is older than 45 years of age).

Cause

- Approximately 95% of cases of Down syndrome are due to maternal meiotic nondisjunction. Nondisjunction is a failure of separation of chromosome pairs in anaphase I or failure of separation of chromosome pairs into chromatids in anaphase II.

- Approximately 4% of cases of Down syndrome are due to a Robertsonian translocation, which is a translocation of the long arm (q) of chromosome 21 to the q arm of another acrocentric chromosome, such as 14 or 22. A Robertsonian translocation does not result in loss of genetic material; it results in loss of the p arm of 21 and the p arm of 14 or 22. However, in acrocentric chromosomes, loss of the p arm is silent. The carrier of a Robertsonian translocation is 45,XX or 45,XY.

- Approximately 1% of cases of Down syndrome are mosaics.

Manifestations of Down syndrome

- Mental retardation.

- Flat facial profile and epicanthal folds.

- Congenital heart defects, which are often endocardial cushion defects such as ostium primum atrial septal defect (most common cardiac defect in Down syndrome), atrioventricular defects, or ventricular septal defects (Figure 6-6).

- Duodenal atresia.

- Early development of Alzheimer disease.

- Increased risk of leukemia—10 to 20 times increased risk for acute lymphoblastic leukemia (ALL) in children with Down syndrome. Also, acute megakaryoblastic leukemia is most commonly associated with patients with Down syndrome.

- Atlantoaxial instability.

- Brushfield spots on iris.

Laboratory studies: Mothers will have an elevated β-human chorionic gonadotropin (β-hCG) and decreased levels of α-fetoprotein.

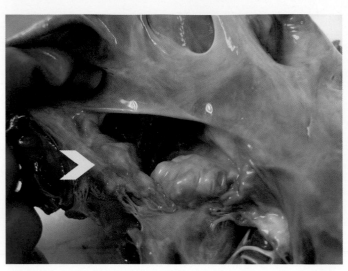

Figure 6-6. Common atrioventricular canal. Patients with Down syndrome commonly have congenital heart disease, and the congenital heart disease often originates from a defect in the endocardial cushions. This defect may manifest as a common atrioventricular canal, a primum atrial septal defect, or a ventricular septal defect. The photograph illustrates a common atrioventricular canal. The defect involves the lower portion of the interatrial septum and the upper portion of the interventricular septum. The arrowhead indicates the cleft anterior leaflet of the mitral valve, a feature that is commonly seen in patients who have this congenital heart defect.

TRISOMY 18 (EDWARD SYNDROME)

Incidence: 1 in 8000 live births.

Manifestations

- Prominent occiput, low-set ears, small jaw, mental retardation, cerebellar and brainstem abnormalities, congenital heart disease, and rocker bottom feet.

- Almost all patients die of apnea in the first year of life.

TRISOMY 13 (PATAU SYNDROME)

Incidence: 1 in 15,000 live births.

Manifestations

- Microphthalmia, holoprosencephaly, mental retardation, microcephaly, polydactyly, congenital heart disease (ventricular septal defect commonly), and rocker bottom feet.

- Almost all patients die in the first year of life.

22q11.2 DELETION

Two forms: DiGeorge syndrome, which has predominantly thymus, parathyroid, and cardiac pathology, and **velocardiofacial syndrome,** which has predominantly palate, facial, and cardiac abnormalities.

Mutation: Unknown gene.

Incidence: 1 in 4000 live births.

Manifestations: Congenital heart disease, abnormal palate, facial dysmorphism, developmental delay, variable T-cell immunodeficiency due to thymic aplasia, and hypocalcemia due to parathyroid gland aplasia; increased incidence of schizophrenia and bipolar disorder. Patients have absent thymic shadow on chest x-ray.

Diagnosis: Requires fluorescent in situ hybridization (FISH).

CRI-DU-CHAT SYNDROME

Mutation: Deletion of 5p.

Features: Microcephaly, mental retardation, high-pitched crying.

SEX CHROMOSOME ABNORMALITIES

KLINEFELTER SYNDROME

Genetic abnormality: A male hypogonadism due to the presence of two or more X chromosomes and one or more Y chromosomes (82% of cases are 47,XXY).

Incidence: 1 in 500 live births.

Mechanism: Increased level of follicle-stimulating hormone (FSH) and decreased level of testosterone.

Manifestations of Klinefelter syndrome

- Hypogonadism (atrophic testes and small penis) and sterility.
- Tall stature due to increase in length between sole and pubic bone (long legs).
- Reduced body hair.
- Most have normal intelligence.
- 20 times increased risk for breast carcinoma.
- Barr body (inactive X chromosome).

TURNER SYNDROME

Genetic abnormality: A female hypogonadism due to the presence of an XO karyotype (57% of cases are XO; 14% have structural abnormality of X chromosomes; 29% are mosaics)—*SHOX* gene involved.

Incidence: 1 in 2000 live births (99% of fetuses with an XO karyotype do not survive gestation).

Manifestations of Turner syndrome

- Short stature and widely spaced nipples.
- Cystic hygromas, webbed neck (Figure 6-7).
- Accelerated loss of oocytes leads to streaked ovaries by the age of 2 years and resultant primary amenorrhea.
- Horseshoe kidney (Figure 6-8).
- Coarctation of the aorta and bicuspid aortic valve.

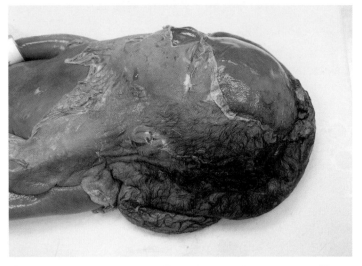

Figure 6-7. Cystic hygroma. The photograph depicts a stillborn fetus with Turner syndrome. The skin slippage and red discoloration of the skin is a feature of stillbirth; however, the redundancy (i.e., folds) of the posterior neck represents a cystic hygroma. Oftentimes, pregnancies involving a fetus with Turner syndrome end with a non-therapeutic abortion.

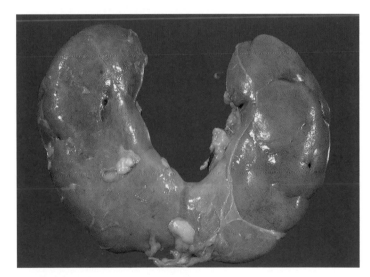

Figure 6-8. Horseshoe kidney. Although horseshoe kidneys are not specific for Turner syndrome, they represent one abnormality that is commonly associated with the syndrome.

FRAGILE X SYNDROME

Genetic abnormality: Trinucleotide (CGG) repeats on the X chromosome; affects *FMR1* gene (Xq27.3).

Manifestations: Long face with large mandible; large testicles; mental retardation.

Important points regarding Fragile X syndrome

- Normal individuals have about 30 repeats; affected individuals have 230+ repeats.

- Individuals with 50 to 230 repeats are referred to as premutations.

- Premutations can expand the number of repeats during oogenesis, but not during spermatogenesis. Therefore, fathers with premutations cannot pass the disease to sons, but repeats will amplify in his daughters and affect his grandsons and granddaughters. Understanding of this potential by parents produces the anticipation effect.

- Fragile X is the most common inherited genetic cause of mental retardation.

DISEASES OF GENOMIC IMPRINTING

PRADER-WILLI AND ANGELMAN SYNDROMES

Genetic abnormality: The gene involved in these disorders is on chromosome 15q—deletion of paternal-derived 15q12 leads to Prader-Willi syndrome, and deletion of maternal-derived 15q12 leads to Angelman syndrome. In other words, a child must receive the paternally derived gene at 15q12 to *not* develop Prader-Willi syndrome, and must receive the maternally derived gene at 15q12 to *not* develop Angelman syndrome.

Manifestations of Prader-Willi syndrome: Include mental retardation, extreme hyperphagia, short stature, obesity, and hypogonadism. Most patients die from complications of obesity.

Manifestations of Angelman ("happy puppet") syndrome: Include ataxic gait, seizures, and inappropriate laughter.

SEXUAL DIFFERENTIATION DISORDERS

TRUE HERMAPHRODITE

Basic description: Possession of both testicular and ovarian tissue.

Mechanism: Possible translocation of *SRY* gene; most cases are 46,XX, but some are mosaics.

FEMALE PSEUDOHERMAPHRODITE

Basic description: Female internal genitalia with ambiguous external genitalia.

Mechanism: Excessive androgens during gestation; common cause is congenital adrenal hyperplasia.

MALE PSEUDOHERMAPHRODITE

Basic description: Male internal genitalia with ambiguous external genitalia.

Mechanism: Many causes; most commonly due to defect in androgen synthesis.

Specific forms (testicular feminization and 5α-reductase deficiency)

1. **Testicular feminization** (also referred to as **androgen insensitivity syndrome**) is the most common form of male pseudohermaphroditism, which is due to a mutation in the androgen receptor gene on Xq11-12. Laboratory findings include increased levels of testosterone, estrogen, and luteinizing hormone (LH).

2. **5α-reductase deficiency**

   Mechanism: 5α-reductase is normally required for conversion of testosterone to dihydrotestosterone.

   Effects of deficiency: Patients have ambiguous genitalia until puberty; then, at puberty, increased levels of testosterone cause masculinization of the genitalia.

FETAL ALCOHOL SYNDROME

Epidemiology: Affects more than 1200 children per year. It is the most common form of preventable mental retardation in the United States.

Mechanism: Potentially due to acetaldehyde crossing the placenta and damaging the fetal brain.

Manifestations: Microcephaly, malformations of the brain, mental retardation, and facial malformations (e.g., short palpebral fissures, maxillary hypoplasia, and smooth philtrum, or upper lip).

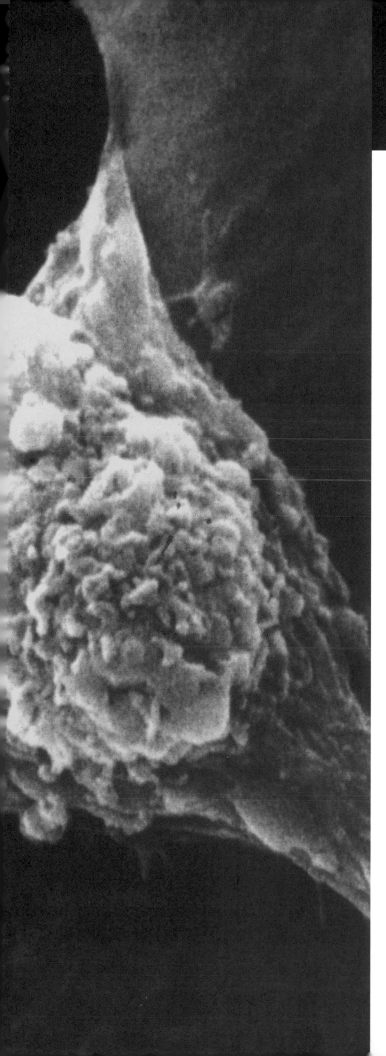

CHAPTER 7

PEDIATRIC PATHOLOGY

OVERVIEW

Although many conditions that affect adults also affect children, pediatric pathology includes many conditions found only in patients younger than 18 years of age. This chapter will address many of these conditions.

One group of conditions involving the infant population is congenital anomalies. Several terms are important to remember when discussing congenital anomalies. A **malformation** is a congenital anomaly due to an intrinsic defect in development. A **disruption** occurs when a normally developing organ is secondarily damaged by another process. For example, in **amniotic band syndrome,** a fragment of the amniotic membrane wraps around a portion of the body and damages or amputates it. A **deformation** is an abnormal development of an organ due to an extrinsic process. A **sequence** is a collection of several anomalies, all of which are due to one malformation, disruption, or deformation. For example, **Potter sequence** is due to oligohydramnios and includes flat facies, small chest, hypoplastic lungs, club foot (**talipes equinovarus**), and nodules in the amniotic sac. Finally, a **syndrome** is a group of related anomalies. Common congenital anomalies include clubfoot, patent ductus arteriosus, ventricular septal defect, and cleft lip or cleft palate. Although most congenital anomalies are diagnosed during infancy, they are present and can cause complications into adulthood.

This chapter will discuss causes of congenital anomalies and major congenital anomalies by organ system. Also discussed are conditions diagnosed in the pediatric population such as prematurity, perinatal infections, hydrops fetalis, sudden infant death syndrome (SIDS), and select pediatric tumors, including neuroblastoma and Wilms tumor.

CAUSES OF CONGENITAL ANOMALIES

Overview: The causes of congenital anomalies are genetic, environmental, and multifactorial; however, the etiology of many congenital anomalies is unknown. Two common environmental causes of congenital anomalies are nicotine and maternal diabetes mellitus.

- **Nicotine:** Use of nicotine when pregnant predisposes the mother to a high risk for spontaneous abortion, placental abruption, premature labor, or placental abnormalities.

2. Cytomegalovirus (CMV) infection

Routes of acquisition

■ Can be congenital due to newly acquired infection in the mother. The highest risk of congenital infection is when maternal infection occurs during the second trimester.

■ Can be perinatal due to cervical or vaginal secretions or from milk.

Features of congenital CMV infection: Include intrauterine growth retardation, hepatosplenomegaly, hemolytic anemia, encephalitis, and microcephaly. Periventricular calcifications are classic findings identified on CT scan. Congenital CMV infection can produce a purpura similar to the **"blueberry muffin baby"** seen in congenital rubella.

3. Congenital rubella

Route of acquisition: Transplacental.

Time period: Fetus is at risk up to week 16 of gestation.

Features of congenital rubella infection: Tetrad of cataracts, heart defect (e.g., patent ductus arteriosus, pulmonary stenosis), deafness, and mental retardation. **"Blueberry muffin"** purpura caused by extramedullary hematopoiesis is a classic finding.

4. Congenital syphilis

Route of acquisition: Transplacental.

Time period: Maternal transmission to fetus occurs during primary or secondary syphilis.

Features of congenital syphilis

■ **Early manifestations:** Nasal discharge ("snuffles") and congestion; desquamative rash.

■ **Late manifestations:** Notched central incisors (**"Hutchison teeth"**), interstitial keratitis with blindness, saddle nose, saber shins, and deafness.

Features of syphilis in adults

■ **Primary stage:** Firm, painless, ulcerated lesion (**chancre**).

■ **Secondary stage:** Occurs 2–10 weeks after primary infection and consists of maculopapular scaly or pustular rash (classically on soles and palms); **condyloma lata** are broad-based plaques on moist skin.

■ **Tertiary stage:** Occurs 5 or more years after secondary stage. Manifestations include progressive "bark-like" dilation of aortic root (**"luetic aneurysm"**), **tabes dorsalis, Argyll-Robertson pupils,** and general paresis. Tabes dorsalis is caused by degeneration of the dorsal columns of the spinal cord, and patients present with broad-based gait, loss of proprioception, and lightening-like pains in the lower extremities. Argyll-Robertson pupils are small and irregular and react to accommodation but not to light.

FETAL HYDROPS

Basic description: Edema occurring during gestation (Figure 7-5 *A* and *B*).

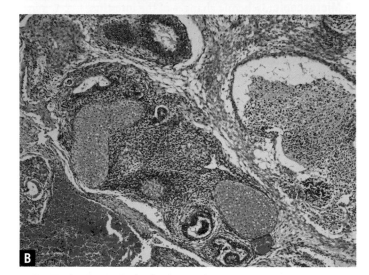

Figure 7-5. Fetal hydrops due to congenital cervical teratoma. **A,** This infant is diffusely and markedly edematous. The fetal hydrops was the result of the large mass in the neck and its pressure on adjacent vessels. **B,** The mass is a congenital cervical teratoma. Note the cartilage interspersed between clusters of immature cells. The most common teratoma associated with a fetus is a sacrococcygeal teratoma. A sacrococcygeal teratoma can impair the birth process by obstructing the transit of the fetus through the birth canal. Hematoxylin and eosin, 200×.

Immune causes of fetal hydrops

▪ Most commonly due to Rh incompatibility. In most cases, it is due to an Rh-negative mother giving birth to her second Rh-positive child.

▪ Occasionally occurs with ABO blood groups and other red blood cell antigens.

Nonimmune causes of fetal hydrops

▪ Cardiovascular malformations.

▪ Chromosomal anomalies (e.g., Turner syndrome).

▪ Fetal anemia (such as occurs in Parvovirus infection).

SUDDEN INFANT DEATH SYNDROME (SIDS)

Basic description: The death of an infant that is unexplained after complete investigation, including autopsy.

Epidemiology: Infant is older than 1 month and younger than 1 year of age, and most commonly between 2 to 4 months of age.

Risk factors for SIDS

▪ **Parental risk factors:** Younger than 20 years of age; maternal cigarette smoking during pregnancy.

▪ **Infant risk factors:** Male gender; prematurity.

▪ **Environmental risk factors:** Prone sleeping position; exposure to second-hand smoke.

Other possible causes of sudden unexpected death at younger than 1 year of age: Myocarditis, suffocation (accidental or homicidal), long QT syndrome, and fatty acid oxidation disorders such as medium chain acyl CoA dehydrogenase deficiency (MCAD).

Morphology of SIDS: Thymic and pleural petechiae (not specific for SIDS) (Figure 7-6).

PEDIATRIC NEOPLASMS

Common pediatric neoplasms: Leukemia, neuroblastoma, Wilms tumor, hepatoblastoma, retinoblastoma, and rhabdomyosarcoma.

Small round cell tumors: General term used to describe many pediatric tumors. The histologic appearance of the neoplastic cells is often not distinctive; hence the generalized name of small round cell tumors. Correct diagnosis is based upon location of the tumor and other ancillary studies, including immunohistochemistry and chromosomal analysis (Table 7-1). Small round cell tumors to be discussed below include Ewing sarcoma and primitive neuroectodermal tumor, rhabdomyosarcoma, Burkitt lymphoma, medulloblastoma, neuroblastoma, and Wilms tumor. Ewing sarcoma is discussed in more detail in Chapter 19, Pathology of the Bones and Joints. Burkitt lymphoma is discussed in more detail in Chapter 12, Hematopathology. Medulloblastoma is discussed in more detail in Chapter 11, Neuropathology.

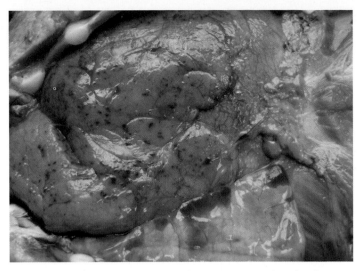

Figure 7-6. Thymic petechiae. The numerous pinpoint hemorrhages (petechiae) were identified in the thymus of this infant who died as a result of sudden infant death syndrome (SIDS). Although thymic petechiae are often identified in infants who have died as a result of SIDS, they are not specific for the condition.

TABLE 7-1. Small Round Cell Tumors

Neoplasm	Genetic Abnormality	Immunostain
Ewing sarcoma and PNET	t(11;22)	CD99 positivity
Rhabdomyosarcoma	t(2;13), t(1;13)	MyoD1
Burkitt lymphoma	t(8;14), t(2;8), t(8;22)	CD10, CD19 positivity
Medulloblastoma	17p deletion	GFAP, synaptophysin positivity
Neuroblastoma	N-*MYC*	Neuron-specific enolase positivity
Wilms tumor	11p13 deletion	

GFAP, glial fibrillary acidic protein; PNET, primitive neuroectodermal tumor.

Ewing sarcoma and primitive neuroectodermal tumor (PNET): Ewing sarcoma and PNET are positive with a CD99 (MIC2) immunostain, and their characteristic chromosomal abnormality is a t(11;22) translocation.

Rhabdomyosarcoma: Rhabdomyosarcoma is positive with a MyoD1 immunostain, and their characteristic chromosomal abnormality is a t(2;13) translocation.

Burkitt lymphoma: Burkitt lymphoma cells are positive for CD10, CD19 and CD20, and their characteristic chromosomal abnormality is a t(8;14) translocation.

Medulloblastoma: Medulloblastoma is positive for either synaptophysin or glial fibrillary acidic protein (GFAP) immunostain, and their characteristic chromosomal abnormality is a 17p deletion or isochromosome 17q.

NEUROBLASTOMA

Epidemiology: Neuroblastomas represent about 7–10% of all pediatric malignancies; the average age at diagnosis is 2 years. The tumor has a male predominance, and is more common in whites than in African Americans.

Location: About 40% are in the adrenal medulla; others occur in the sympathetic chain.

Morphology of neuroblastoma

- **Gross:** Soft, gray-tan mass.
- **Microscopic:** Small round blue cells with background of neuropil. The neoplastic cells are positive for neuron-specific enolase immunostain, and can form **Homer-Wright rosettes** (a circle of neoplastic cells around a space with neuropil) (see Figure 7-7).

Clinical Course: Some neuroblastomas are asymptomatic, and some spontaneously mature to become a ganglioneuroblastoma (neuroblastoma cells admixed with mature ganglion cells) and further mature to a ganglioneuroma (mature ganglion cells admixed with Schwannian stroma).

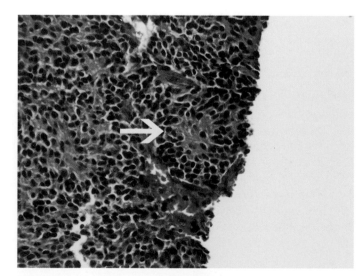

Figure 7-7. Neuroblastoma. Neuroblastoma is one of the small round cell tumors of childhood and frequently arises within the adrenal gland. The arrow indicates a Homer-Wright rosette, a histologic feature that is characteristic of a neuroblastoma. Hematoxylin and eosin, 400×.

Prognostic factors for neuroblastoma

- **Age:** If diagnosed at younger than 1 year of age, the patient has an excellent prognosis. Children diagnosed between 1 and 5 years of age have an intermediate prognosis.
- **N-*MYC* amplification:** Presence of N-*MYC* amplification is a poor prognostic indicator, while absence of N-*MYC* amplification is a good prognostic indicator.
- **Histology**
  - **Good prognosis:** Schwannian stroma, calcification, and low mitotic rate.
  - **Poor prognosis:** No Schwannian stroma, no calcification, and high mitotic rate.
- **Other prognostic factors**
  - Hyperdiploid or near triploid is a good prognostic indicator, whereas diploid or near diploid is a poor prognostic indicator.
  - Stage.

Laboratory studies: About 85% of these tumors secrete catecholamines into the blood. Urinalysis reveals elevated levels of vanillylmandelic acid (VMA) and homovanillic acid (HVA).

Clinical presentation of neuroblastoma: Neuroblastomas usually present before age 5. The classic clinical signs include **opsoclonus-myoclonus syndrome** ("dancing eyes-dancing feet"), which is present in only 2% of patients, and periorbital ecchymoses ("raccoon eyes") secondary to metastasis to the orbits.

WILMS TUMOR

Epidemiology of Wilms tumor: Average age at diagnosis is between 2 to 5 years of age.

Location of Wilms tumor: Kidney; 5–10% of cases have involvement of both kidneys, either synchronous (at same time) or metasynchronous (one after the other).

Precursor lesion: Nephrogenic rests.

Morphology of Wilms tumor

- **Gross:** Soft, tan mass.
- **Microscopic:** Triphasic (epithelial, stromal, and blastemal). Triphasic Wilms tumors are fairly readily diagnosed histologically; however, Wilms tumor can be monophasic, with only one of the three above listed histologic architectures. A blastemal Wilms tumor can be difficult to distinguish from other small round cell tumors (see Figure 7-8).

Associated conditions with high risk for Wilms tumor

1. **WAGR syndrome**
   - **Features:** Wilms tumor, aniridia, genital anomalies, mental retardation.
   - **Gene involved:** 11p13 del (*WT1*).

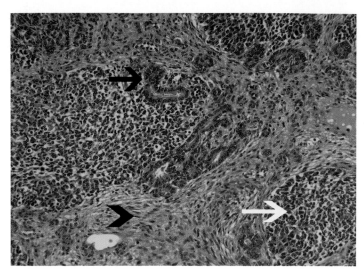

Figure 7-8. Wilms tumor. This photomicrograph illustrates the characteristic triphasic histologic appearance of Wilms tumor. Epithelial (*black arrow*), stromal (*black arrowhead*), and blastemal (*white arrow*) components are all readily identified. A monophasic Wilms tumor, composed only of blastemal cellular architecture, can easily be confused histologically with some of the other small round cell tumors of childhood. Hematoxylin and eosin, 200×.

EDEMA

Basic description: Accumulation of fluid within the cells, interstitial tissue, and body cavities.

Mechanisms of edema formation: Include increased vascular hydrostatic pressure, decreased plasma osmotic pressure, lymphatic obstruction, and inflammation. Increased vascular hydrostatic pressure is usually due to impaired venous return or arteriolar dilation.

Causes of increased vascular hydrostatic pressure

- **Heart failure:** The heart is not pumping blood as effectively as it should, so there is a back up of blood into the veins.

- **Cirrhosis:** Fibrous scarring of the liver that impairs return of blood through the portal vein, thereby increasing venous pressure in portal vein tributaries and causing fluid to leak into the peritoneal cavity.

- **Venous obstruction:** For example, a tumor pushing on a vein will cause back up of blood, eventually with leakage of fluid into the interstitium.

Causes of decreased plasma osmotic pressure

- **Decreased production of albumin by the liver** (e.g., in cirrhosis or other forms of generalized liver damage). A decreased level of albumin results in edema through decreased plasma osmotic pressure. Also, the decreased intravascular volume that accompanies edema stimulates an elevated level of aldosterone. The elevated level of aldosterone, along with several complex changes within the kidney, promotes sodium and water retention. However, because the patient with cirrhosis is hypoalbuminemic, the retained water enters the interstitial space, further contributing to the formation of edema.

- **Increased loss of protein by the kidney** (e.g., certain glomerular diseases) **or in the gut** (e.g., protein-losing gastroenteropathy).

- **Malnutrition.**

Causes of lymphatic obstruction: Lymphoma compressing the thoracic duct or lymphatic channels; certain parasitic infestations, such as elephantiasis.

Inflammation: An important component of acute inflammation is increased vascular permeability, which causes edema.

Effects of edema depend upon organ involved

- **In soft tissues of the extremities:** Edema usually produces no clinically significant damage. Over time, edema can cause changes in skin, but these are usually only cosmetic.

- **In the lungs:** Edema fluid fills the alveoli and pleural cavities, **impairing the ability of the lung to oxygenate** the red blood cells (Figure 8-1 *A* and *B*).

- **In the brain:** The brain is in a rigid compartment; edema causes the brain to swell, producing **increased intracranial pressure** (Figure 8-2). When the brain swells, there are only a few places into which it can expand. These expansions of the brain through available spaces are called **herniations.** Types of herniation include subfalcine, uncal, and cerebellar tonsillar (see Chapter 11 for further discussion of herniation).

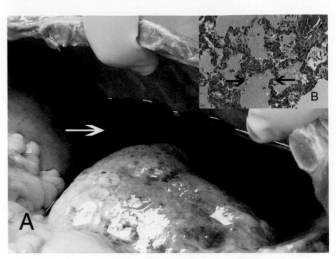

Figure 8-1. Pleural effusion with pulmonary edema. **A,** Accumulation of fluid in the pleural cavities, or pleural effusions (*arrow*), may cause respiratory problems by limiting expansion of the lungs. **B,** Microscopic section from a patient with pulmonary edema. The edema fluid (*arrows*) stains light pink in this hematoxylin and eosin stained section and fills the alveolar spaces. The presence of fluid within the alveoli interferes with proper oxygenation of blood in the alveolar capillaries. Hematoxylin and eosin, 200×.

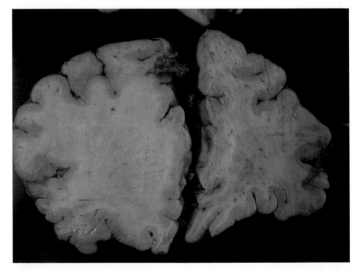

Figure 8-2. Cerebral edema. This patient had a neoplasm on the left side of the brain. The edema of the brain was confined to the left cerebral hemisphere (the site of the tumor), and serves to illustrate the appearance of an edematous versus nonedematous brain. Expansion of the cerebral parenchyma, as seen in the section on the left side of the image, displaces the nonedematous right hemisphere in this case. Various herniation patterns may also occur in this condition. Note the flattening of the crests of the cortical gyri, caused by pressure on the brain from the inner surface of the skull.

Important concepts and terms

- **Transudate:** Protein and cell-poor fluid that has a specific gravity < 1.012. Cardiac failure or decreased protein levels cause a transudate.

- **Exudate:** Protein and cell-rich fluid that has a specific gravity > 1.020. Inflammation causes an exudate.

- **Dependent edema:** Occurs in the extremities and areas of the body where accumulation of fluid is dependent upon gravity. Dependent edema is most commonly associated with heart failure.

- **Pitting edema:** When the skin and underlying soft tissues of a leg with edema are compressed with fingers, the impressions remain. This type of edema is most commonly associated with heart failure and is usually a transudate (Figure 8-3 A and B).

- **Anasarca:** Generalized edema of the entire body that is most commonly associated with glomerular protein loss by the kidneys.

HYPEREMIA AND CONGESTION

Basic descriptions

- **Hyperemia:** Active accumulation of blood within vessels, such as would occur in vasodilation due to acute inflammation.

- **Congestion:** Passive accumulation of blood within vessels, such as would occur in the lungs due to left-sided heart failure, or in the liver and extremities due to right-sided heart failure.

- **Acute passive congestion:** Passive congestion that developed recently.

- **Chronic passive congestion:** Passive congestion that has been occurring over time and is often associated with hemosiderin-laden macrophages and organ damage.

Morphology of hyperemia and congestion

- **Hyperemia and acute passive congestion:** Blood vessels are dilated by red blood cells; to differentiate the two would require knowledge of the scenario in which it is occurring.

- **Chronic passive congestion:** A condition due to multiple episodes of acute passive congestion. Red blood cells break down, leaving hemosiderin and stimulate mild inflammation, which results in scarring.

Chronic passive congestion of the lung

- **Cause:** Left-sided heart failure, which causes blood to back up into the lungs because the left ventricle is not pumping the blood out as quickly or as efficiently as it should.

- **Gross morphology of chronic passive congestion of the lung:** Darkly pigmented, heavy and firm lungs.

- **Microscopic morphology of chronic passive congestion of the lung:** Hemosiderin in macrophages (**"heart failure cells"**) and fibrosis of the alveolar septae (Figure 8-4).

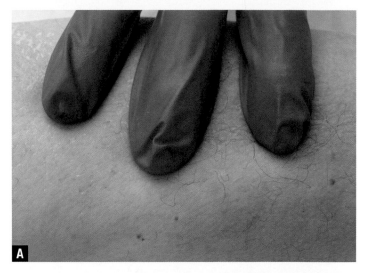

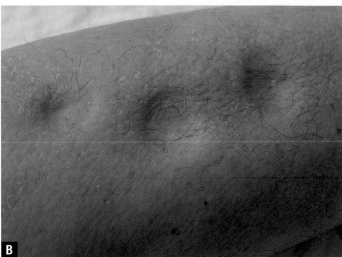

Figure 8-3. Pitting edema. Compression of the tissue with fingertips (**A**) leads to temporary impressions (**B**). This form of edema is commonly associated with left-sided congestive heart failure and occurs most often in the lower extremities.

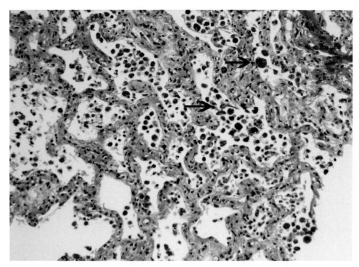

Figure 8-4. Chronic passive congestion of the lung. The section illustrates the two features of chronic passive congestion of the lung, alveolar septal fibrosis and hemosiderin-laden macrophages (*arrows*), also called "heart-failure cells." Hematoxylin and eosin, 200×.

Chronic passive congestion of the liver

■ **Cause:** Right-sided heart failure, which causes blood to back up into the liver because the right ventricle is not pumping the blood out as quickly or as efficiently as it should.

■ **Mechanism of chronic passive congestion of the liver:** In this condition, passive congestion of the blood with sinusoidal dilation is associated with a component of hypoxic injury. The sinusoidal dilation and hypoxic injury lead to atrophy and sometimes necrosis of the centrilobular hepatocytes.

■ **Gross morphology of chronic passive congestion of the liver: Nutmeg liver** (shrunken and congested centrilobular areas with raised, tan portal areas) (Figure 8-5).

■ **Microscopic morphology of chronic passive congestion of the liver:** Atrophy of the centrilobular hepatocytes associated with sinusoidal dilation. Fibrosis may be present around the central veins. In cases of severe heart failure or shock caused by other conditions, the centrilobular hepatocytes are frankly necrotic.

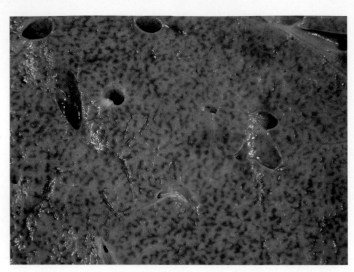

Figure 8-5. Chronic passive congestion of the liver. Shrunken and congested centrilobular areas impart the characteristic "nutmeg" appearance to the liver. This finding is most commonly associated with right-sided congestive heart failure.

HEMORRHAGE

Basic description: Leakage of blood from vessels.

Types of hemorrhage

1. **Petechiae**
   • **Gross morphology:** Pinpoint hemorrhages.
   • **Causes:** Include platelet dysfunction and increased vascular pressure (Figure 8-6).

2. **Purpura**
   • **Gross morphology:** Larger than petechiae and usually raised.
   • **Causes:** Commonly associated with vasculitis.

3. **Ecchymoses**
   • **Gross morphology:** Larger than purpura (> 1.0 cm).
   • **Causes:** Trauma.

Complications of hemorrhage

■ **Important point:** To understand the complications of hemorrhage, think about the location of the hemorrhage. For example, a cut in the skin that causes 250 mL of blood loss is usually not clinically significant (the average blood donation is about 450 mL), but a 5-mL hemorrhage in the brainstem can be fatal. To die solely from just the amount of the hemorrhage itself, an individual must lose 40% or more of their blood volume, or about 2000 mL.

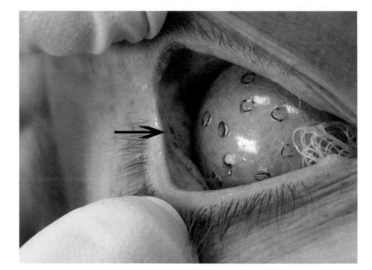

Figure 8-6. Petechial hemorrhages. The pinpoint hemorrhages (*arrow*) in the palpebral conjunctivae are petechiae. Petechiae are commonly the result of platelet dysfunction or increased vascular pressures. The clear yellow plastic cap and underlying fibrous material were placed after removal of the corneae for transplantation purposes.

ADDITIONAL BASIC TERMINOLOGY ASSOCIATED WITH HEMORRHAGE

Hematoma: A space-occupying hemorrhage.

Hemothorax, hemopericardium, and hemoperitoneum: Hemorrhage within the pleural cavity, the pericardial sac, or the peritoneal cavity, respectively (Figure 8-7 *A* and *B*).

HEMOSTASIS AND THROMBOSIS

Basic description of hemostasis: Physiologic coagulation of blood with the purpose of preventing bleeding.

Basic description of thrombosis: Pathologic coagulation of blood resulting in the formation of a solid mass within a chamber of the heart or within a blood vessel.

THROMBUS

Factors predisposing to thrombus formation (i.e., Virchow triad)

- **Stasis of blood** (e.g., due to congestive heart failure, obesity, immobilization). Stasis is a particularly common predisposing condition in patients who develop **venous** thrombi.

- **Hypercoagulability:** Hypercoagulable states may contribute to the development of thrombi in any location, and include hereditary conditions as well as various acquired states.

- **Endothelial damage:** Endothelial damage plays a major role in many **arterial** thrombi.

Important hereditary conditions predisposing to thrombosis (i.e., primary hypercoagulable states)

- **Factor V Leiden mutation:** A mutation in the factor V gene removes the cleavage site for protein C from factor V; therefore, protein C is no longer able to cleave activated factor V. The incidence of factor V Leiden mutations is 2–15% of the Caucasian population.

- **Prothrombin gene mutation:** Causes an elevated level of prothrombin. Patients with the prothrombin gene mutation have a threefold risk of having venous thromboses. The incidence is 1–2% of the general population.

Acquired states predisposing to thrombosis (i.e., secondary hypercoagulable states)

- Myocardial infarct, tissue damage (e.g., surgery, trauma, burns), cancer, prosthetic cardiac valves, disseminated intravascular coagulation (DIC), heparin-induced thrombocytopenia, and anti-phospholipid antibody syndrome.

Fates of thrombi: Propagation, organization, recanalization, dissolution, and embolization.

Complications of thrombi: Occlusion of the blood vessel, which leads to ischemia. Ischemia causes cell injury and cell death (necrosis). The region of necrotic cells is referred to as an **infarct.**

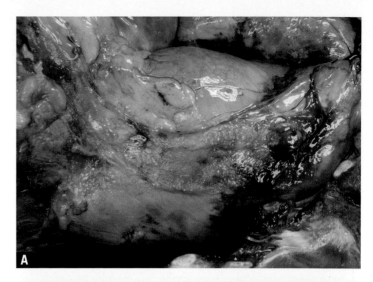

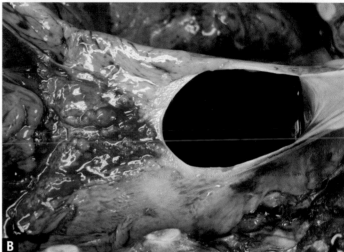

Figure 8-7. Hemopericardium. The decedent sustained a transected aorta after a motor vehicle collision, causing a hemopericardium. In (**A**), the pericardial sac is intact (the sternum has been removed), and the blue discoloration visible through it is blood within the pericardial sac. A small amount of blood (200–300 mL) in this location is potentially lethal because of its impairment of the ability of the heart to fill with blood during diastole. In (**B**), the pericardial sac has been opened, revealing the blood within.

Morphology of recent thrombi

◼ **Gross morphology:** Solid red to red-tan mass occluding or partially occluding the lumen of the blood vessel or lining the wall of a cardiac chamber.

◼ **Microscopic morphology:** Have **Lines of Zahn,** which are alternating layers of red blood cells, platelets, and fibrin within the thrombus (Figure 8-8).

EMBOLUS

Overview: An embolus is a substance that forms within or enters the vascular system at one site and is carried through the blood stream to another area of the body, where it lodges in a blood vessel and produces its effects (usually infarcts). If a thrombus breaks free from where it forms and goes to another part of the body, it becomes a thromboembolus. Substances besides thrombi, such as cardiac valvular vegetations, foreign bodies, fat, and air, can also embolize.

Types of emboli

1. **Pulmonary thromboembolus** (Figure 8-9)

Source: Deep venous thrombi.

Risk factors for formation of deep venous thrombi: Immobility due to obesity, injury, or recent surgery; hereditary hypercoagulable states such as factor V Leiden; oral contraceptives; and neoplasms.

Complications of pulmonary thromboemboli

◼ **Sudden death:** If a pulmonary thromboembolus obstructs more than 60% of the pulmonary vasculature (most often a saddle embolus at the bifurcation of the pulmonary trunk), sudden death of the patient can result.

◼ **Pulmonary infarct:** Due to occlusion of the blood vessel and resultant ischemic injury of the lung parenchyma. Pulmonary infarcts typically occur when a patient has a thromboembolus in combination with a condition that compromises the bronchial circulation (e.g., congestive heart failure) or in combination with pneumonia (Figure 8-10). The classic radiologic finding of **"Hampton hump,"** a wedge-shaped pleural infiltrate in the lower lobes, is rarely seen.

◼ **Pulmonary hypertension:** Obstructive lesions compromising a significant percentage (usually > 60%) of the pulmonary arterial circulation increase the work of the right ventricle, leading to pulmonary hypertension.

Gross morphology of pulmonary thromboembolus: Branching thrombi within the pulmonary vasculature. The branching represents a cast of the vein in which the thrombus formed.

Clinical presentation of a pulmonary thromboembolus

◼ **Symptoms and signs:** Sudden onset of chest pain and dyspnea; tachypnea; cough with or without hemoptysis is present in 50% of cases; and hypoxia (arterial pO_2 is < 80%), respiratory alkalosis, and A-a gradient > 45. The most common electrocardiogram finding is tachycardia. The classic deep S wave in lead I, Q wave, and inverted T wave in lead III (S1-Q3-T3) is uncommon.

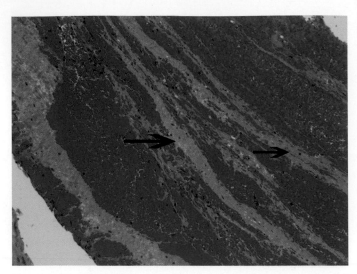

Figure 8-8. Lines of Zahn. Lamellae of platelets and fibrin (*arrows*) separated by red blood cells are indicative of a thrombus and are not seen in postmortem "clots." Hematoxylin and eosin, 200×.

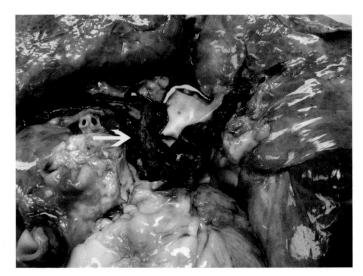

Figure 8-9. Pulmonary thromboembolus. The pulmonary trunk and proximal right and left pulmonary artery have been opened, revealing a tangled, branching red-tan mass within (*arrow*). A thromboembolus at this location (a "saddle" thromboembolus) is still a relatively common and often undiagnosed cause of sudden death in a patient in the hospital.

Diagnosis: Determined by history and physical examination, blood gases, ventilation-perfusion scan of the lung, pulmonary angiography, and spiral CT scans.

2. Fat embolus

Source: Bone marrow; adipose tissue.

Risk factors for formation of fat embolus: Most commonly associated with long bone fractures after motor vehicle accidents and with orthopedic procedures.

Complications of fat emboli: High mortality rate.

Microscopic morphology of fat embolus: Cleared spaces (vacuoles) in blood vessels that stain positive with an oil-red-O stain for fat in frozen sections (Figure 8-11).

Clinical presentation of fat embolus (clinical triad)

- Axillary petechiae from emboli lodging in cutaneous vasculature and causing extravasation of blood.

- Altered mental status from emboli to the brain.

- Dyspnea from emboli filling the pulmonary vasculature and impairing the oxygenation of red blood cells.

3. Amniotic fluid embolus

Source: Amniotic fluid.

Risk factors for development of amniotic fluid embolus: Pregnancy causes dilation and distension of pelvic veins. During delivery, these veins can tear, allowing amniotic fluid to enter them.

Complications of amniotic fluid embolus: About 80% mortality rate due to development of shock and DIC.

Microscopic morphology of amniotic fluid embolus: Anucleate squamous cells in the maternal vasculature.

4. Air embolus

Source: A small amount of air injected into the arteries (1–2 mL) can cause complications. For example, if air enters the coronary arteries, even a small amount can cause an infarct of the heart. If air is injected into the veins, a larger amount is required to cause complications (100–200 mL).

Risk factors for formation of air embolus: Iatrogenic (medically induced) or traumatic injuries of arteries or veins (e.g., incised wound of the neck).

Complications: Infarcts, death.

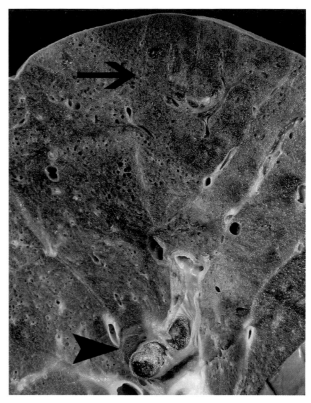

Figure 8-10. Pulmonary thromboembolus causing red "hemorrhagic" infarct. This superior- to inferior-oriented cross-section of the lung reveals a wedge-shaped pulmonary infarct in the upper lobe (*arrow*) and a thromboembolus near the hilum (*arrowhead*).

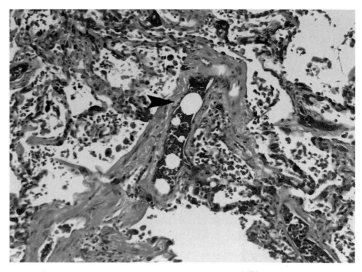

Figure 8-11. Fat embolus. The vessel in the center of this section has several well-defined clear spaces within the blood (*arrowhead*), which are fat emboli. As is evident from the photomicrograph, patients with fatty emboli have dyspnea as well as mental status changes and axillary petechial hemorrhages. Hematoxylin and eosin, 200×.

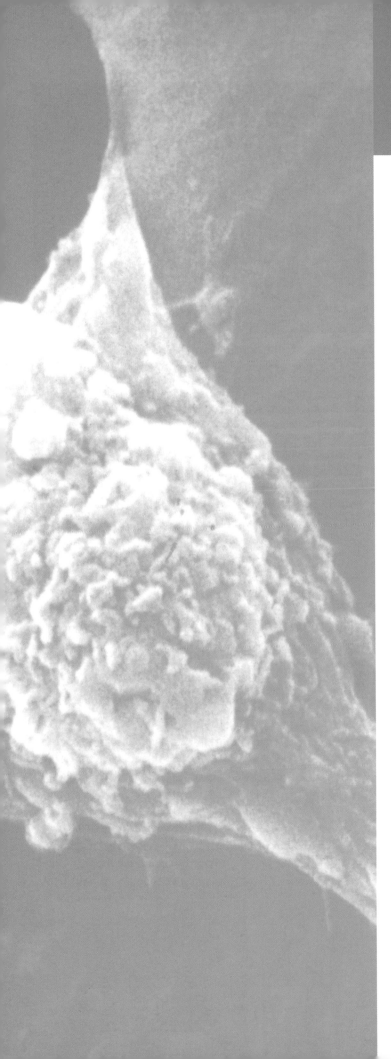

CHAPTER 9

VASCULAR PATHOLOGY

OVERVIEW

Vessels are the conduits by which blood is distributed to and from the organs. Obstruction or occlusion of vessels leads to ischemia of the organs, which causes cell death (necrosis). The most common cause of obstruction or occlusion of vessels is **arteriosclerosis** ("hardening of the arteries").

Pressure within the vessels is determined by a combination of contraction of cardiac muscle and resistance created by the vessels themselves. Changes in this system (e.g., increased vascular resistance) can lead to hypertension, which can cause irreversible damage of the vessels. Examples of structural changes include narrowing of the lumen and dilations of vessels (i.e., aneurysms). Other disorders (e.g., vasculitis) as well as hypertension can cause vascular injury. This chapter will discuss arteriosclerosis and atherosclerosis, systemic hypertension, aortic dissection, pulmonary hypertension, aneurysms, vasculitis, and vascular proliferations.

ARTERIOSCLEROSIS

Overview: Arteriosclerosis is also known as "hardening" or sclerosis of the arteries and occurs in three main forms, Mönckeberg medial calcification, arteriolosclerosis, and atherosclerosis.

Mönckeberg medial calcification: A condition of little clinical significance because the changes are nonstenotic. It is characterized by medial calcification ("pipestem rigidity") of the muscular arteries (often radial and ulnar arteries) in elderly men.

Arteriolosclerosis: Thickening of arterioles (see the discussion below on systemic hypertension).

ATHEROSCLEROSIS

Pathogenesis of atherosclerosis

1. Chronic endothelial cell injury by hyperlipidemia, hypertension, toxins in cigarette smoke, elevated levels of homocysteine, and hemodynamic forces (e.g., turbulent blood flow) leads to endothelial cell dysfunction.

Microscopic morphology of pulmonary hypertension

Grade 1: Medial hypertrophy.
Grade 2: Intimal and medial hypertrophy.
Grade 3: "Pipestem" fibrosis of arteries.
Grade 4: Plexiform lesions.
Grade 5: Fibrinoid necrosis.

Clinical presentation of pulmonary hypertension: Exertional dyspnea (60% of patients) and weakness (19% of patients), cyanosis, digital clubbing, jugular venous distention, and chest pain. Pulmonary hypertension of grades I–III is potentially reversible.

ANEURYSMS

Basic description of a true aneurysm: Dilation of the wall of a blood vessel involving all layers. The three types of true aneurysms are saccular, fusiform, and mycotic.

Types of true aneurysms

- **Saccular aneurysm:** Saccular outpouching from one side of the affected vessel.

- **Fusiform aneurysm:** Generalized dilation of the entire circumference of the affected vessel.

- **Mycotic aneurysm:** An aneurysm that occurs as the result of an infection from septic emboli or an aneurysm that has subsequently become infected. A mycotic abdominal aortic aneurysm is commonly due to *Salmonella* infection from gastroenteritis.

Basic description of a false aneurysm (i.e., **pseudoaneurysm**): A defect in the wall allows blood to escape the vessel or organ (e.g., the heart) and accumulate outside the wall. If the extravasated blood is contained, it appears like a saccular dilation but it is not. False aneurysms can result from trauma or rupture of a vessel.

PATHOGENESIS OF AN ANEURYSM

Aneurysms can have several etiologies, including atherosclerosis, cystic medial degeneration, and tertiary syphilis.

- The primary intimal changes of atherosclerosis weaken the media and can result in an aneurysm. Atherosclerosis is the most common cause of aneurysms, and such aneurysms most commonly occur in the abdominal aorta (Figure 9-9). Atherosclerosis also causes thoracic aortic aneurysms and aneurysms of other vessels. Contributing factors are matrix metalloproteinases that are secreted by macrophages and contribute to damage of the wall. Aneurysms have a decreased level of tissue inhibitors of metalloproteinases (TIMP).

- Cystic medial degeneration can lead to true aneurysms as well as to the previously described aortic dissection.

- **Luetic aortic aneurysm of tertiary syphilis**

  - **Mechanism:** Syphilis causes obliterative endarteritis of the vasa vasorum, which results in ischemia of the vessel's media. The ischemia of the media leads to scarring and loss of elastic recoil, so the vessel dilates.

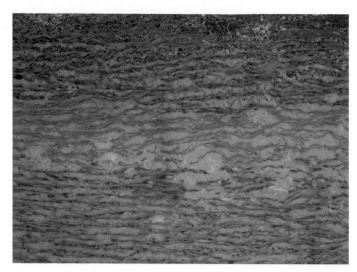

Figure 9-8. Cystic medial degeneration. The acellular, myxoid (blue) material dividing the collagen fibers in the media of this aorta is cystic medial degeneration. Cystic medial degeneration is commonly seen in patients with Marfan syndrome, but can be seen in the aorta of patients with hypertension. The changes produced by cystic medial degeneration may predispose individuals to develop an aortic dissection. Hematoxylin and eosin, 100×.

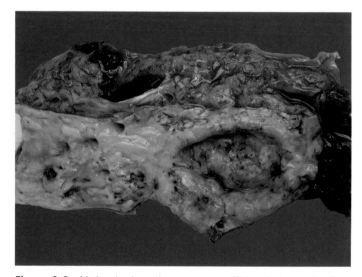

Figure 9-9. Abdominal aortic aneurysm. This photograph of an aorta opened longitudinally (proximal end at left side of image, and distal end at right side of image) illustrates an aortic aneurysm, just distal to the ostia of the renal arteries.

Location: Thoracic aorta (aortic root and arch).

Complications of syphilitic aortitis

- Aortic insufficiency as a result of dilation of the aortic valve annulus, which can cause congestive heart failure.

- Compression of the lungs and airways, causing respiratory difficulties.

- Compression of the esophagus, causing dysphagia.

- Compression of the recurrent laryngeal nerve, causing cough.

- Rupture: Not common; the wall is scarred, and scars do not tear easily.

Morphology of syphilitic aortitis

- **Gross:** "Tree-barking" of the intima is a result of irregular scarring of the media, causing contraction of intima.

- **Microscopic: Obliterative endarteritis** is obliteration of the vasa vasorum by intimal changes and scarring. The wall of the vessel has a variably dense plasma cell infiltrate.

Others causes of aneurysms: Congenital weakness of the wall (e.g., berry aneurysms), trauma.

Complications of aneurysms

- Emboli from atherosclerotic plaques that form within the aneurysm.

- Thrombosis: Aneurysm allows for stagnation of blood and formation of thrombi, with or without resultant emboli.

- Rupture of aneurysm with resultant hemorrhage (Figure 9-10).

- Obstruction of branch vessels.

- Impingement on neighboring structures.

Gross morphology of aneurysms: Outpouching of the vessel wall (i.e., saccular), or generalized dilation of the vessel wall (i.e., fusiform).

Clinical presentation of aneurysm: Presentation as a pulsatile mass. Abdominal aortic aneurysms may be palpated by physical examination.

Clinical presentation of ruptured aneurysm

- **Triad:** Abdominal pain, hypotension, and pulsatile abdominal mass.

- **Important point:** Abdominal aortic aneurysms larger than 5 cm have a greatly increased risk of rupture (10% per year). Abdominal aneurysms larger than 4.0 cm and thoracic aneurysms larger than 6.0 cm should be considered for repair.

ARTERIOVENOUS FISTULA

Basic description: Abnormal connection between an artery and a vein.

Pathogenesis: Can be developmental and can develop after trauma.

Complications: High-output cardiac failure; rupture with hemorrhage.

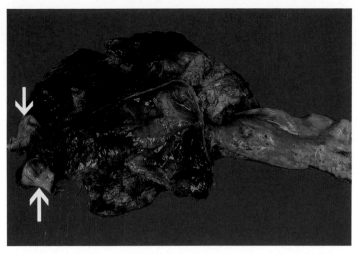

Figure 9-10. Ruptured abdominal aortic aneurysm. This photograph shows an aorta with a large (> 6.0 cm) abdominal aortic aneurysm. The proximal aorta is located at the right side of the image and has been opened longitudinally. The arrows indicate the left and right iliac arteries (also opened longitudinally). The aneurysm has been previously opened for examination and folded closed for the photograph. The hemorrhage in the retroperitoneal tissue, which resulted from the rupture of the aneurysm, is easily identifiable.

VASCULITIS

Overview: Vasculitis is inflammation of the vessels, which most commonly has an infectious or immune-mediated cause. Infectious causes of vasculitis include *Neisseria*, *Rickettsiae*, and syphilis. Immune-mediated vasculitis occurs due to one of three mechanisms include immune-complex deposition, ANCA-mediated, or direct antibody interaction, and will be discussed below. In many cases, the pathogenesis of vasculitis is unknown, but most likely it is an immune-mediated mechanism.

IMMUNE COMPLEX DEPOSITION–MEDIATED VASCULITIS

Mechanism: Antibodies induced by the disease process bind antigens. This interaction forms a complex that deposits within the vessel wall. The immune complex causes vasculitis through activation of complement.

Diseases associated with immune complex deposition–mediated vasculitis: Patients with hepatitis B and hepatitis C infections and systemic lupus erythematosus can develop an immune complex deposition–mediated vasculitis. Drug-induced vasculitis, which often involves the skin, is due to immune-complex deposition.

ANCA-MEDIATED VASCULITIS

Basic description: ANCAs are antineutrophil cytoplasmic antibodies.

Mechanism: Unknown for certain; however, one possible explanation is that ANCAs cause degranulation of neutrophils. The degranulation of the neutrophils releases substances that have toxic effects on vessels and surrounding tissue.

Two types of ANCA

- **c-ANCA:** Antibody against PR-3.
- **p-ANCA:** Antibody against myeloperoxidase.

Disease associations: Patients with Wegener granulomatosis can have c-ANCA. Patients with microscopic polyarteritis and Churg-Strauss syndrome can have p-ANCA.

DIRECT ANTIBODY INTERACTION–MEDIATED VASCULITIS

Mechanism: Antibodies bind directly to the antigens in the target organ.

Disease associations: Goodpasture syndrome, which is caused by antibodies to the glomerular basement membrane, and Kawasaki syndrome, which has antiendothelial antibodies.

MAJOR VASCULITIDES (TABLE 9-2)

Overview: The major forms of vasculitis, which will be discussed below, are giant cell arteritis, Takayasu arteritis, polyarteritis nodosa, Wegener granulomatosis, Buerger disease, Kawasaki disease, microscopic polyarteritis, and Churg-Strauss syndrome.

TABLE 9-2. Important Points Regarding Specific Vasculitides

Disorder	Vessels Affected	Important Points
Giant cell arteritis	Branches of carotid artery and aorta	Affects females >50 years of age; causes headaches; diagnosis determined with biopsy; treatment is steroid therapy
Takayasu arteritis	Aorta	Affects females <50 years of age; causes weak pulses in upper extremities
Polyarteritis nodosa	Small and medium-sized arteries; spares pulmonary arteries	Histologic lesions are temporally heterogeneous; patients present with multitude of symptoms
Wegener granulomatosis	Small vessels	Classic clinical triad of chronic sinusitis, pneumonitis, and renal disease; patients are positive for c-ANCA
Kawasaki disease	Coronary arteries	Causes coronary artery aneurysms
Buerger disease	Small and medium-sized arteries	Associated with tobacco use; patients develop ulcers of fingers and toes

GIANT CELL ARTERITIS (TEMPORAL ARTERITIS)

Vessels affected: Aorta and branches of the carotid arteries (ophthalmic, temporal).

Complications: Thoracic aortic aneurysms.

Epidemiology: Women older than 50 years of age.

Microscopic morphology: Granulomatous inflammation of vessel wall with disruption of elastic lamellae (Figure 9-11).

Clinical presentation of giant cell arteritis: Includes visual disturbances (e.g., diplopia and visual loss) and unilateral temporal headache and jaw claudication. Patients can have an elevated erythrocyte sedimentation rate.

Diagnosis: Definitive diagnosis requires biopsy.

Treatment of giant cell arteritis: Steroid therapy.

TAKAYASU ARTERITIS

Vessels affected: Aorta, branch vessels to upper extremities, and pulmonary arteries. The condition is also called **"pulseless disease."**

Complications: Thoracic aortic aneurysms.

Epidemiology: Women younger than 50 years of age; Asians.

Morphology of Takayasu arteritis

- **Gross:** Vessel wall with near occlusion of lumen by thick intima.

- **Microscopic:** Varies from a mononuclear inflammatory infiltrate to granulomatous inflammation. Intimal proliferation and fibrosis is present.

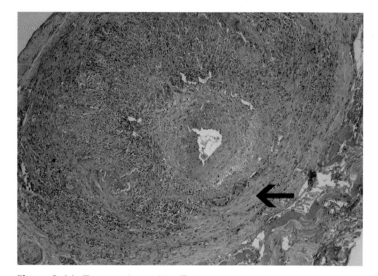

Figure 9-11. Temporal arteritis. This temporal artery has a wall that is thickened by an inflammatory infiltrate. The inflammatory infiltrate includes giant cell formation (*arrow*). Hematoxylin and eosin, 200×.

CHAPTER 10

CARDIAC PATHOLOGY

OVERVIEW

Diseases of the heart fit into several general categories: congenital heart disease, ischemic heart disease, valvular diseases, and diseases of the myocardium (i.e., cardiomyopathies). Pericardial diseases and cardiac tumors are an additional small subset of conditions affecting the heart. A common manifestation of many different forms of heart disease is **congestive heart failure** (CHF). In general terms, congestive heart failure is the inability of the heart to pump enough blood to supply the body's oxygen requirements. It can represent failure of cellular adaptation (e.g., decompensated hypertrophy due to hypertension or chamber dilation due to regurgitant valves) or the outcome of myocardial damage caused by other diseases (e.g., scarring due to ischemic injury, inflammation, or accumulation of iron in hemochromatosis).

Classic symptoms of heart disease are chest pain or discomfort, **dyspnea** (including **orthopnea** and **paroxysmal nocturnal dyspnea**), palpitations, syncope, and edema. Dyspnea is an uncomfortable awareness of breathing. Orthopnea is dyspnea when in the recumbent position due to increased venous return and increased pulmonary venous pressure. Patients with orthopnea sleep upright on pillows to avoid becoming short of breath. Paroxysmal nocturnal dyspnea is when patients awaken with dyspnea 2–4 hours after falling asleep (due to central redistribution of peripheral edema).

An understanding of heart sounds is important in the clinical evaluation of heart disease. The S_1 sound is caused by closing of the mitral and tricuspid valves, and the S_2 sound is caused by closing of the aortic and pulmonary valves. In a patient with hypertension (systemic or pulmonary), closing of the associated valve (aortic or pulmonic) is accentuated (louder); in a patient with stenosis, the closing is diminished in strength (softer sound). S_2 is physiologically split during inspiration (aortic, A_2, first and pulmonic, P_2, second)—increased venous return to the right side of the heart delays closure of the pulmonic valve and decreased return to the left side speeds closure of the aortic valve. Wide splitting of S_2 is caused by a greater than normal delay in pulmonic closure (e.g., right bundle branch block, pulmonic stenosis) or earlier aortic valve closure due to decreased left ventricular volume (e.g., mitral regurgitation, ventricular septal defect). Paradoxical splitting (P_2 first and A_2 second) occurs with delayed closure of the aortic valve

Gross morphology: Prior to 12 hours of age, unable to see myocardial infarct; at 1 to 3 days, neutrophil infiltrate causes yellow discoloration; at 3 to 7 days, macrophages engulfing dead cells cause shrinkage of tissue; and by 8 weeks, only a dense scar is present (Figures 10-10, 10-11, and 10-12).

REPERFUSION OF MYOCARDIAL INFARCT

Basic description: Term applied when blood flow is reestablished to a previously ischemic region.

Complications of reperfusion

Calcium influx into the cells causes hypercontraction of the myofibrils.

Generation of reactive oxygen species, which can further damage the cells.

Leakage of blood from vessels previously damaged by ischemia (see Figure 10-9).

Microscopic morphology of reperfusion: Hemorrhage and contraction band necrosis.

MECHANICAL, STRUCTURAL, AND ELECTRICAL COMPLICATIONS OF A MYOCARDIAL INFARCT

Overview: There are many possible complications of a myocardial infarct. Many of these complications can be divided into the three categories of mechanical, structural, and electrical (Table 10-2).

1. **Mechanical complications of myocardial infarct**

   Left ventricular failure.

   Right ventricular failure.

   Cardiogenic shock: Most common cause of death inside the hospital. Cardiogenic shock requires death of more than 40% of the myocardium for it to develop (Figure 10-13).

2. **Structural complications of myocardial infarct**

   Rupture: Ruptures usually occur 3–7 days after a myocardial infarct, when the cells are dead and macrophages have removed debris. The three areas that can rupture with different subsequent complications are the free wall, the interventricular septum, and the papillary muscles.

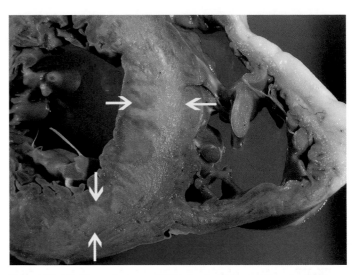

Figure 10-10. Recent myocardial infarct of interventricular septum. The yellow discoloration in the interventricular septum and inferior wall of the left ventricle (*arrows*) is a myocardial infarct of approximately 2–4 days of age.

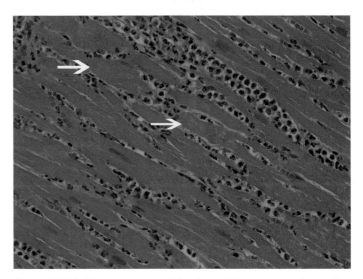

Figure 10-11. Recent myocardial infarct. This microscopic section of the infarct pictured in Figure 10-10 exhibits coagulative necrosis and a prominent neutrophilic infiltrate, consistent with 2–4 days of age. Occasional necrotic myocytes contain contraction bands (*arrows*). The punctate brown pigment is lipofuscin. Hematoxylin and eosin, 200×.

- **Complications of rupture:** Free wall rupture leads to a hemopericardium, which causes cardiac tamponade (Figures 10-14 *A* and *B*); interventricular septum rupture leads to a left-to-right shunt; papillary muscle rupture (or simply death of the papillary muscle) leads to acute mitral insufficiency (see Figure 10-13).
- **Risks for rupture:** Women, younger than 60 years of age, preexisting hypertension, and no prior infarcts (fibrosis of the myocardium caused by a prior infarct protects against rupture).

Aneurysm: A grossly visible aneurysm is a late term pathologic condition, which requires formation of a scar and subsequent bulging outward of the scar (Figure 10-15). Aneurysms can be seen immediately clinically because the necrotic tissue will bulge outward with contraction of the heart.

Pseudoaneurysm: Rupture of the free wall, which is sealed by the pericardium. The hematoma outside of the wall of the heart imitates an aneurysm.

3. **Electrical complications of myocardial infarcts**

Arrhythmia (bradyarrhythmias, ventricular ectopy, tachyarrhythmias, sudden cardiac death): Arrhythmias are the most common cause of death outside the hospital. Most deaths are due to sustained ventricular tachycardia or ventricular fibrillation.

Conduction abnormalities: Heart block, bundle branch blocks.

Other complications of myocardial infarcts: Some complications of a myocardial infarct do not fit easily within the mechanical, structural, or electrical categories (see Table 10-2).

Pericarditis (two patterns)

1. Pericarditis occurring within days of the infarct: Caused by the acute inflammation associated with a transmural infarct.

2. Pericarditis occurring within 1 to 2 months after the infarct (referred to as **Dressler syndrome**): Attributed to probable autoimmune reaction; patients also have systemic symptoms (e.g., fever, malaise).

Mural thrombi: Adjacent inflammation of the wall and abnormal contraction of the wall can cause stasis of the blood and result in thrombi, which line the wall of the ventricle. Mural thombi can embolize (see Figures 10-13 and 10-14*B*).

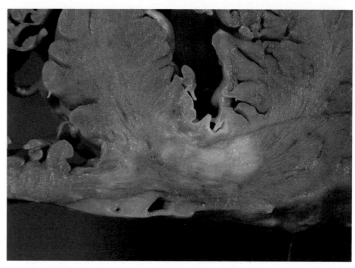

Figure 10-12. Remote myocardial infarct. The inferior wall of the left ventricle has a subendocardial scar (white fibrous area), with focal fatty degeneration (adjacent yellow area). A white fibrous scar indicates that the myocardial infarct is 2 or more months of age.

TABLE 10-2. Complications of Myocardial Infarct

Category of Complication	Types of Complications
Mechanical	Left and right ventricular failure Cardiogenic shock
Structural	Aneurysms Rupture
Electrical	Arrhythmias Conduction abnormalities
Other	Pericarditis Mural thrombi Right ventricular infarct Infarct extension Infarct expansion

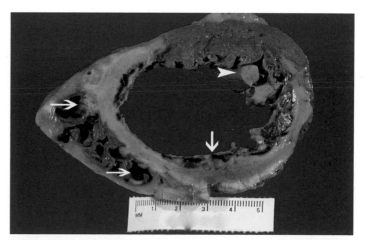

Figure 10-13. Mural thrombi and acute mitral insufficiency following a myocardial infarct. This patient sustained a transmural myocardial infarct involving more than 40% of the myocardium of the left ventricle (the area of the infarct is the yellow tissue). The left ventricle is dilated, consistent with cardiogenic shock. The patient also had mural thrombi (*arrows*), as well as mitral insufficiency due to a necrotic papillary muscle (*arrowhead*).

Right ventricular infarct: Infarcts solely of the right ventricle are rare, but inferoseptal infarcts of the left ventricle frequently (20% of cases) extend to involve the right ventricle.

Infarct extension: Increase in size of the infarct beyond its original borders; due to retrograde propagation of thrombus, vasospasm, or impaired contractility.

Infarct expansion: Outward bulging of the infarcted segment; due to stretching, thinning, and dilation of infarcted segment (see Figure 10-14 *B*).

SUDDEN CARDIAC DEATH

Overview: Sudden cardiac death is due to cardiac pathology. The time frame required to call a death "sudden cardiac death" is < 24 hours if the patient is untreated, and < 1 hour if patient is treated). Most cases are due to an arrhythmia, usually ventricular tachycardia or fibrillation.

Mechanism of sudden cardiac death: Most cases of sudden cardiac death are associated with either atherosclerotic coronary artery disease or structural heart disease such as dilated or hypertrophic cardiomyopathy. The strongest predictor of sudden cardiac death is left ventricular dysfunction of any cause. Ischemia due to obstruction of a vessel makes myocytes irritable and irritable myocytes are prone to arrhythmias, some of which can be lethal. Patients with congenital arrhythmias such as long QT syndrome are also at increased risk for sudden cardiac death.

CHRONIC ISCHEMIC HEART DISEASE

Overview: Chronic ischemic heart disease is a condition resulting from ischemic injuries occurring over time (i.e., in multiple episodes). Patients may have a few or many myocardial infarcts, or they may have diffuse severe atherosclerosis with chronic ischemia, which damages the heart over time, leading to structural changes such as hypertrophy and dilation (Figure 10-16).

Complications: Congestive heart failure.

HYPERTENSIVE CARDIOVASCULAR DISEASE

Basic description: Cardiac disease occurring because of long-standing hypertension.

Gross morphology of hypertensive cardiovascular disease

Cardiac hypertrophy: Increase in the weight of the heart and thickness of the wall of the left ventricle (**concentric hypertrophy**).

The disease is often accompanied by significant coronary artery atherosclerosis.

Complications of hypertensive cardiovascular disease: CHF, lethal cardiac arrhythmias, and atrial fibrillation secondary to left atrial dilation. The hypertrophic myocardium is more susceptible to ischemic injury.

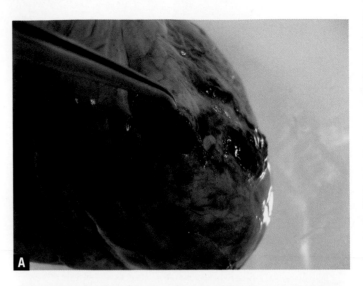

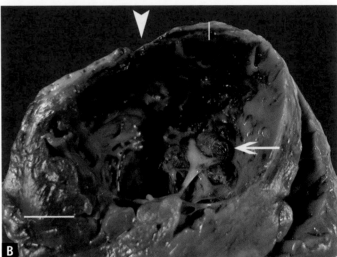

Figure 10-14. Ruptured myocardial infarct. **A,** A full-thickness tear in the anterior wall of the left ventricle, which resulted in a hemopericardium. **B,** A cross-section of the left ventricle at the level of the tear (*arrowhead*). The lumen of the left ventricle is expanded anteriorly in the area of the infarct and the infarcted myocardium is thinned (*shorter white line*) compared to a non-necrotic segment of the ventricle (*longer white line*); these changes represent infarct expansion. The *arrow* indicates mural thrombi.

CONGESTIVE HEART FAILURE

Basic description: The heart can no longer pump out enough blood to supply the body's needs.

Types and terminology of CHF: Most cases of CHF are systolic, low output, and either left sided or biventricular.

Systolic dysfunction: The heart cannot generate enough force to pump enough blood.

Diastolic dysfunction: The heart cannot dilate adequately to fill with enough blood to pump out.

Left-sided heart failure: CHF due to a condition involving or affecting the left side of the heart.

Right-sided heart failure: CHF due to a condition involving or affecting the right side of the heart.

○ **Most common cause of right-sided heart failure:** Left-sided heart failure.

○ **Other causes of right-sided heart failure:** Pulmonary disease (e.g., obstructive and restrictive lung diseases; pulmonary hypertension).

High-output failure: *Not* due to a problem intrinsic to the heart. The heart can pump an adequate amount of blood under normal circumstances, but some process extrinsic to the heart places additional demands upon the heart. Causes include anemia, hyperthyroidism, arteriovenous malformation, and thiamine deficiency (**wet beriberi**).

Low-output failure: The heart simply cannot pump a sufficient amount of blood.

Acute or chronic failure: Depends on rapidity of the development of symptoms.

Morphology of CHF: The mechanism of the morphologic changes and signs and symptoms is primarily increased hydrostatic pressure; however, other mechanisms also play a role, including activation of the renin-angiotensin-aldosterone system and other intrarenal mechanisms for sodium retention. Therefore, although the following morphologic changes and the signs and symptoms are listed under one type of CHF (right or left sided), the changes are not 100% specific (i.e., pitting edema can occur with left-sided heart failure).

Morphology of left-sided heart failure: Recurrent bouts of pulmonary edema and increased pulmonary venous pressure lead to hemorrhage and hemosiderin-laden macrophages (i.e., "**heart failure cells**") in the lung.

Morphology of right-sided heart failure

○ Hepatosplenomegaly: Increased venous pressure due to increased resistance to portal flow results in passive congestion of blood in the liver and spleen.

○ Ascites and peripheral pitting edema.

Symptoms of CHF: Dyspnea on exertion due to lack of increased cardiac output with exercise in patients with heart failure; orthopnea, as the result of pooling of blood in the lungs in the supine position due to increased venous pressure; and paroxysmal nocturnal dyspnea. Patients also have cough (because of interstitial pulmonary edema), fatigue, and nocturia (because

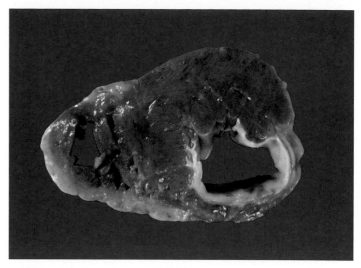

Figure 10-15. Ventricular aneurysm caused by a transmural myocardial infarct. This patient had a myocardial infarct involving the full thickness of the wall of the left ventricle, which healed, becoming a thin, but dense fibrous scar. With contraction of the heart, this noncontractile, scarred area expanded, producing an aneurysmal sac. The endocardium is thicker than normal.

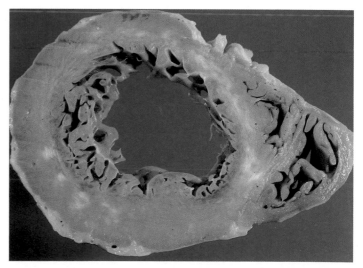

Figure 10-16. Chronic ischemic heart disease. This heart contains multiple remote myocardial infarcts (all the dense white scars, most prominent in the interventricular septum). Although each infarct may have been undiagnosed clinically due to its small size, the cumulative loss of myocytes in such cases can eventually cause congestive heart failure.

the kidney attempts to reduce the volume of fluid that is mobilized when the patient is recumbent).

Signs of CHF occurring as result of compensatory mechanisms

- Increased heart rate due to increased sympathetic tone.
- Narrowed pulse pressure due to peripheral vasoconstriction.

Signs of CHF most commonly associated with right-sided heart failure

- Pitting peripheral edema.
- Increased right atrial pressure (i.e., distention of right internal jugular vein > 4 cm above the sternal angle).
- **Kussmaul sign:** Increase in venous pressure and jugular venous distention with inspiration. Normally, inspiration causes negative intrathoracic pressure, which causes blood to drain into the thorax, thereby reducing venous pressure. In right-sided heart failure, inspiration presents a venous load that a failing right ventricle cannot handle, resulting in an increase in jugular venous pressure and jugular venous distention.
- **Hepatojugular reflux:** Seen in right-sided heart failure, pressure applied over the congested liver returns blood to the heart and increases the right atrial pressure, resulting in increased jugular venous pressure and distention.

Signs of CHF most commonly associated with left-sided heart failure

- Crackles in the lung are indicative of pulmonary edema.
- S_3 is consistent with systolic dysfunction.

Laboratory findings of CHF: β-natriuretic peptide (BNP) is elevated in patients with symptomatic left ventricular dysfunction.

GENERAL VALVULAR DISEASE

Overview: Conditions specifically related to the aortic and mitral valve will be discussed later; endocarditis (inflammation of the cardiac valves) and rheumatic fever will be discussed in this section.

ENDOCARDITIS

Basic description: Infection (usually bacterial) involving the valve cusps or the adjacent endocardium, or both (Figure 10-17).

Risks for bacteremia: Dental and gastrointestinal procedures. In patients with known valve abnormalities, prosthetic valves, or congenital heart defects, these procedures require antibiotic prophylaxis to reduce the risk of endocarditis (Figures 10-18 and 10-19). Rheumatic valvular disease, while less common today, is still a predisposing factor in as many as 20% of patients with infective endocarditis.

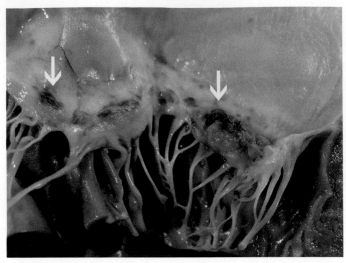

Figure 10-17. Endocarditis of the mitral valve. The leaflets of the mitral valve have several soft, tan-red vegetations (*arrows*).

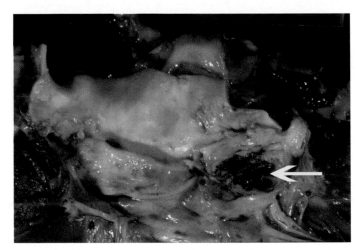

Figure 10-18. Endocarditis of a bicuspid aortic valve. This patient had a congenital bicuspid aortic valve, and subsequently developed endocarditis (endocarditis commonly involves abnormal valves). The infectious agent perforated one cusp (*arrow*), which can result in acute valvular regurgitation.

Types of endocarditis

Infective endocarditis: Traditionally, the terminology of endocarditis was based upon the virulence of the causative organism and was divided into acute and subacute types. With effective antimicrobial therapy, the types are less well-defined and the general term **infective endocarditis** is preferred.

Nonbacterial thrombotic endocarditis (marantic endocarditis)

○ **Microscopic morphology of nonbacterial thrombotic endocarditis:** Bland; vegetations contain fibrin but no neutrophils or bacteria.

○ **Causes of nonbacterial thrombotic endocarditis:** Nonbacterial thrombotic endocarditis forms in the background of sepsis and cancer (especially mucinous adenocarcinoma of the pancreas and gastrointestinal tract).

Complications of infective endocarditis

Sepsis: Bacterial endocarditis sheds bacteria into the blood, which results in sepsis.

Septic emboli with resultant distant abscesses and "mycotic" arterial aneurysms.

Valvular regurgitation: Acute regurgitation as a result of perforation of the leaflet(s) or rupture of the chordae tendineae; or chronic regurgitation due to fibrosis occurring as result of repair of infective endocarditis (see Figure 10-18).

Ring abscess: Inflammation of the valve ring.

Other complications of infective endocarditis: Glomerulonephritis, pericarditis, and local myocarditis.

Gross morphology of infective endocarditis: Vegetations on the cusp or leaflet (i.e., friable excrescences associated with variable degrees of valve destruction).

Microscopic morphology of infective endocarditis: Vegetations are composed mostly of fibrin and bacterial organisms with few neutrophils (Figure 10-20).

Clinical presentation of infective endocarditis

Symptoms: Fever, chills, night sweats, arthralgias, weakness, and shortness of breath are the most common symptoms.

Signs: New cardiac murmur; other findings include **Osler nodes** (i.e., raised tender lesions on the fingers); **Roth spots** (i.e., pale lesions in the retina surrounded by hemorrhage); **Janeway lesions** (i.e., erythematous nontender lesion on palm or sole); and splinter hemorrhages in nail beds.

Diagnosis of infective endocarditis: Persistently positive blood cultures in combination with fever and appropriate clinical history and physical examination. Transesophageal echocardiography identifies vegetations in 75–95% of patients with infective endocarditis.

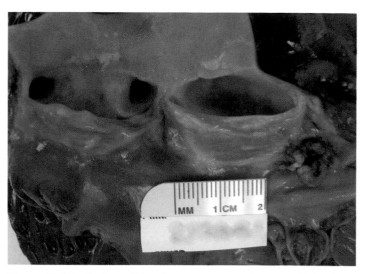

Figure 10-19. Endocarditis of a bicuspid aortic valve. This aortic valve is an uncommon true bicuspid valve, in which the cusps are of equal size and neither has a midline raphe. To the right of the ruler, at the junction of the noncoronary cusp and anterior leaflet of the mitral valve, is a vegetation. Patients with abnormal cardiac valves (e.g., a bicuspid aortic valve) are at greater risk for the development of endocarditis. Courtesy of Dr. Janis Townsend-Parchman, Dallas County Medical Examiner's Office, Dallas, TX.

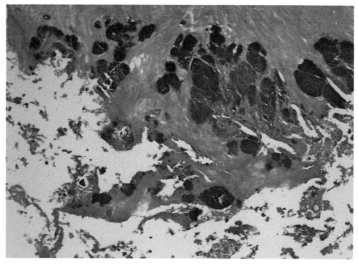

Figure 10-20. Endocarditis. This photomicrograph shows the components of a vegetation. The punctate blue material is bacterial organisms. The acellular pink material is fibrin. Only occasional neutrophils are present due to the absence of local blood vessels. This composition gives the vegetations little support, allowing small fragments to easily break free in the blood stream and embolize to distant sites. Hematoxylin and eosin, 40×.

PERICARDIAL EFFUSION

Basic description: Accumulation of fluid in the pericardial sac.

Causes of pericardial effusion: Same as pericarditis.

Clinical presentation of pericardial effusion

Symptoms: Pressure in chest; symptoms due to compression of adjacent structures (e.g., dysphagia, dyspnea).

Signs: Muffled heart sounds; diminished QRS voltages; variation of amplitude of QRS from beat-to-beat (called **QRS alternans**).

CARDIAC TAMPONADE

Basic description: Compression of the heart due to an increase in fluid within the pericardial sac.

Clinical presentation of cardiac tamponade

Symptoms: If slowly developing, dyspnea and fatigue; if rapidly developing, cardiogenic shock.

Signs

- **Pulsus paradoxus,** which is an exaggerated decrease in systolic pressure with inspiration. Systolic pressure normally decreases by as much as 10 mm Hg with inspiration due to negative intrathoracic pressure; the right ventricle distends but compression of the left ventricle is minimal. With cardiac tamponade, expansion of the right ventricle pushes on the interventricular septum more since the right ventricle cannot push into the pericardial sac. This additional pressure on the left ventricle by the right ventricle reduces systolic pressure.

- QRS alternans.

- Pulseless electrical activity (the heart generates electrical impulses but does not contract accordingly).

CARDIAC TUMORS

Overview of cardiac tumors: Primary cardiac tumors are rare. Neoplasms with a propensity for cardiac metastases include malignant melanoma.

IMPORTANT POINTS REGARDING CARDIAC TUMORS

Atrial myxoma

Most common primary tumor in adults.

Usually benign.

Usually in the left atrium.

Complications: Embolization of fragments; obstruction of the mitral valve.

Rhabdomyoma

Benign tumor of skeletal muscle.

Associated with tuberous sclerosis.

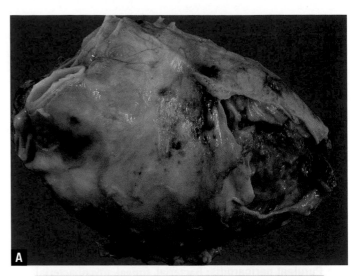

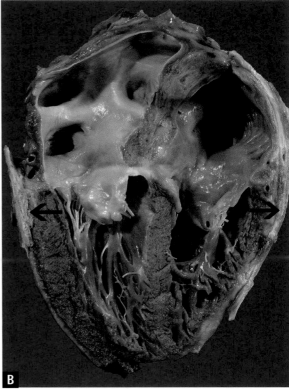

Figure 10-32. A and **B**. Constrictive pericarditis. This patient had systemic lupus erythematosus, and presumably experienced multiple episodes of acute pericarditis. These episodes resulted in the formation of a dense fibrous and partially calcified band around the heart (**A**, and *arrows* in **B**). Because of the constrictive nature of the pericarditis, these patients can present with hemodynamic abnormalities similar to those seen in a restrictive cardiomyopathy.

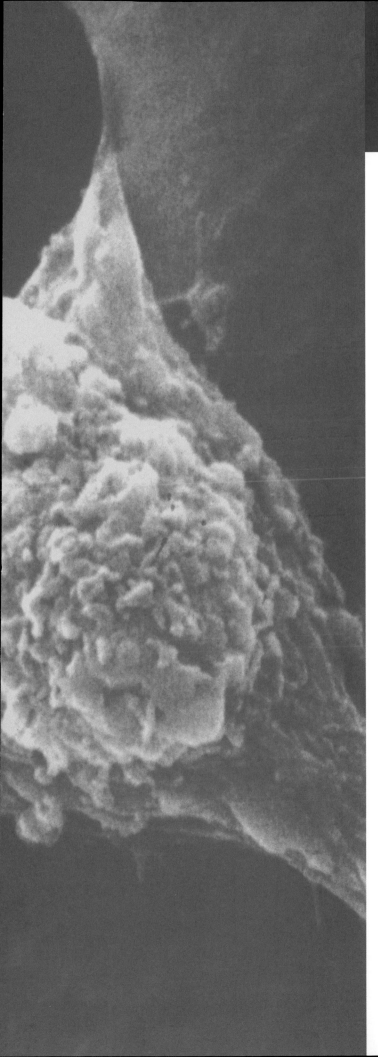

CHAPTER 11

NEUROPATHOLOGY

OVERVIEW

The central nervous system (CNS) is the body's major communication network. Because of localization of functions, neurologic deficits related to disease processes are variable in their presentation. In certain locations of the brain, a lesion will cause minimal or no symptoms, whereas in other areas, it will cause major neurologic deficits. CNS disease can present in many ways, including changes in consciousness, focal neurologic deficits (e.g., aphasia and amnesia, motor and sensory defects), headaches, dizziness, and seizures. Knowledge of the various neurologic pathways will allow a physician to localize the cause of the patient's symptoms.

CNS diseases are classified within one of many categories, including vascular diseases (e.g., infarcts and spontaneous hemorrhages), trauma, infections, neoplasms, degenerative diseases, toxic and metabolic disorders, and demyelinating diseases. Because the pathology of nervous system diseases is intimately related to their neurologic manifestations, this chapter will begin with a discussion of clinical presentations of central nervous system disorders. This will be followed by a discussion of basic pathologic changes, malformations, vascular diseases, traumatic disorders, infections of the CNS, neoplasms, degenerative diseases, demyelinating disorders, and, finally, a few basic peripheral nerve and skeletal muscle disorders.

DISORDERS OF CONSCIOUSNESS

Requirement for consciousness: Intact and functioning brainstem reticular activating system and its cortical projections.

Terminology for impaired levels of consciousness, in order of increasing severity

- **Confusion:** Impairment of the capacity to think with normal speed and clarity, associated with inattentiveness and disorientation. Delirium is a special example of an acute confusional state in which impaired attention and reasoning are associated with agitation, hallucinations, and in some cases, tremor and convulsions.

- **Drowsiness:** Inability to remain awake without external stimulation; often associated with some degree of confusion.

■ **Stupor:** State in which only vigorous external stimulation can arouse the patient; once aroused, responses remain markedly impaired.

■ **Coma:** Deep sleep-like state; patient cannot be aroused even with vigorous or repeated external stimulation.

Causes of change in consciousness

1. **With abnormal CT scan**

   • Hemispheric mass lesions that cross the midline or impinge upon the brainstem.

   • Brainstem lesions that directly affect the reticular formation.

   • Subarachnoid hemorrhage.

2. **With normal CT scan**

   • Inflammatory disorders, such as bacterial meningitis and viral encephalitis.

   • Exogenous toxins, such as sedative drugs, alcohols, opioids, and carbon monoxide.

   • Endogenous metabolic insults, such as global hypoxic-ischemic insults, hypoglycemia, hyperammonemia, and hypercalcemia.

   • Postictal state.

   • Selective brainstem ischemia.

Diagnosis of cause of changes in consciousness: Establishing a differential diagnosis for the cause of a patient's change in consciousness requires evaluation of the history preceding the change, the physical examination, and the effectiveness of initial empirical therapy.

Categories of cause of changes in consciousness

■ **Toxic and metabolic** (e.g., opiate overdose, alcohol).

■ **Infectious** (e.g., meningitis, encephalitis, septic shock).

■ **Cerebrovascular** (e.g., stroke).

■ **Trauma.**

■ **Other** (e.g., seizures, neoplasms).

Role of history in diagnosis of changes in consciousness

■ Preceding headache suggests meningitis, subarachnoid hemorrhage, or encephalitis.

■ Preceding intoxication, confusion, or delirium suggests a diffuse process such as meningitis, endogenous metabolic insults, or exogenous toxins.

■ Sudden onset of coma suggests brainstem infarct or hemorrhage (e.g., subarachnoid hemorrhage).

Role of physical examination in diagnosis of changes in consciousness

■ **Localizing signs:** Suggest focal lesion.

■ **No localizing signs:** Suggests encephalopathy as a result of either an exogenous toxin or an endogenous metabolic insult.

STRUCTURAL VERSUS METABOLIC CAUSES OF COMA

Asymmetrical or reflex functioning of the motor system indicates a focal mass lesion. Changes in pupillary size and reflexes are also useful in assessing the cause of coma.

- A unilaterally dilated nonreactive pupil suggests oculomotor nerve (CN III) compression by an expanding hemispheric mass.
- Pinpoint minimally reactive pupils suggests compromise of the pontine tegmentum (e.g., in a pontine hemorrhage); may also be seen in opiate intoxication. Small but reactive pupils are a feature of many metabolic encephalopathies.
- Minimally reactive pupils in a mid or slightly dilated position suggests a midbrain lesion.
- Bilaterally dilated, nonreactive pupils can be seen in cases of damage to the midbrain tectum or in global ischemic brain injury. It may also be caused by atropine and similar anticholinergic agents.

LOCALIZED CORTICAL DEFECTS

Overview: Focal lesions within the brain can cause symptoms that help the physician localize the lesion to a specific site. These localizing cortical defects include weakness, visual changes, decreased sensation, and a few specialized conditions such as aphasia and amnesia, and others conditions including agnosia and apraxia. Aphasia and amnesia are described in this section.

APHASIA

Basic description: Aphasia is impairment or loss of language function due to damage to language centers in the dominant hemisphere (usually the left). In addition to the two forms of aphasia (Broca and Wernicke aphasia) described below, there are many other forms, such as conduction aphasias caused by lesions to the arcuate fasciculus and global aphasia.

1. **Broca (expressive) aphasia**

Basic description: Disorder of fluency of speech affecting both speech and writing. Patients speak with "broken sentences" but comprehension is intact.

Association: Contralateral arm and face weakness due to the proximity of Broca's area to the motor cortex.

Area involved to produce Broca aphasia: Dominant hemisphere (usually left), inferior frontal lobe.

2. **Wernicke (receptive) aphasia**

Basic description: Impairment of comprehension of written and spoken language. Patient can speak but sentences are meaningless (i.e., "wordy sentences").

Area involved to produce Wernicke aphasia: Inferior superior temporal cortex of the dominant hemisphere.

AMNESIA

Overview: In general terms, amnesia indicates the presence of a memory deficit. With **anterograde amnesia,** patients cannot form new memories. This type of amnesia commonly occurs

Noncommunicating (obstructive) hydrocephalus

■ **Mechanism:** An obstruction exists somewhere within the ventricular system.

■ **Causes:** Include a tumor in the third ventricle or one that obstructs the foramen of Munro; a tumor of the cerebral aqueduct; or, in infants, a malformed or stenotic aqueduct.

Hydrocephalus ex vacuo

■ **Mechanism:** A compensatory dilation of the ventricles in response to a loss of cerebral parenchyma. Not typically associated with increased intracranial pressure.

■ **Causes:** Include Alzheimer disease or a stroke.

Normal pressure hydrocephalus: Patients have dilated cerebral ventricles associated with a normal intracranial pressure. Normal pressure hydrocephalus causes dementia.

Pseudotumor cerebri: Classically seen in young obese females; presents as severe headache with papilledema and elevated intracranial pressure.

CEREBRAL EDEMA AND HERNIATION

Overview: Because of the rigid nature of the cranial vault and dural reflections, the brain has only a limited space in which to expand. Expansion of the brain is associated with a variety of mechanical deformations, including flattening of the gyri (Figure 11-3) and several types of herniation patterns. Although cerebral edema can be a generalized process, expansion of the brain can occur as a local process due to a wide variety of causes, including neoplasms and hemorrhage.

TYPES OF CEREBRAL EDEMA

Overview: The two types of cerebral edema are vasogenic and cytotoxic edema, both of which are explained below. However, in many clinical situations, edema is caused by both cytotoxic and vasogenic mechanisms.

1. **Vasogenic edema**
   - **Basic description:** Edema occurring as a result of disruption of the integrity of the blood-brain barrier, allowing fluid to escape into the interstitial tissue. The brain has no lymphatics.
   - **Examples:** Neoplasms, abscesses, infarcts.

2. **Cytotoxic edema**
   - **Basic description:** Increase in intracellular fluid due to cellular injury.
   - **Examples:** Generalized ischemic injury, infarcts.

Complications of cerebral edema

■ **Cerebellar tonsillar herniation** (Figure 11-4): Cerebellar tonsils herniate down the foramen magnum and press on the brainstem. A cerebellar tonsillar herniation is almost always associated with damage to adjacent brainstem structures that control respiration and heart beat, and for that reason, this type of herniation is associated with a high mortality rate.

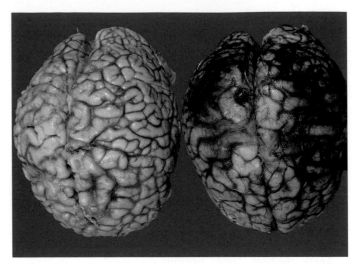

Figure 11-3. Cerebral edema due to subarachnoid hemorrhage versus the normal brain. The brain on the right side had a subarachnoid hemorrhage, which caused cerebral edema. Note the flattened gyri and narrowed sulci. In comparison, the gyral surfaces of the normal brain on the left are gently rounded, and the intervening sulci are well preserved.

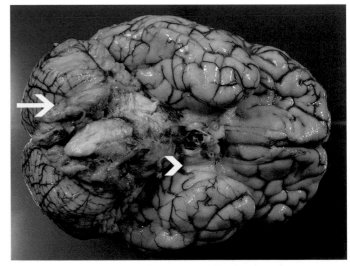

Figure 11-4. Cerebellar tonsillar and uncal herniation. Increased intracranial pressure in this case has displaced the ventral portion of the cerebellum downward through the foramen magnum, compressing the cerebellar tonsils (*arrow*). The tonsillar parenchyma is soft and fragmented due to ischemic injury associated with mechanical compression. In addition, the uncal gyri, located on the medial aspect of each temporal lobe, have been pushed against the free leaflet of the tentorium cerebelli, causing prominent grooves to form in these structures (*arrowhead*).

■ **Uncal (transtentorial) herniation** (see Figure 11-4): The uncus (on the medial aspect of the temporal lobe) herniates under the tentorium cerebelli. The *uncus can compress the oculomotor nerve (CN III), compromising the parasympathetic fibers and resulting in ipsilateral pupillary dilation with associated ophthalmoplegia ("down and out").* The uncus can also compress the posterior cerebral artery, causing an ipsilateral occipital lobe infarct (Figure 11-5). **Cheyne-Stokes respirations** are commonly seen with mesial temporal transtentorial herniation.

■ **Cingulate (subfalcine) herniation:** The cingulate gyrus herniates under the falx cerebri. The anterior cerebral artery may be compressed, causing an infarct of the frontal or parietal lobe in the midline.

■ **Transcalvarial herniation:** When cerebral edema develops in a patient after surgery or trauma, the brain can herniate through the surgical defect in the skull.

Associated condition: Secondary brainstem **(Duret)** hemorrhage.

■ **Mechanism of formation of Duret hemorrhage:** Kinking of branches of the basilar artery during downward displacement of the brainstem.

■ **Gross morphology:** Midline and paramedian streak-like hemorrhage in the brainstem, oriented dorsal to ventral (Figure 11-6).

MALFORMATIONS

Overview: Most CNS malformations are classified in one of several categories, including neural tube defects, malformations associated with hydrocephalus (Chiari types I and II), disorders of forebrain development, and disorders of neuronal migration. Each of these categories will be discussed below, with examples of each.

NEURAL TUBE DEFECTS

Risk factors: Include maternal folate deficiency, incompletely defined geographic and other environmental factors, and gender (incidence is greater in females than in males).

Laboratory testing: Increased level of α-fetoprotein.

Examples of neural tube defects: anencephaly and spina bifida

1. **Anencephaly** (Figure 11-7)

Mechanism of formation: Failure of closure of the anterior neuropore.

Manifestation: Failure of development of the brain and the calvarium.

Incidence: 2–3 in 1000 live births.

2. **Spina bifida**

Mechanism of formation: The more severe forms of spina bifida are the result of failure of closure of the posterior neuropore. Less severe forms, such as **spina bifida occulta,** are the result of failure of secondary neurulation and failure of tail bud formation.

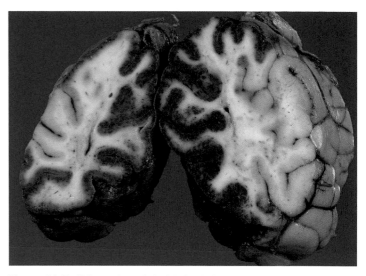

Figure 11-5. Bilateral occipital lobe infarcts due to uncal herniation. The red discoloration of the medial gray matter of both occipital lobes is secondary to ischemia induced by compression of the posterior cerebral arteries. Uncal herniation compresses the posterior cerebral arteries, and can also impinge upon the oculomotor nerve (CN III), damaging the parasympathetic nerves and causing ipsilateral pupillary dilation.

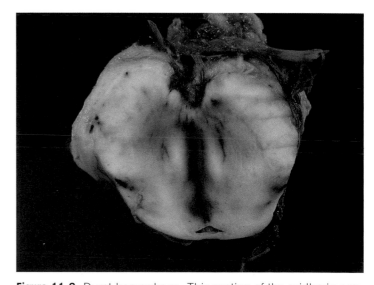

Figure 11-6. Duret hemorrhage. This section of the midbrain contains a secondary brainstem, or Duret hemorrhage, visible here as a midline linear focus of hemorrhage. A secondary brainstem hemorrhage is believed to result from downward displacement of the brainstem, resulting in kinking of branches of the basilar artery and hemorrhagic necrosis of the brainstem parenchyma supplied by these branches.

Morphology of diffuse axonal injury

◼ **Gross:** Punctate hemorrhages in the corpus callosum or the dorsolateral brainstem.

◼ **Microscopic:** Axonal spheroids (globular, eosinophilic structures), which stain with β-amyloid precursor protein (Figure 11-22).

Clinical presentation of diffuse axonal injury: Abrupt loss of consciousness following head trauma.

CONCUSSION

Basic description: Head injury causing temporary loss of consciousness and reflexes; can have residual amnesia. There are no visible pathologic injuries (considered grade O diffuse axonal injury).

CNS INFECTIONS

Overview: The three main forms of CNS infections are meningitis, brain abscesses, and encephalitis. The routes by which the brain and meninges can become infected include hematogenous, direct implantation, local extension, and spread along the peripheral nervous system.

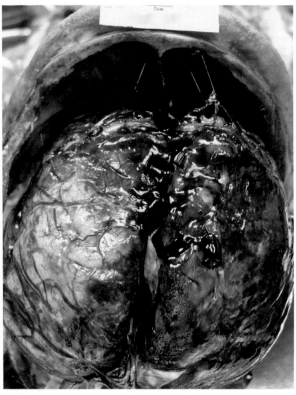

Figure 11-19. Subarachnoid hemorrhage. In contrast to the subdural hemorrhage in Figure 11-18, the hemorrhage in this photograph is tightly applied to the brain because it is under the arachnoid mater. Compared to an acute subdural hemorrhage, in a subarachnoid hemorrhage, the amount of blood required to cause death is far less. Subarachnoid hemorrhages often do not cause significant mass effect; instead, presumably because of the irritating and compressive nature the subarachnoid blood has on cerebral vessels, they cause vasoconstriction and resultant ischemia.

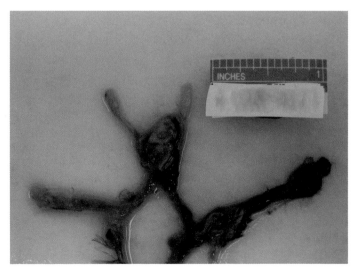

Figure 11-20. Berry (saccular) aneurysm. Arising from the junction of the anterior communicating cerebral artery and the left anterior cerebral artery is an approximately 1.0 cm aneurysm. Most berry aneurysms occur within the cerebral vessels derived from the internal carotid system, and most commonly arise at arterial branch points.

MENINGITIS

Basic description: Inflammation of the leptomeninges and subarachnoid space.

Types and causes of meningitis

- **Acute purulent (pyogenic) meningitis:** Usually bacterial in origin. Causes by age group are listed in Table 11-2.

- **Acute lymphocytic (aseptic) meningitis:** Viral in origin; commonly echovirus, coxsackie, mumps, or human immunodeficiency virus (HIV).

- **Chronic meningitis** (bacterial or fungal): Causes include tuberculosis, *Cryptococcus*, or dimorphic fungi.

- **Chemical meningitis:** Causes include an irritating parameningeal process such as a tumor or abscess, or a foreign substance such as air, or medications.

Complications of meningitis

- **Bacterial meningitis:** Scarring with resultant communicating hydrocephalus, mental retardation, seizures, or focal cranial nerve deficits. Acute bacterial meningitis can cause death.

- **Viral meningitis:** Usually resolves with no complications, unless accompanied by encephalitis.

Important points regarding meningitis

- In children, *Haemophilus influenzae* was at one time the most common cause of bacterial meningitis; however, the development of an effective vaccine has greatly reduced its incidence.

- Meningitis usually remains localized to the meninges and does not involve the cerebral parenchyma, unless the pia or blood-brain barrier is damaged (e.g., old head injuries).

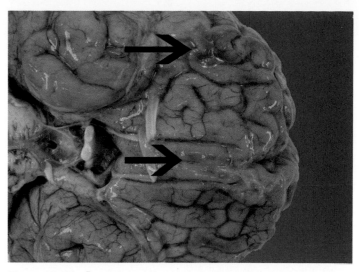

Figure 11-21. Remote cerebral contusions. The arrows indicate shallow, irregular depressions on the inferior surface of the left and right frontal lobes. The yellow-brown discoloration of the rims of the depressions is from hemosiderin deposition. Based upon the location, these lesions most likely represent remote contrecoup contusions, occurring as a result of a fall and landing on the back of the head.

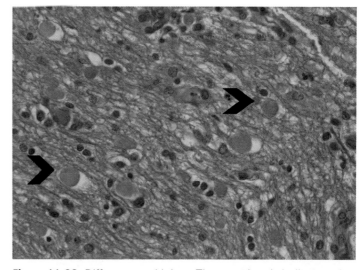

Figure 11-22. Diffuse axonal injury. The arrowheads indicate spheroids. Spheroids are axonal swellings associated with diffuse axonal injury. Diffuse axonal injury is most commonly associated with severe head injury; however, spheroids can also occur as a result of ischemic, infectious, and various other processes. Hematoxylin and eosin, 400×.

TABLE 11-2. Causative Organisms of Meningitis by Age Group

Age Group	Causative Organism
Neonate	*Escherichia coli*, group B *Streptococcus, Listeria monocytogenes*
Children, young and old adults	*Streptococcus pneumoniae, Haemophilus influenzae*
Epidemics in young adults in crowded living conditions (e.g., college dormitories and military barracks)	*Neisseria meningitidis*

Gross morphology of meningitis: The morphology can depend upon the pathogen, as described below.

▪ **Acute bacterial meningitis:** In *Streptococcus pneumoniae*, purulent exudates on the cerebral convexities (Figure 11-23 A and B); *H influenzae* is classically associated with basal exudates; and *Neisseria* meningitis often has considerably less exudates grossly than meningitis caused by *S pneumoniae* infection. *N meningitidis* infection is often associated with a cutaneous petechial rash and hemorrhage into the adrenal glands (referred to as **Waterhouse-Friderichsen syndrome**).

▪ **Tuberculous meningitis and meningitis caused by dimorphic fungi:** Classically associated with a thick basilar exudate, and often accompanied by acute infarcts of underlying brain parenchyma.

▪ **Cryptococcal meningitis:** Gelatinous slick material in leptomeninges; usually no associated exudate.

▪ **Acute lymphocytic meningitis:** Parenchyma may be edematous; leptomeninges are usually clear.

Microscopic morphology of meningitis: As with the gross morphology, the microscopic morphology depends upon the pathogen.

▪ **Bacterial:** Neutrophilic infiltrate.

▪ **Mycobacterial and dimorphic fungal:** Can have granulomas and giant cells; commonly associated with inflammation and thrombosis of the penetrating arteries.

▪ **Cryptococcal meningitis:** Numerous budding yeasts with little if any associated inflammation. Mucicarmine stain is used to identify organisms in tissue sections (Figure 11-24). India ink is used in CSF smears.

▪ **Viral:** Lymphocytic infiltrate; many organisms have associated parenchymal inflammation (encephalitis).

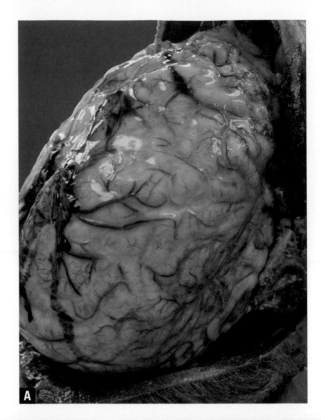

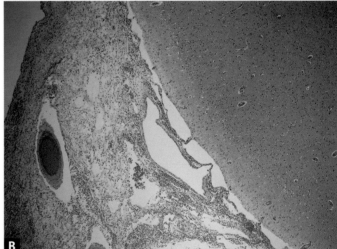

Figure 11-23. Acute purulent bacterial meningitis. **A,** The yellow-green discoloration centered around the vessels at the convexity of the right cerebral hemisphere represents an acute bacterial meningitis caused, in this case by *Streptococcus pneumoniae*. **B,** This low-power photomicrograph depicts the cortical surface and meninges. The meninges are expanded by a cellular infiltrate, which is composed predominantly of neutrophils. Hematoxylin and eosin, 40×.

Important points regarding morphology of meningitis

- **Tuberculosis** (and dimorphic fungi): Usually basilar in location (Figure 11-25). Heal with fibrosis, which can involve the brain (**meningoencephalitis**), cranial nerves, and blood vessels (**obliterative endarteritis**), with resultant complications (e.g., ischemia from obliterative endarteritis).

- ***S pneumoniae*** usually involves the convexities.

Symptoms of meningitis: In general, meningeal irritation causes headache, neck stiffness, photophobia, and altered mental status.

- **Bacterial meningitis:** Headache, fever, meningismus, photophobia; can have cranial nerve deficits.

- **Viral meningitis:** Can have the same symptoms as with bacterial meningitis.

- **Fungal meningitis:** Infections are more indolent. Patients may have only headache and a decreased level of consciousness. In cryptococcal meningitis, in particular, classic "meningeal" symptoms and signs are often absent.

Signs of meningitis: Passive flexion of the neck results in reflex flexion of one or both knees (**Brudzinski sign**); neck pain with knee extension while the hip is flexed (**Kernig sign**).

Diagnosis of meningitis: Analysis of CSF obtained by lumbar puncture (Table 11-3).

Brain abscess (Figure 11-26)

Causes

- **Hematogenous dissemination** (e.g., from bacterial endocarditis, or in patients with cyanotic congenital heart disease with right-to-left shunt, which allows infectious emboli to bypass lungs, a phenomenon known as **"paradoxical embolism"**).
  - **Organisms:** *Staphylococcus*, *Streptococcus*.
  - **Locations:** Frontal lobe more commonly than the parietal lobe, which is affected more commonly than the cerebellum.

- **Local extension** (e.g., from sinusitis, otitis media).

- **Implantation.**

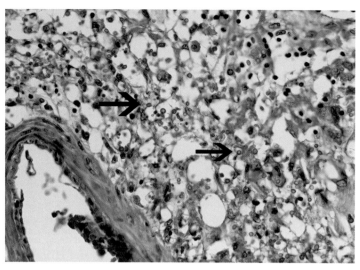

Figure 11-24. Cryptococcal meningitis. This high-power photomicrograph of the meninges, stained with mucicarmine, highlights encapsulated and budding yeast forms. In cryptococcal meningitis, an opportunistic disorder most commonly associated with HIV infection, there is minimal inflammatory reaction. The capsule of *Cryptococcus neoformans* stains with mucicarmine (*arrows*). Mucicarmine, 400×.

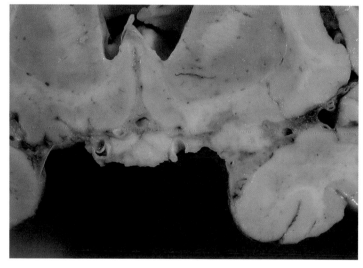

Figure 11-25. Basilar meningitis. The vessels and cranial nerves are encased by a thick white-tan inflammatory exudate. Basilar meningitis is most commonly associated with *Mycobacterium tuberculosis*; however, dimorphic fungi can also produce a similar picture. The causative agent in this case was *Coccidioides immitis*.

VASCULAR DEMENTIA

Clinical presentation: Stepwise decline in cognitive function.

Pathogenesis of vascular dementia: Small microinfarcts and/or strategic infarcts (i.e., infarcts affecting the hippocampus and other areas specifically involved with memory function).

NORMAL PRESSURE HYDROCEPHALUS

Clinical presentation: Clinical triad of dementia, gait instability, and urinary incontinence ("wacky, wobbly, and wet").

Important points: Lumbar puncture and shunting may be therapeutic. Most commonly seen in elderly patients, and is one of the few reversible causes of dementia. CT shows dilated ventricles; normal intracranial pressure. Treatment is with CSF shunt.

OTHER NEURODEGENERATIVE DISEASES

Overview: In addition to the neurodegenerative diseases that cause dementia and affect mainly the cerebral cortex, there are many other neurodegenerative diseases that affect other parts of the brain, including the basal ganglia and brainstem, causing movement disorders. The features of some of these other neurodegenerative disorders, including Huntington chorea, idiopathic Parkinson disease, progressive supranuclear palsy, and amyotrophic lateral sclerosis, will be discussed here.

HUNTINGTON CHOREA

Clinical findings

- Involuntary writhing motions (i.e., **choreiform**) when presenting in adults during the fourth or fifth decades; seizures and rigidity when presenting at a younger age.

- Depression and cognitive impairment (i.e., dementia).

- Patients often commit suicide because of the prognosis.

Mutation

- Huntingtin gene on chromosome 4.

- Mutation is an increase in the number of CAG repeats in the huntingtin gene. Transcription of the expanded CAG repeats results in the accumulation of excess numbers of polyglutamine residues in the huntingtin protein. There is an inverse relationship between the number of CAG repeats and the age of onset of disease. The CAG repeats increase in number during spermatogenesis, which results in the disease presenting earlier in successive generations (referred to as **anticipation**).

Inheritance pattern: Autosomal dominant.

Morphology of Huntington chorea

- **Gross:** Bilateral atrophy of caudate nuclei and putamen.

- **Microscopic:** Loss of medium spiny GABA-ergic neurons in the caudate and putamen; associated with gliosis.

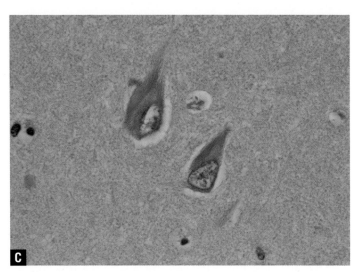

Figure 11-34. (*Continued*) **C,** Both neurons in this section contain neurofibrillary tangles, which appear in this H&E stained section as compact filamentous basophilic inclusions within the cytoplasm of the neurons. Like the dystrophic neurites in senile plaques, neurofibrillary tangles are rich in hyperphosphorylated tau protein. The morphologic diagnosis of Alzheimer disease is based upon the identification of large numbers of senile plaques and neurofibrillary tangles in the cerebral neocortex. Hematoxylin and eosin, B and C, 400×.

IDIOPATHIC PARKINSON DISEASE

Basic description: Degenerative disease with impairment of motor function; 20% of patients have dementia. Idiopathic Parkinson disease represents a spontaneous systems degeneration (i.e., it is *not* caused by an exogenous insult). Similar clinical abnormalities ("parkinsonism") may be caused by certain exogenous insults, however, as discussed below.

Pathogenesis of idiopathic Parkinson disease: Reduced level of dopamine because of loss of dopamine-containing neurons, particularly in the substantia nigra.

Mutations: Mutations of α-synuclein and parkin (substrate of α-synuclein) occur in rare hereditary cases.

Clinical findings of parkinsonism: Cogwheel rigidity (ratchet-like movements), bradykinesia, flat affect, "masked facies," and pill-rolling tremor plus a shuffling gait. Parkinson disease is a movement disorder; however, 20% of patients have a dementia component. The dementia may be the result of associated Alzheimer disease, or it may occur as a component of diffuse Lewy body disease.

Morphology of idiopathic Parkinson disease (Figure 11-35 *A* and *B*)

- **Gross:** Pallor of substantia nigra and locus ceruleus.
- **Microscopic:** Lewy bodies, which are round well demarcated intracytoplasmic eosinophilic inclusions that stain with antibodies to ubiquitin and α-synuclein.

Important point regarding idiopathic Parkinson disease: The diagnosis of idiopathic Parkinson disease is determined based upon the clinical findings.

SECONDARY PARKINSONISM

Basic description: Parkinsonian symptoms caused by an exogenous insult.

Causes: Medications (e.g., antipsychotic agents), toxins (e.g., carbon monoxide), MPTP (1-methyl-4-phenyl-1,2,3,6-tetrahydropyridine) toxicity, encephalitis (e.g., West Nile virus), and hypoxic-ischemic injury.

PROGRESSIVE SUPRANUCLEAR PALSY

Epidemiology: Occurs in the fifth to seventh decades; male predominance, with a male to female ratio of 2:1.

Microscopic morphology of progressive supranuclear palsy: Neuronal loss in the globus pallidus, subthalamic nucleus, and dentate nucleus of cerebellum. Progressive supranuclear palsy is associated with the accumulation of tau-rich globose neurofibrillary tangles and tau-rich aggregates in glial cells (progressive supranuclear palsy represents yet another member of a growing list of degenerative diseases associated with accumulation of the abnormal tau protein. Other examples include Alzheimer disease, Pick disease, and frontotemporal dementia associated with parkinsonism).

Clinical presentation: Progressive supranuclear palsy shares some of the features of Parkinson disease. Patients have truncal rigidity, disequilibrium (with resultant falls), pseudobulbar

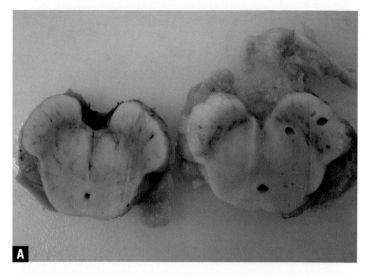
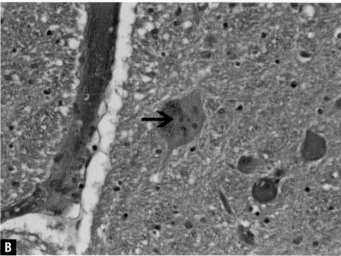

Figure 11-35. Idiopathic Parkinson disease. **A,** The brainstem on the left side of the image has a pale substantia nigra compared to the age-matched control on the right side of the image. A grossly pale substantia nigra is characteristic of Parkinson disease, and is caused by a selective loss of pigmented dopamine-secreting neurons in this nucleus. The well-circumscribed defects near the substantia nigra in the brainstem on the right side are artifacts, due to early decomposition and gas formation. **B,** The neuron in the center of the image has several Lewy bodies, visible in this section as basophilic homogeneous cytoplasmic inclusions surrounded by a clear halo (*arrow*). Lewy bodies are the hallmark of Parkinson disease, and are rich in a protein known as α-synuclein. Hematoxylin and eosin, 400×.

palsy, abnormal speech, and ocular disturbances (e.g., loss of voluntary eye movements with preservation of oculocephalic reflex eye movements).

AMYOTROPHIC LATERAL SCLEROSIS (ALS; LOU GEHRIG DISEASE)

Basic description: Neurogenic muscle atrophy (i.e., amyotrophy) occurs because of loss of lower motor neurons, and hyperreflexia occurs because of loss of upper motor neurons.

Epidemiology: Usually occurs in the fifth decade or later; male predominance. Most cases are sporadic; however, hereditary forms account for a minority of cases (5–10%). Some familial cases have been linked to mutations in the superoxide dismutase (SOD)-1 gene.

Morphology of ALS

- **Gross:** Atrophic anterior spinal nerve roots.

- **Microscopic:** A loss of neurons in the anterior horn is associated with gliosis. Residual motor neurons may contain eosinophilic **Bunina bodies** and ubiquitin-rich filamentous aggregates. There is loss of some brainstem motor nuclei and neurons in the primary motor cortex and degeneration of corticospinal tracts caused by the upper motor neuron loss.

Clinical presentation of ALS

- **Upper motor neuron signs:** Spasticity, hyperreflexia, and Babinski sign.

- **Lower motor neuron signs:** Weakness, fasciculations, and muscle atrophy.

SPINAL MUSCULAR ATROPHY, INCLUDING WERDNIG-HOFFMANN DISEASE

Basic description: Condition caused by degeneration of the anterior horn cells of the spinal cord.

Important point: Spinal muscular atrophy is the second most common lethal autosomal recessive disease (cystic fibrosis is the most common).

Mutation: 5q11.2-13.3; deletions or point mutations in the survival motor neuron (SMN) locus in this region account for more than 98% of cases.

Clinical presentation of spinal muscular atrophy: Severe and progressive weakness and hypotonia in early infancy. Most infants do not survive beyond 1 year of age. Tongue fasciculations are classic but not specific.

Microscopic morphology of spinal muscular atrophy: Groups of rounded and atrophic fibers associated with fibers of normal diameter and hypertrophied type I fibers; loss of neurons in the anterior horn of the spinal cord.

DEMYELINATING DISEASES

Overview: Demyelinating diseases are due to a process that affects the oligodendroglia cells or the myelin sheath itself, resulting in loss of myelin. May be primary (e.g., leukodystrophies) or acquired (e.g., multiple sclerosis). Multiple sclerosis, acute disseminated encephalomyelitis, acute necrotizing hemorrhagic encephalomyelitis, progressive multifocal leukoencephalopathy, and central pontine myelinolysis are discussed in this section.

MULTIPLE SCLEROSIS (MS)

Basic description: Most common demyelinating disorder of the CNS.

Epidemiology: Young adults (< 40 years); occurs in 1 in 1000 individuals (in the U.S. and Europe). Female to male ratio is 2:1. Generally more common in northern regions of the United States and Europe than in the southern regions.

Pathogenesis of MS: Almost certainly an autoimmune disorder. There is presence of CD4$^+$ T$_H$1 and CD8$^+$ T cells in lesions, which are reactive against myelin basic protein. Environmental and hereditary factors also likely to play a role.

Forms of MS: Although most of the discussion in this section pertains to classic MS, there are a few other forms, including Devic disease, acute MS, and Baló disease, that are also discussed.

- **Devic disease (neuromyelitis optica)**
  - **Manifestations:** Bilateral optic neuritis and spinal cord involvement.
  - **Clinical course:** Rapidly progressive.
- **Acute MS (Marburg):** Widespread myelin injury; affects younger patients and has a fulminant, monophasic course.
- **Baló disease (concentric sclerosis):** Rare, rapidly progressive variant associated with the development of lesions containing concentric rings of myelinated and demyelinated white matter.

Morphology of MS (Figure 11-36 *A* and *B*)

- **Gross:** Gray-white translucent areas (i.e., **plaques**) occurring in white matter. Common sites of occurrence include the corner of the lateral ventricles, optic nerves, and spinal cord. **Acute plaques** are soft and slightly pink, and **remote plaques** are more firm, pearly gray, and relatively circumscribed.
- **Microscopic**
  - **Active plaque:** Sharply defined collections of foamy macrophages, associated with relative preservation of neurons.
  - **Remote (inactive) plaques:** Gliosis.
  - **Shadow plaques:** Axons with a thin layer of myelin at the edge (i.e., evidence of partial demyelination or remyelination); not sharply circumscribed.

Clinical presentation of MS

- **Symptoms:** The symptoms are highly variable from patient to patient and depend upon location of plaques, and may involve both upper and lower motor neurons. **Unilateral optic neuritis** (i.e., eye pain with an acute change in visual acuity) and **transverse myelitis** are common and highly suggestive of MS. Other symptoms include diplopia, ataxia, spasticity, and weakness. The course of MS in most patients is relapsing and remitting (with intervals from weeks to months to years).

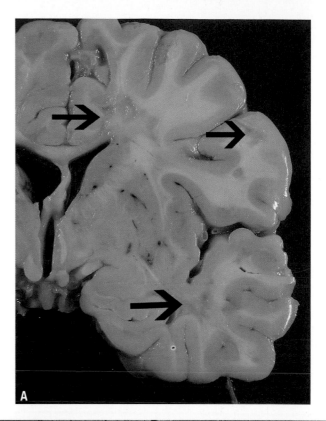

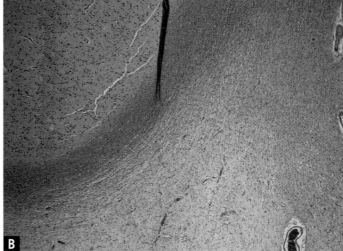

Figure 11-36. Multiple sclerosis. **A,** This section of the brain contains several opaque vaguely gelatinous areas in the white matter, which represent areas of demyelination, also known as plaques (*arrows*). As in the two on the left side of this image, the plaques are characteristically found at the corner of the cerebral ventricles. **B,** In the left upper corner of this image is gray matter. The purple band immediately adjacent to it is normally staining white matter. The remainder of the image (right lower half of photomicrograph) is white matter, which is poorly stained due to the loss of myelin. This image is a photomicrograph of an inactive plaque. Luxol-fast blue, 40×.

- **Laboratory studies:** Evaluation of CSF can reveal myelin basic protein during active myelin breakdown, oligoclonal bands because of proliferation of B cells, and elevated CSF IgG index (CSF IgG/CSF albumin divided by serum IgG/serum albumin). The antibodies produced are not shown to directly initiate the disease process.

ACUTE DISSEMINATED ENCEPHALOMYELITIS

Basic description: Immune-mediated demyelinating disease that follows a viral illness (often measles or chickenpox) or occasionally follows a vaccination.

Clinical course of acute disseminated encephalomyelitis

- Monophasic illness of abrupt onset (in contrast to classical MS, which is relapsing and remitting and chronic in nature).
- **Symptoms:** Seizures, coma, focal neurologic deficits.
- **Important point:** The disease has an acute onset and fulminant course, and is fatal in about one fourth of cases.

Microscopic morphology: Collections of foamy macrophages, comparable to those seen in MS plaques.

ACUTE NECROTIZING HEMORRHAGIC ENCEPHALOMYELITIS

Basic description: Immune-mediated demyelinating disease that follows an upper respiratory tract infection (usually *Mycoplasma pneumoniae*).

Epidemiology: Affects children and young adults.

Clinical course of acute necrotizing hemorrhagic encephalomyelitis: Acute onset; fulminant course.

Microscopic morphology: More extensive than acute disseminated encephalomyelitis; has white and gray matter necrosis, neutrophilic infiltrate, and fibrin deposition.

PROGRESSIVE MULTIFOCAL LEUKOENCEPHALOPATHY

Basic description: Demyelination as result of viral infection involving oligodendroglial cells.

Causes: JC virus (a member of the papovavirus family) in association with immunosuppression (most commonly HIV infection).

Morphology of progressive multifocal leukoencephalopathy

- **Gross:** Gelatinous foci at junction between gray and white matter.
- **Microscopic:** Demyelination associated with enlarged oligodendroglial cells whose nuclei contain smudgy purple inclusions. Atypical astrocytes are also quite common.

CENTRAL PONTINE MYELINOLYSIS

Basic description: Demyelinating disorder involving the central area of the basal pons.

Causes: Uncertain; associations include rapid correction of hyponatremia and alcoholism.

PERIPHERAL NERVE PATHOLOGY

Overview: Neuropathies are conditions involving primary injury to the axon, nerve cell body, or myelin sheath. Some specific types of peripheral neuropathies discussed in this section include axonal neuropathy, demyelinating neuropathy, immune neuropathy (e.g., Guillain-Barré syndrome), metabolic and toxic neuropathy, and infectious neuropathy.

Axonal neuropathy: Primary injury of the axonal process, associated with the formation of fragmented axonal processes and myelin debris (**"myelin ovoids"**). Most cases evolve as a dying-back process with distal to proximal degeneration. A special form of axonal degeneration, termed **Wallerian degeneration,** represents degeneration of the distal axonal process following transection, as might occur in a patient with segmental ischemic nerve injury associated with vasculitis. The most common types of neuropathies are axonal.

Demyelinating neuropathy: Primary damage is to Schwann cells, typically in a multifocal segmental distribution along the length of the axon. It is characterized by selective myelin injury and relative preservation of the axon; secondary axonal injury may occur in some cases, however. Chronic cases are associated with concentric layers of Schwann cell cytoplasm and collagen (so-called **"onion bulbs"**) around residual axons.

Immune neuropathy

Overview: Although there are several immune neuropathies, one of the most important is Guillain-Barré syndrome, which will be discussed in detail.

Incidence of Guillain-Barré syndrome: 1–3/100,000 of the general population.

Clinical presentation of Guillain-Barré syndrome

- **Course:** Usually begins with weakness in the distal extremities and progresses to involve the proximal muscle groups (the progression is referred to as ascending paralysis); respiratory muscles may be involved.

- **Predisposing factor:** Two thirds of cases follow an influenza-like illness. Guillain-Barré syndrome is also associated with *Campylobacter jejuni*, CMV, and Epstein-Barr virus (EBV) infections.

Microscopic morphology of Guillain-Barré syndrome: Inflammation and demyelination of nerves.

Metabolic and toxic neuropathies

- **Diabetes mellitus** (various types of neuropathy): Distal symmetric sensory or sensorimotor, autonomic, and focal or multifocal asymmetric.

- **Other causes:** Vitamin deficiencies, malignancy, heavy metals.

Infectious neuropathy: Causes include leprosy, diphtheria, and varicella-zoster virus.

Clinical presentation of anemia

- **General features:** Pale skin, fatigue, dyspnea on exertion, chest pain, syncope, and dizziness. Chest pain, syncope, and dizziness are all due to inadequate oxygenation of the heart and brain.

- **Laboratory studies:** Most important are MCV, reticulocyte count, and peripheral smear. The reticulocyte count is critical in distinguishing primary failure of red blood cell production (which has decreased reticulocytes or no reticulocytes) from increased red cell destruction (which has increased numbers of reticulocytes). Accurate assessment of the reticulocyte count requires a corrected count (reticulocyte count multiplied by the patient's Hct/normal Hct). If the reticulocyte count is decreased, consider primary bone marrow disorders or deficiency of iron, vitamin B$_{12}$, or folate. If the reticulocyte count is increased, consider hemolysis or blood loss as the source of the anemia.

Types of anemia based upon morphologic classification: There are three types of anemia based upon the patient's MCV: microcytic, normocytic, and macrocytic.

- MCV < 80 femtoliter (fL) is microcytic.
- MCV from 80 to 100 fL is normocytic.
- MCV > 100 fL is macrocytic.

MICROCYTIC ANEMIAS

Overview: MCV < 80 fL. Types include iron deficiency anemia, thalassemias, and anemia of chronic disease.

Iron deficiency anemia

- **Causes:** In the United States, iron deficiency anemia is most commonly the result of chronic loss of blood due to gastrointestinal hemorrhage or menstruation. Therefore, it is often an anemia due to two mechanisms: chronic blood loss and subsequent decreased production. Other causes include dietary iron deficiency (rare in the U.S.), malabsorption of iron, or increased demands for iron (such as occur in pregnancy).

- **Laboratory findings in iron deficiency anemia** (Table 12-2): Decreased ferritin (storage form of iron), decreased serum iron, decreased iron in bone marrow on biopsy, increased total iron-binding capacity (TIBC), increased RDW, and decreased transferrin saturation (transferrin saturation is the ratio of serum iron to TIBC, which is normally > 20%). In iron deficiency anemia, transferrin saturation is normally < 10%.

- **Microscopic morphology of iron deficiency anemia:** Prominent central pallor of red blood cells due to greatly reduced hemoglobin; "pencil cells" (i.e., elongated red blood cells); and marked anisocytosis of red blood cells (i.e., variation in size), which corresponds to high RDW (Figure 12-1).

TABLE 12-2. Laboratory Studies Used to Differentiate Microcytic Anemias

Type of Microcytic Anemia	Ferritin Concentration	Serum Iron Concentration	TIBC	Transferrin Saturation
Iron deficiency anemia	↓	↓	↑	↓
Thalassemia	N	N	N	N
ACD	↑	↓	↓	↑

TIBC, total iron binding capacity; N, normal; ACD, anemia of chronic disease.

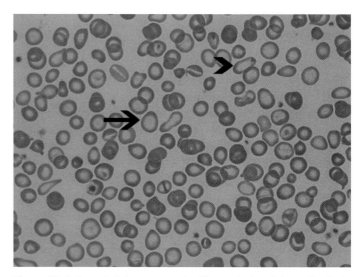

Figure 12-1. Iron deficiency anemia. The majority of the red cells in this photomicrograph exhibit central pallor (*arrow*). Also present is a characteristic "pencil cell" (*arrowhead*). Wright-Giemsa, 1000×.

THALASSEMIAS

Basic description: Deficient production of hemoglobin due to mutation or complete loss of a globin chain. There are four copies of the α-globulin chain gene and two copies of the β-globulin chain gene; the types are **α-thalassemia** and **β-thalassemia**.

α-Thalassemia

■ **Basic description:** Condition is due to complete loss of one or more of the four copies of the α-globulin chain gene. The loss of one copy of the gene is silent (the patient is a carrier), and the loss of two copies is asymptomatic (called **α-Thal trait**). The loss of three copies of the gene (called **HbH disease**) and of four copies (called **hydrops fetalis**) produces symptoms.

■ **Epidemiology:** Prevalent in Africans and Asians.

■ **Important points regarding α-thalassemia**

○ Loss of three copies of the gene results in elevated levels of HbH (β_4) and HbBart (four γ chains).

○ β_4 tetramers are relatively soluble and *do not* damage cells as do α chain tetramers.

○ Loss of four α chains usually results in death in utero (hydrops fetalis).

β-Thalassemia

■ **Basic description:** Malfunction of the gene is due to a mutation in the promoter sequence or to a mutation that causes chain termination or splicing defects, unlike in α-thalassemia, in which the disease is due to complete loss of one or more of the α-globulin chain genes. Mutations producing chain termination result in complete loss of protein (β^0). Mutations in the promoter sequence may result in decreased production of the protein (β^+). Mutations causing splicing defects can cause no splicing to occur (β^0), or form new splice sites with some normal protein being produced (β^+). Patients who are β^+/β^+ or β^0/β^0 have **thalassemia major;** patients who are β^+/β or β^0/β have **thalassemia minor;** and patients who are β^+/β^+ (minor variants, not severe enough to cause thalassemia major) or β^+/β^0, have **thalassemia intermedia.**

■ **Important points regarding β-thalassemia**

○ α-Chains are insoluble and damage red blood cells, resulting in intravascular hemolysis and ineffective erythropoiesis (apoptosis of red blood cells in marrow).

○ Patients with β-thalassemia have elevated HbA$_2$.

■ **Epidemiology:** Common in Mediterranean countries (where patients have a worse form of the disease) and in parts of Africa and Southeast Asia.

■ **Complications**

○ Thalassemia major requires blood transfusions from about the time of birth, eventually leading to secondary hemochromatosis.

○ Bone marrow expansion leads to skeletal abnormalities.

Laboratory findings in thalassemia (see Table 12-2): Iron deficiency anemia and thalassemia are both hypochromic

Associated condition: pernicious anemia

- **Basic description:** Pernicious anemia is another term for autoimmune gastritis, which secondarily causes vitamin B_{12} deficiency because of loss of parietal cells and, thus, of intrinsic factor (IF).

- **Pathogenesis of pernicious anemia:** Autoimmune condition due to antibodies against parietal cells, or blocking antibodies that prevent binding of vitamin B_{12} to IF, or antibodies against the vitamin B_{12}-IF complex. Any of these three antibodies prevents the absorption of vitamin B_{12}.

FOLATE DEFICIENCY

Important point: The megaloblastic anemia caused by folate deficiency is clinically indistinguishable from that caused by vitamin B_{12} deficiency without testing of the levels of each vitamin. There are, however, some important differences between the two deficiencies.

Differences between deficiencies of folate and vitamin B_{12}
(Table 12-3)

- Folate deficiency does *not* cause neurologic deficits.

- In the United States, folate deficiency is often due to dietary deficiency.

- Folate deficiency is *not* associated with pernicious anemia.

Microscopic morphology of megaloblastic anemia

- **Peripheral blood smear:** Oval macrocytes and hypersegmented neutrophils; pancytopenia (Figure 12-3).

- **Bone marrow biopsy:** Hyperplasia; patients have **ineffective erythropoiesis** in which cells are dividing, but they undergo apoptosis in the bone marrow due to impaired DNA synthesis.

OTHER FORMS OF ANEMIA ASSOCIATED WITH DECREASED PRODUCTION

Overview: When comparing the initial outline of mechanisms of anemia to the classification of anemia based upon morphology, with the exception of aplastic anemia, infiltration of bone marrow (i.e., myelophthisic anemia), and pure red cell aplasia, most anemias due to decreased production can be categorized as microcytic or macrocytic. As microcytic and macrocytic anemias have been discussed in their own sections, this section will discuss aplastic anemia, myelophthisic anemia, and pure red cell aplasia.

APLASTIC ANEMIA

Basic description: Anemia due to absence (or near absence) of red blood cells in the bone marrow (Figure 12-4). Aplastic anemia also involves other hematopoietic cells, unless it is pure red cell aplasia, a disease associated with thymomas.

Causes of aplastic anemia

- Idiopathic (> 50% of cases).

- Secondary to drug therapy: May be a dose-dependent response (as seen with use of alkylating agents), or an idiosyncractic response (as seen with use of chloramphenicol).

TABLE 12-3. Comparison and Contrast of Vitamin B_{12} and Folate Deficiencies

Feature	Vitamin B_{12} Deficiency	Folate Deficiency
Form of anemia caused	Megaloblastic anemia	Megaloblastic anemia
Cause of neurologic deficits	Yes	No
Common cause of vitamin deficiency	Pernicious anemia	Dietary

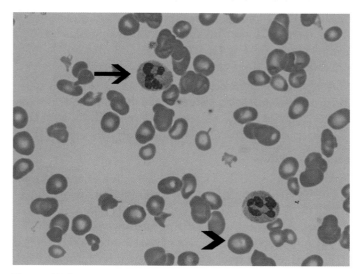

Figure 12-3. Megaloblastic anemia. This photomicrograph illustrates the two characteristic cells of megaloblastic anemia, hypersegmented neutrophils (*arrow*) and oval macrocytes (*arrowhead*). Wright-Giemsa, 1000×.

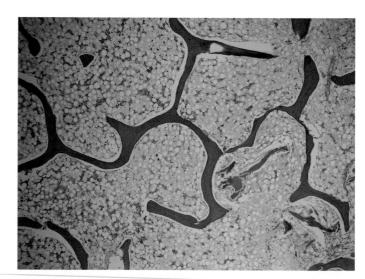

Figure 12-4. Aplastic anemia. This low-power photomicrograph of the bone marrow exhibits only a small amount of hematopoiesis. Hematoxylin and eosin, 40×.

- Secondary to toxins: Benzene.

- Secondary to infections: Parvovirus B19, Epstein-Barr virus (EBV), human immunodeficiency virus (HIV), and hepatitis (not hepatitis A, B, or C).

- Radiation.

- Genetic (e.g., **Diamond-Blackfan syndrome**).

Pathogenesis of aplastic anemia: Possibly due to suppression of stem cell function, or because the inciting agent exposes new antigens on the red blood cells, which are acted upon by the immune system.

Important point: No splenomegaly.

Laboratory findings for aplastic anemia

- Two of three findings are needed to determine a diagnosis of aplastic anemia: Neutrophil count < 500/μL, platelet count < 20,000/μL, or anemia with corrected reticulocyte count of < 1%.

- Bone marrow: Cellularity < 25%.

Clinical presentation: Can be insidious. Symptoms include weakness, fatigue, dyspnea, palpitations, gingival bleeding, epistaxis, and recurrent bacterial infections.

MYELOPHTHISIC ANEMIA

Basic description: Anemia due to space-occupying disease of the bone marrow (Figure 12-5); often associated with extramedullary hematopoiesis (i.e., hematopoiesis outside the bone marrow, often in the liver or spleen).

Causes of myelophthisic anemia: Metastatic tumor or idiopathic fibrosis of bone marrow.

PURE RED CELL APLASIA

Overview: May be primary or secondary. Secondary causes of pure red cell aplasia include thymoma (Figure 12-6), large granular lymphocytic leukemia, and autoimmune diseases.

HEMOLYTIC ANEMIAS

Overview: All hemolytic anemias have increased red blood cell destruction (either intravascular or extravascular), increased erythropoiesis (elevated erythropoietin and reticulocytosis), and increased iron deposition in tissues (mainly in the spleen and liver). Some patients have pigment gallstones and occasional extramedullary hematopoiesis.

Laboratory findings for hemolytic anemia: Patients with intravascular hemolysis have decreased plasma haptoglobin, increased unconjugated bilirubin, increased lactate dehydrogenase (LDH), positive urine hemosiderin, and positive urine hemoglobin. Patients with extravascular hemolysis have decreased haptoglobin and increased unconjugated bilirubin, but they do not have positive results for urine hemosiderin or urine hemoglobin.

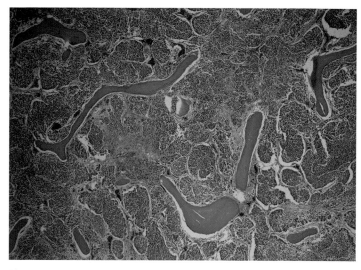

Figure 12-5. Myelophthisic anemia. Myelophthisic anemia is due to a space-occupying lesion in the bone marrow, which hinders hematopoiesis. In this photomicrograph, the bone marrow space is expanded and the hematopoietic cells are obliterated by metastatic small cell lung carcinoma. Hematoxylin and eosin, 40×.

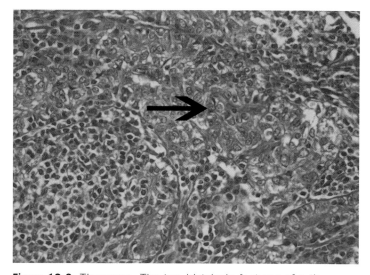

Figure 12-6. Thymoma. The two histologic features of a thymoma are lymphocytes (left lower corner) and epithelial cells (*arrow*). Thymomas are associated with pure red cell aplasia. Hematoxylin and eosin, 400×.

OVERVIEW OF LEUKEMIA AND LYMPHOMA

Overview: The neoplastic process represents a monoclonal proliferation resulting from one transformed cell. Thus, testing such as immunoglobin heavy-chain rearrangement or analysis of κ or λ light chains will reveal only one type. About 80–85% of leukemias and lymphomas are B cell in origin.

Surface markers expressed by myeloid and lymphoid cells (can be used to analyze origin of neoplastic cell)

- B-cell markers: CD10, CD19, and CD20
- T-cell markers: CD2, CD3, CD4, CD7, and CD8
- Lymphoblast: TdT
- Myeloid markers: CD13, CD14, CD15, and CD64
- Stem cell marker: CD34

Signs and symptoms: The signs and symptoms listed below apply mainly to leukemia, since most lymphomas present as a painless mass. However, in advanced states where there is metastases and extensive bone marrow involvement, lymphomas can present with many of the listed signs and symptoms.

- Damage to bone marrow by leukemias and metastatic lymphomas causes anemia, which will produce pallor, dyspnea, and fatigue; leukopenia, which causes the patient to be susceptible to infections, fever, and sepsis; and thrombocytopenia, which causes abnormal bleeding (e.g., petechial hemorrhages, ecchymoses) (Figure 12-9 *A* and *B*).

- The neoplasms are disorders of the immune system; therefore, the neoplastic cells may be responsible for a hypogammaglobulinemia or autoimmune complications.

- Acute leukemias usually have a sudden onset of a few months from symptoms to diagnosis, whereas chronic leukemias may be an incidental diagnosis determined in patients who are hospitalized for other reasons.

- Bone pain from expansion of marrow; lymphadenopathy and splenomegaly are due to infiltration of lymph nodes and the spleen by neoplastic cells.

- Hypertrophy of gingivae is due to infiltration with leukemic cells.

- Meningismus and cranial nerve deficits are due to infiltration of meninges with leukemic cells.

- Occlusion of blood vessels leads to priapism; central nervous system (CNS) symptoms (e.g., headache, blurring of vision), and strokes.

Microscopic morphology of leukemia

- **Lymphoid leukemias:** High nuclear to cytoplasmic ratio; few nucleoli.
- **Myeloid leukemias:** More prominent cytoplasm; more prominent nucleoli.
- **Acute leukemias:** Composed of immature cells (i.e., blasts) that are using their chromatin, so it will be euchromatin and the nucleus will have a smooth texture.
- **Chronic leukemias:** Composed of mature cells (e.g., myelocytes) that are *not* using their chromatin, so it will be more heterochromatin and the nucleus will have a more granular texture.

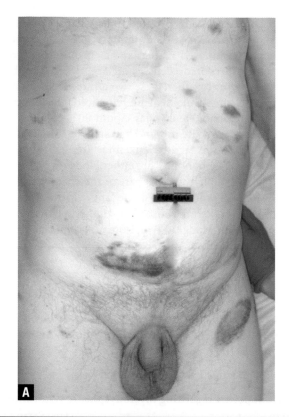

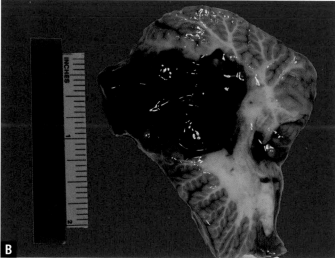

Figure 12-9. Hemorrhage due to leukemia. This patient has multiple cutaneous hemorrhages (ecchymoses) due to a coagulopathy associated with leukemia. **A**, Note the large hemorrhages on the anterior surface of the left thigh and on the right lower quadrant of the abdomen, as well as other smaller hemorrhages on the upper torso. **B**, Cerebellar hemorrhage, which was the cause of death of this patient. Courtesy of Dr. Gary Dale, Forensic Science Division, Montana State Department of Justice, Missoula, MT.

LEUKEMIA

Overview: Risk factors for leukemia include high-dose radiation and benzene. The clinical presentation of acute leukemia is usually due to complications of bone marrow failure (i.e., anemia, infections, bleeding), and proliferating blasts can produce bone pain. There are four types of leukemia: acute lymphoid leukemia, chronic lymphoid leukemia, acute myeloid leukemia, and chronic myeloid leukemia (see below). The four types of leukemia are each associated with specific cell markers and genetic abnormalities (Table 12-6).

ACUTE LYMPHOID LEUKEMIA (ALL) (SEE TABLE 12-6)

Basic description: Neoplastic monoclonal proliferation of lymphoid cells, predominantly present in the blood. The neoplastic proliferation is composed of lymphoblasts. ALL is subdivided into several categories, based upon the CD markers present on the cell. Most are **precursor B-cell type** (CD10 positive); some are **early precursor B-cell type** (CD10 negative); and others are **pre-B cell type**, which is defined by the presence of cytoplasmic Ig.

Epidemiology: ALL occurs more commonly in children and represents 70% of all childhood leukemias. An increased incidence is seen in patients with Down syndrome.

Markers: Most cases of ALL are precursor B-cell type and cells are positive for CD19, CD20, and CD10; however, 20% are precursor T-cell type.

- Precursor B-cell leukemia presents with leukemia and extensive bone marrow involvement.
- Precursor T-cell leukemia/lymphoma (see below): Male predominance; thymic involvement.

Good prognostic factors for ALL

- Hyperdiploid (> 50 chromosomes per cell).
- Age of patient: 2–10 years.
- CD10 positive.
- t(12;21) involving *TEL1* and *AML1*.
- Low white blood cell count.

TABLE 12-6. Cell Markers and Genetic Abnormalities for Leukemia

Form of Leukemia	Cell Markers		Genetic Abnormality
Acute lymphoid (lymphoblastic) leukemia (ALL)	Precursor B-cell	CD 10+	t(12;21)–*TEL1/AML1* t(9;22)–*bcr-abl*
	Early precursor B-cell Pre–B-cell	CD10- Cytoplasmic Ig+	
Chronic lymphocytic leukemia (CLL)	CD 19,20,23, and 5 positive		del 13q12-14 and del 11q trisomy 12
Acute myelogenous leukemia (AML)	CD 13,15, 64 positive		t(15;17)–*PML/RARA* t(8;21)–*CBFα/ETO*
Chronic myelogenous leukemia (CML)			t(9;22)–*bcr-abl*

HODGKIN LYMPHOMA-NODULAR SCLEROSIS TYPE

Microscopic morphology: The parenchyma is divided by bands of sclerosis (i.e., fibrosis) into nodules (Figure 12-16); rare Reed-Sternberg cells are present. Hodgkin lymphoma-nodular sclerosis type has **lacunar cells**, which are characterized by clearing around the mononuclear Reed-Sternberg cell variants.

Epidemiology: Female predominance. Nodular sclerosis is the most common type of Hodgkin lymphoma (60–70% of cases).

Markers of nodular sclerosis Hodgkin lymphoma: Cells are positive for CD15 and CD30; Reed-Sternberg cells are negative for EBV.

MIXED CELLULARITY HODGKIN LYMPHOMA

Microscopic morphology: Reed-Sternberg cells are more easily found in the tumor than in the nodular sclerosis type. The background cells are reactive and include eosinophils, neutrophils, and lymphocytes (Figure 12-17).

Epidemiology: Older patients (> 50 years). Mixed cellularity Hodgkin lymphoma represents 25% of cases of Hodgkin lymphoma.

Markers of mixed cellularity Hodgkin lymphoma: Cells are positive for CD15 and CD30; 70% of Reed-Sternberg cells are positive for EBV.

LYMPHOCYTE PREDOMINANT HODGKIN LYMPHOMA

Microscopic morphology: Vaguely nodular; has Reed-Sternberg cell variants, which are referred to as L&H, or popcorn cells.

Epidemiology: Younger males (age 35).

Markers of lymphocyte predominant Hodgkin lymphoma: Cells are negative for CD15 and CD30; cells are positive for CD20 and EMA.

Important points regarding lymphocyte predominant Hodgkin lymphoma

- Very benign and often cured with local excision.

- Often present with cervical or axillary lymphadenopathy.

Important points regarding Hodgkin lymphoma

- **Staging:** HL staging is based upon the number of lymph nodes involved (stage I is one lymph node) and the location of lymph nodes in relation to the diaphragm. Stage II is two or more lymph nodes on the same side of the diaphragm; stage III is two or more lymph nodes on opposite sides of the diaphragm; and stage IV represents disseminated disease.

- HL spreads node-to-node and is often localized at the time of presentation.

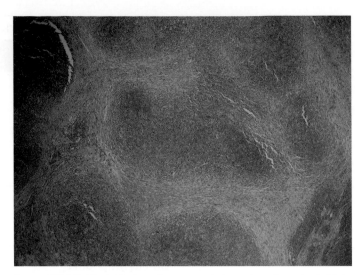

Figure 12-16. Hodgkin lymphoma, nodular sclerosis variant. Note the nodules of lymphocytes and other hematopoietic cells divided by broad fibrous septae. Hematoxylin and eosin, 40×.

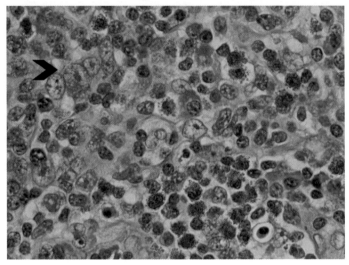

Figure 12-17. Hodgkin lymphoma, mixed cellularity variant. Note the Reed-Sternberg cell (*arrowhead*). The other cell types in this image are reactive (only the Reed-Sternberg cell is neoplastic) and include neutrophils, lymphocytes, and, prominently in this image, eosinophils. Hematoxylin and eosin, 400×.

NON-HODGKIN LYMPHOMA

Overview (see Table 12-8)

■ **Epidemiology:** Varies with types. Some are more common in childhood, and others are more common in adulthood.

■ **Lymph node involvement:** Discontinuous groups, so non-Hodgkin lymphoma cannot be effectively surgically excised. Extranodal involvement is common and more so among aggressive subtypes of non-Hodgkin lymphoma. Non-Hodgkin lymphoma can involve the spleen (Figure 12-18).

■ **Neoplastic cells:** Most non-Hodgkin lymphomas are derived from B cells, and others are from T cells.

■ **Important points:** Non-Hodgkin lymphoma is often disseminated at the time of diagnosis; aggressive lymphomas have a propensity for involving the leptomeninges.

■ **Clinical presentation of non-Hodgkin lymphoma**

  ○ Painless lymphadenopathy (most commonly, neck, inguinal, and axillary regions).

  ○ Approximately 20% of patients have constitutional symptoms (e.g., fever, weight loss, and/or night sweats) called "B" symptoms. These symptoms are more common in patients with aggressive lymphomas.

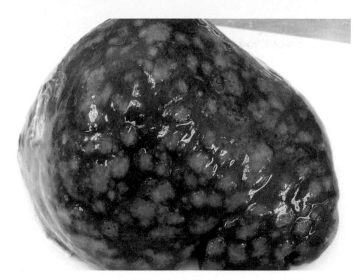

Figure 12-18. Spleen, non-Hodgkin lymphoma. This spleen exhibits uniform multicentric involvement of the white pulp by a malignant lymphoma. These changes contribute to generalized splenomegaly.

TWO GENERAL TYPES OF NON-HODGKIN LYMPHOMA: INDOLENT AND AGGRESSIVE

Overview: Indolent (low-grade) lymphomas have a longer survival curve, but patients are never cured. Aggressive (high-grade) lymphomas have a rapid drop off of the survival curve, but the curve then flattens out because patients can be cured. Mantle cell lymphoma has the worst prognosis of both types: a more rapid drop off of the survival curve, with no patients being cured.

■ Indolent lymphomas have a longer survival interval with no hope of cure, and include follicular lymphoma and small lymphocytic lymphoma.

■ Aggressive lymphomas have a shorter survival interval; however, with correct treatment, a cure is possible with indefinite survival. Includes Burkitt lymphoma and diffuse large B-cell lymphoma.

WHO classification of lymphoid neoplasms

■ Precursor B-cell neoplasms.

■ Peripheral B-cell neoplasms (CLL/SLL, lymphoplasmacytic lymphoma, mantle cell lymphoma, follicular lymphoma, hairy cell leukemia).

■ Precursor T-cell neoplasms.

■ Peripheral T-cell and NK-cell neoplasms (anaplastic large cell lymphoma).

TYPES OF NON-HODGKIN LYMPHOMA

Overview: Although there are many types of non-Hodgkin lymphoma, only the more common types will be discussed below. These include follicular lymphoma, small lymphocytic lymphoma, diffuse large B-cell lymphoma, Burkitt lymphoma, precursor T-cell lymphoblastic leukemia and lymphoma, mantle cell lymphoma, MALToma, hairy cell leukemia, and mycosis fungoides and Sézary syndrome.

FOLLICULAR LYMPHOMA (FIGURE 12-19 *A* AND *B*)

Epidemiology: Older patients; male to female ratio is equal; 40% of cases of non-Hodgkin lymphoma are diagnosed as follicular lymphoma.

Cytogenetic abnormality: t(14;18), which moves *bcl-2* gene adjacent to the Ig heavy-chain gene. Bcl-2 inhibits apoptosis; by moving its location adjacent to the Ig heavy-chain gene (a gene often transcribed), more bcl-2 is produced. Occasionally, follicular lymphomas have translocations involving *bcl-6* on 3q27.

Markers of follicular lymphoma: Neoplastic cells are positive for CD19, CD20, CD10, surface Ig, and bcl-2 (normal follicle center cells are negative for bcl-2).

Prognosis: Patients can survive 7–9 years, and most progress to develop diffuse large B-cell lymphoma or to Burkitt lymphoma.

Microscopic morphology of follicular lymphoma: Back-to-back follicles of the same size, composed of small cells or large cells. Bone marrow involvement (seen in 85% of cases) is usually peritrabecular.

Clinical presentation of follicular lymphoma

- Painless lymphadenopathy.
- Fever, night sweats, and fatigue.
- Most patients (80–90%) present with advanced stage III or stage IV disease.

SMALL LYMPHOCYTIC LYMPHOMA (SLL)

Microscopic morphology: SLL has proliferation centers, which are clusters of mitotically active prolymphocytes.

Important point: SLL and CLL are essentially the same process; however, in SLL the involvement of the lymph nodes is the most prominent, and in CLL the involvement of the bone marrow and blood is the most prominent.

DIFFUSE LARGE B-CELL LYMPHOMA (DLBCL)

Epidemiology: Most patients are older than 60 years of age; however, DLBCL represents 15% of childhood lymphomas. Overall, DLBCL represents 50% of cases of adult NHL. It occurs in males slightly more commonly than in females.

Cytogenetic abnormality: Approximately 10–20% of cases have t(14;18), a translocation involving *bcl-2*; 30% of cases have a translocation involving 3q27 (*bcl-6*).

Markers: Neoplastic cells are positive for CD19, CD20, CD79a, and surface Ig.

Microscopic morphology: Monotonous sheets of large cells with prominent nucleoli (Figure 12-20).

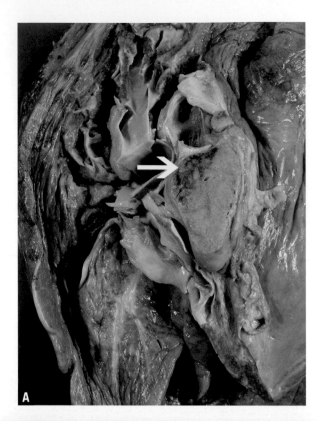

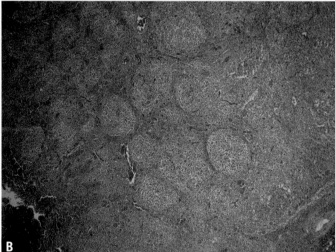

Figure 12-19. Follicular lymphoma. **A,** Follicular lymphoma involves this hilar lymph node. The black material (*arrow*) represents normal lymphoid parenchyma with anthracotic pigment displaced to one side by the expanding tan lymphomatous process. **B,** This lymph node exhibits the characteristic low power features of follicular lymphoma, tightly packed lymphoid follicles of approximately equal size. Hematoxylin and eosin, 40×.

Important points regarding DLBCL

- Some cases of DLBCL are associated with EBV (in HIV and immunosuppressed patients).
- Human herpesvirus 8 (HHV-8) is associated with a form of DLBCL called **primary effusion lymphoma,** which occurs in body cavities.

BURKITT LYMPHOMA

Epidemiology: Represents 30% of cases of childhood non-Hodgkin lymphoma.

Forms of Burkitt lymphoma: Sporadic and endemic

- **Sporadic type:** Occurs in the United States. Presents in the abdomen near the ileocecal valve, in the ovaries, or in the retroperitoneum; 15–20% of sporadic-type Burkitt lymphomas are associated with EBV infection.
- **Endemic type:** Occurs in Africa. Commonly presents in the jaw. All endemic-type Burkitt lymphomas are associated with EBV infection.

Cytogenetic abnormality: *MYC* (chr 8) translocated adjacent to the Ig heavy-chain gene on chromosome 14 (t(8;14) is the most common; or *MYC* is translocated adjacent to Ig light-chain gene (κ on chromosome 2 [t(2;8)] or λ on chromosome 22 [t(8;22)]).

Markers of Burkitt lymphoma: Neoplastic cells are positive for CD10, CD19, CD20, bcl-6, and surface Ig.

Microscopic morphology: Tumor is composed of diffuse sheets of cells. There is a "starry-sky" pattern produced by macrophages engulfing cellular debris (Figure 12-21).

Important points regarding Burkitt lymphoma

- Burkitt lymphoma has the highest turnover rate of any human malignancy, and carries an extremely high risk of tumor lysis syndrome.
- **Tumor lysis syndrome** is caused by chemotherapy, and is characterized by metabolic acidosis, hyperuricemia, hyperkalemia, and hyperphosphatemia. Acute renal failure is the most common complication. Treatment with allopurinol or rasburicase before chemotherapy is preventative.

PRECURSOR T-CELL LYMPHOBLASTIC LEUKEMIA AND LYMPHOMA

Epidemiology: Adolescent males aged 15–20 years.

Markers: Cells are positive for TdT, CD2, and CD7.

Cytogenetic abnormality: Most common is translocation involving *TAL1.*

Gross morphology: Usually presents as a mediastinal mass.

Microscopic morphology: Lymphoblasts with irregular nuclear contours, small nucleoli, and scant cytoplasm.

Important points: Propensity for involving bone marrow and propensity to relapse and involve the leptomeninges.

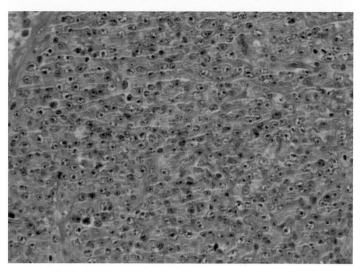

Figure 12-20. Diffuse large B-cell lymphoma. The photomicrograph shows a sheet of monotonous large neoplastic cells with prominent nucleoli. Hematoxylin and eosin, 200×.

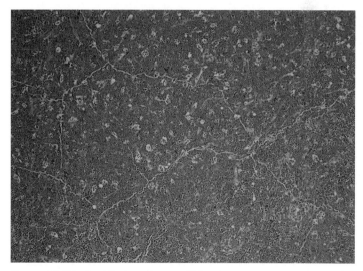

Figure 12-21. Burkitt lymphoma. This photomicrograph illustrates the characteristic low power features of Burkitt lymphoma, a sheet of neoplastic cells interspersed with punctate clearings ("starry sky pattern"). The punctate clearings are macrophages engulfing cellular debris. Burkitt lymphoma is an aggressive rapidly growing neoplasm with abundant cellular turnover, hence the presence of the macrophages. Hematoxylin and eosin, 40×.

MANTLE CELL LYMPHOMA

Epidemiology: Older males.

Cytogenetic abnormality: t(11;14), in which cyclin *D1* on chromosome 11 is translocated adjacent to the Ig heavy-chain gene.

Markers of mantle cell lymphoma: Neoplastic cells are positive for CD19, CD20, CD5, and surface Ig, and are negative for CD 23.

Microscopic morphology: Vaguely nodular or diffuse pattern composed of small cells (some are deeply cleft); usually there are no large cells.

Important points regarding mantle cell lymphoma

- Survival is 3–5 years; *there is no cure.*

- Cells are CD5 positive, although it is a neoplasm of B cells, which indicates aberrant expression of CD5, similar to that seen in CLL.

- Can involve gastrointestinal tract producing polyps (i.e., **lymphomatoid polyposis**).

MALTOMA (ALSO REFERRED TO AS MARGINAL ZONE LYMPHOMA)

Basic description: Lymphoma arising from mucosa-associated lymphoid tissue (MALT).

Cytogenetic abnormalities: t(1;14) involving *bcl-10*; t(11;18) involving *MALI* and *IAP2*.

Conditions associated with MALTomas: *Helicobacter pylori* infection of the stomach, Hashimoto thyroiditis, and Sjögren syndrome.

Important points: MALTomas may regress if the inciting agent is removed; MALTomas remain localized for long periods of time.

HAIRY CELL LEUKEMIA (FIGURE 12-22)

Clinical triad: Older male with pancytopenia and splenomegaly.

Markers: Neoplastic cells are positive for CD19, CD20, CD25, CD11c, and CD103.

Additional clinical finding: Positive for tartrate-resistant acid phosphatase (TRAP).

ADULT T-CELL LEUKEMIA/LYMPHOMA

Basic description: Associated with infections with human T-cell leukemia virus-1 (HTLV-1).

MYCOSIS FUNGOIDES AND SÉZARY SYNDROME

Basic description: Mycosis fungoides is a T-cell lymphoma with infiltration of the epidermis and dermis. It is a chronic condition. Sézary syndrome is a generalized exfoliative dermatitis with leukemic spread.

Microscopic morphology: Cerebriform nuclei (Sézary cells) and Pautrier microabscesses.

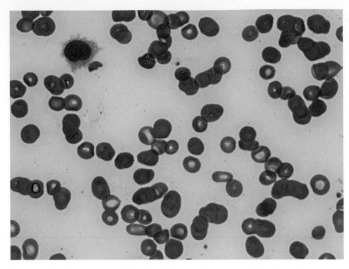

Figure 12-22. Hairy cell leukemia. In the upper left corner is a single neoplastic lymphoid cell. Note the fine hair-like projections from its surface. Wright-Giemsa, 1000×.

PLASMA CELL DYSCRASIAS

Overview: Plasma cell dyscrasias are a group of disorders characterized by a monoclonal proliferation of plasma cells. In many types, this proliferation of cells results in an overproduction of one clone of Ig, producing an **M spike** in the γ region on serum protein electrophoresis. The neoplastic plasma cells can secrete light and heavy chains along with complete immunoglobulin; sometimes they secrete only free light or heavy chains. Free light chains are called **Bence Jones proteins.** The types of plasma cell dyscrasias discussed in this section are multiple myeloma, monoclonal gammopathy of undetermined significance, plasmacytoma, lymphoplasmacytic lymphoma, and heavy chain disease.

MULTIPLE MYELOMA

Epidemiology: 50–60 years of age. Multiple myeloma is the most common tumor arising within bone.

Complications of multiple myeloma

▪ The most common bones involved are the vertebrae, skull, and ribs.

  ○ Bone pain due to expansion of marrow.

  ○ Lytic lesions in bone due to the expansion of plasma cells, which can predispose to pathologic fractures. Production of IL-6 by neoplastic cells stimulates osteoclasts through the RANK ligand.

  ○ Hypercalcemia due to bone resorption.

▪ Decreased levels of functional immunoglobin predispose patients to recurrent infections (e.g., *Staphylococcus aureus*, *Streptococcus pneumoniae*, and *Escherichia coli*).

▪ Overproduction of the light chains, which collect in the kidney as casts in the distal convoluted tubules and collecting tubules. The light chains can cause renal insufficiency.

▪ Amyloidosis due to overproduction of light chains.

Cytogenetic abnormalities: t(4;14) in which fibroblast growth factor receptor gene is translocated adjacent to the Ig heavy-chain gene; also, 13q deletions.

Important points regarding multiple myeloma

▪ Almost 99% of multiple myelomas secrete Ig. There is no M spike in nonsecretory myelomas.

▪ Approximately 60% of multiple myelomas produce IgG; 20–25% produce IgA; and 15–20% produce light chains only (κ or λ).

▪ The main cause of death is infection, and the second most common cause of death is renal failure.

▪ Approximately 20% of patients with multiple myeloma do not have a detectable M protein, but they do have free light chains in the urine.

Microscopic morphology of multiple myeloma (Figure 12-23 *A* and *B*)

▪ More than 30% of bone marrow cells are plasma cells.

▪ Accumulation of immunoglobins in plasma cells (**Russell bodies**).

▪ On peripheral blood smear, cells stack (i.e., rouleaux) like a roll of coins.

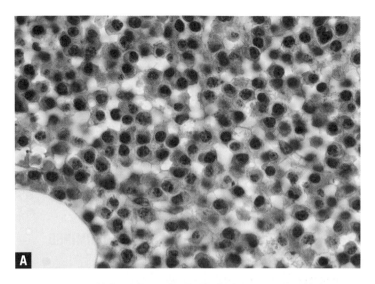
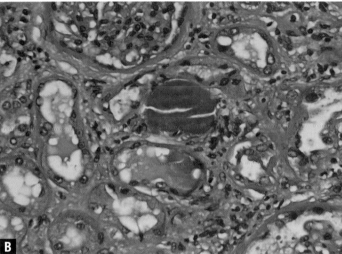

Figure 12-23. Multiple myeloma. **A**, The photomicrograph is of a bone-marrow aspirate from a patient with multiple myeloma. Note that almost all cells present are plasma cells (with "clock-face" chromatin). **B**, The photomicrograph illustrates the changes in the kidney that occur in multiple myeloma. In the center of the image is a tubule plugged with Bence Jones proteins (note the clefts). Hematoxylin and eosin, A and B, 400×.

Complications: Stroke, deep venous thrombosis, limb ischemia, and myocardial infarction.

Important point: Heparin causes a transient thrombocytopenia in 25% of all patients. This is a non–immune-mediated and usually self-limited adverse effect.

Other causes of immune-mediated thrombocytopenias

- **Iso-immune thrombocytopenia:** Development of antiplatelet antibodies due to previous blood or platelet transfusion.
- Collagen vascular disease.
- Drug induced.
- Infectious (HIV).

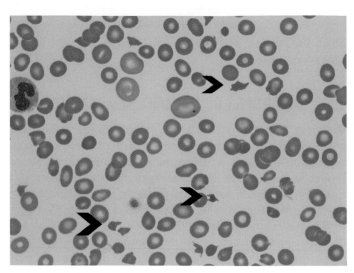

Figure 12-24. Thrombotic thrombocytopenic purpura (TTP). Patients with TTP form platelet microthrombi in their vasculature. Red blood cells impacting these platelet thrombi can be damaged and, hence, the formation of schistocytes (*arrowheads*). Wright-Giemsa, 1000×.

NON–IMMUNE-MEDIATED DESTRUCTION OF PLATELETS

Overview: Causes of non–immune-mediated destruction of platelets include thrombotic thrombocytopenic purpura (TTP), hemolytic uremic syndrome (HUS), DIC, and giant hemangiomas. TTP, HUS, and DIC are discussed below.

THROMBOTIC THROMBOCYTOPENIC PURPURA (TTP)

Clinical presentation of TTP: The classic pentad of signs and symptoms is fever, thrombocytopenia, renal failure, neurologic changes, and microangiopathic hemolytic anemia.

Mechanism: Genetic, autoimmune, or acquired deficiency in ADAMTS-13, an enzyme that degrades very high-weight multimers of von Willebrand factor (vWF).

Laboratory findings of TTP: Microangiopathic hemolytic anemia (with schistocytes); normal PT and PTT.

Microscopic morphology of TTP: Microthrombi (platelets surrounded by fibrin) in capillaries. Schistocytes are seen on peripheral blood smears (Figure 12-24).

HEMOLYTIC UREMIC SYNDROME (HUS)

Clinical presentation of HUS: Similar to TTP, but renal dysfunction is more prominent and neurologic symptoms are less likely. HUS is most commonly associated with O157:H7 *E coli* infections in children, but it also occurs during the postpartum period.

Laboratory findings: See TTP.

Microscopic morphology: See TTP.

DISSEMINATED INTRAVASCULAR COAGULATION (DIC)

Basic description: A condition with widespread activation of both the coagulation system and the fibrinolytic system.

Mechanism: Release of tissue factor and widespread damage to endothelial cells.

Causes of DIC

- **Obstetric conditions:** Placental abruption, retained fetus, septic abortion, and amniotic fluid embolus.
- **Infectious:** Sepsis, meningococcemia, and Histoplasmosis.

- **Neoplastic:** Carcinomas of the pancreas, prostate, and lung, and acute promyelocytic leukemia.
- **Other:** Massive trauma and thermal injury, acute pancreatitis, and liver disease.

Complications of DIC

- Widespread thrombi, which produce ischemia.
- Activation of fibrinolysis and depletion of coagulation factors and platelets leads to bleeding.

Laboratory findings of DIC

- Low number of platelets and elevated PT and PTT.
- Increased fibrin split products.
- Schistocytes on blood smear.

Forms of DIC

- **Acute DIC:** Form most often associated with obstetric and infectious etiologies and with bleeding complications.
- **Chronic DIC:** Form most often associated with neoplastic and hepatic disease and with thrombotic complications.

Microscopic morphology of DIC: Microthrombi in the kidney, heart, lung, and liver (Figure 12-25).

OTHER PLATELET DISORDERS

Overview: In addition to immune-mediated and non–immune-mediated destruction of platelets, the other categories of platelet disorders are decreased production of platelets and platelet dysfunction. Each of these categories will be discussed briefly below.

Causes of decreased production of platelets

- General conditions that cause depletion of all marrow elements (e.g., aplastic anemia, leukemia, lymphoma, and metastatic carcinoma).
- Conditions that selectively cause thrombocytopenia (e.g., alcohol use, thiazide diuretics, measles, and HIV).
- Ineffective megakaryopoiesis (e.g., in megaloblastic anemia).

PLATELET DYSFUNCTION

Overview: The number of platelets is adequate, but the platelets themselves are not functioning correctly.

Causes

- Aspirin therapy, which impairs cyclooxygenase, which in turn impairs production of thromboxane, a factor that is necessary for primary hemostasis.
- Uremia.

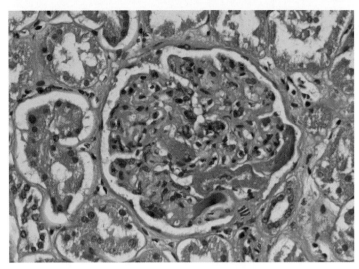

Figure 12-25. Kidney, with disseminated intravascular coagulation (DIC). In DIC, patients have widespread activation of both the clotting and fibrinolytic systems. One result is multiple microthrombi, which can lodge in small vessels. In this glomerulus, the capillaries of the glomerular tuft have several microthrombi (serpentine eosinophilic smudged structures from the 3-o'clock to the 6-o'clock position). Hematoxylin and eosin, 400×.

DISORDERS OF SECONDARY HEMOSTASIS

Overview: Disorders of secondary hemostasis most commonly are due to an inherited defect in the clotting cascade. Although there are many disorders of secondary hemostasis, three of the more common conditions, von Willebrand disease, hemophilia A and hemophilia B, will be discussed below.

VON WILLEBRAND DISEASE

Mechanism: Due to deficiency (quantitative or qualitative) of vWF, which impairs platelet binding to exposed collagen. VWF serves two roles: to bind platelets to the collagen underlying a damaged vessel wall, and to act as a carrier for factor VIII.

Inheritance pattern: Some forms are autosomal dominant (such as type I), and others are autosomal recessive.

Clinical presentation of von Willebrand disease

- **Symptoms:** Bleeding in mucous membranes, epistaxis, increased bleeding after trauma, and menorrhagia.
- **Laboratory findings:** Elevated bleeding time and partial thromboplastin time (PTT); increased ristocetin factor assay.

HEMOPHILIA A

Mechanism: Due to deficiency of factor VIII.

Inheritance pattern: X-linked recessive (30% of cases are new mutations).

Clinical presentation

- **Symptoms:** Hemorrhage after trauma or surgery and hemorrhage into joints and soft tissue. Complications include recurrent hemarthroses, which leads to joint destruction, and intracranial bleeding. Intracranial bleeding is the most common cause of death in hemophiliacs.
- **Laboratory findings:** Elevated PTT with normal PT, bleeding time, and fibrinogen levels.

HEMOPHILIA B

Basic description: Similar characteristics as hemophilia A, but the mechanism is a deficiency of factor IX.

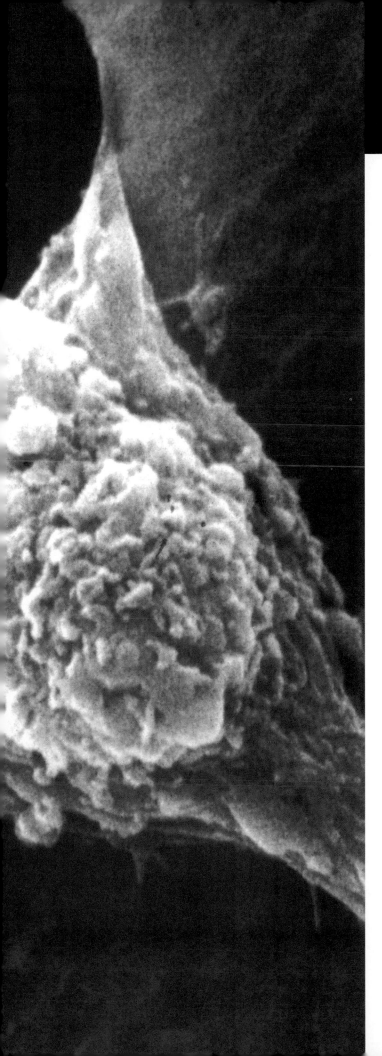

CHAPTER 13

PULMONARY PATHOLOGY

OVERVIEW

Diseases of the lung can be classified into four general categories: (1) obstructive lung disease; (2) restrictive lung disease; (3) infectious disease; and (4) neoplastic disease (Table 13-1). The key clinical difference between obstructive and restrictive lung disease is the forced expiratory volume at one second (FEV_1) and the forced vital capacity (FVC) ratio, which is decreased in obstructive lung disease and normal in restrictive lung disease. In obstructive lung disease, air is trapped within the parenchyma; in restrictive lung disease, airway filling is impaired due to fibrosis of alveolar septae. The four main types of obstructive lung disease are **emphysema, asthma, bronchiectasis,** and **chronic bronchitis.** Restrictive lung disease can be divided into acute and chronic forms, and chronic forms can be subdivided by etiology (i.e., work related, drug induced, autoimmune, and idiopathic).

The seven major forms of infectious lung disease (i.e., pneumonia) are (1) community-acquired typical (e.g., bacterial); (2) community-acquired atypical (e.g., viral, others); (3) nosocomial; (4) aspiration; (5) necrotizing pneumonia; (6) chronic pneumonia (e.g., fungal, mycobacterial); and (7) pneumonia in immunocompromised hosts. Neoplastic disease can be divided into **small cell lung carcinoma** and **non–small cell lung carcinoma.** The designation of non–small cell carcinoma versus small cell carcinoma is of utmost importance when determining treatment options. Small cell carcinoma is assumed at the time of diagnosis to have already metastasized.

This chapter will discuss acute respiratory failure, atelectasis, obstructive lung disease, restrictive lung disease, causes of chronic restrictive lung disease, diffuse pulmonary hemorrhage, pulmonary hypertension, pulmonary infections, pulmonary neoplasms, miscellaneous pleural conditions (including pleural effusions and mesothelioma), and upper respiratory tract conditions.

ACUTE RESPIRATORY FAILURE

Overview: There are two types of acute respiratory failure: hypoxemic acute respiratory failure and hypercapnic acute respiratory failure.

HYPOXEMIC ACUTE RESPIRATORY FAILURE

Basic description: Respiratory failure with pO_2 of < 60 mm Hg.

Causes: Pulmonary edema, **acute respiratory distress syndrome (ARDS)**, pneumonia.

HYPERCAPNIC ACUTE RESPIRATORY FAILURE

Basic description: Respiratory failure with pCO_2 of > 45 mm Hg.

Causes: Obstructive lung disease (e.g., **chronic obstructive pulmonary disease [COPD]**, asthma), upper respiratory obstruction, decreased compliance of the chest wall (e.g., kyphoscoliosis), and hypoventilation.

ATELECTASIS

Overview: Atelectasis is collapse of the pulmonary parenchyma. Because of atelectasis, airways and alveoli are unable to fill, and blood is shunted from the arteries to the veins without adequate oxygenation. The four common types of atelectasis discussed below are compressive, obstructive, microatelectasis, and contraction atelectasis.

COMPRESSIVE ATELECTASIS (FIGURE 13-1)

Mechanism: A condition or lesion external to the lungs (i.e., in the pleural cavity) compresses the lung and impairs filling of the alveoli upon respiration.

Causes of compressive atelectasis: Blood in the pleural cavity (i.e., **hemothorax**), air in the pleural cavity (i.e., **pneumothorax**), and fluid in the pleural cavity (e.g., pulmonary edema).

Mediastinal shift: Away from the source of the atelectasis.

OBSTRUCTIVE ATELECTASIS (RESORPTIVE ATELECTASIS)

Mechanism: An obstruction in the airway impairs filling of alveoli. All air in the alveoli is eventually resorbed and the alveoli collapse.

Causes of obstructive atelectasis: Aspirated foreign body, tumor, and mucus (e.g., in chronic bronchitis and cystic fibrosis).

Mediastinal shift: Toward the source of the atelectasis.

MICROATELECTASIS

Mechanism: Loss of surfactant.

Causes: Prematurity, interstitial inflammation, postsurgical.

CONTRACTION ATELECTASIS

Mechanism: Due to localized or generalized fibrosis impairing the ability of the alveoli to expand and contract.

Cause: Pulmonary fibrosis and scarring.

OBSTRUCTIVE LUNG DISEASE

Overview: Obstructive lung disease is a disease of the lungs that impairs the ability of air to leave the alveoli during expiration,

TABLE 13-1. General Categories of Pulmonary Disease

Category	Subcategories or Specific Conditions
Obstructive lung disease	Emphysema Asthma Chronic bronchitis Bronchiectasis
Restrictive lung disease	Autoimmune Idiopathic Work related Drug related
Infectious lung disease	Community-acquired typical pneumonia Community-acquired atypical pneumonia Nosocomial pneumonia Aspiration pneumonia Necrotizing pneumonia Chronic pneumonia Pneumonia in immunocompromised
Neoplastic lung disease	Non–small cell lung carcinoma Small cell lung carcinoma

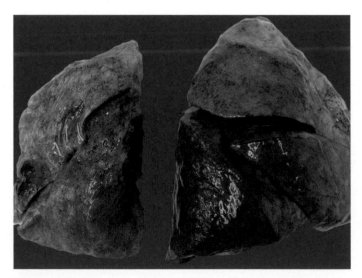

Figure 13-1. Atelectasis. This photograph shows atelectasis as the result of a left-sided hemothorax due to a gunshot wound. The blood in the left pleural cavity caused compressive atelectasis of the left lung. Note the smaller size of the left lung and its wrinkled pleural surface (due to collapse), compared to the smooth pleural surface of the right lung.

trapping it. It is clinically defined by the decreased FEV_1/FVC ratio. The residual volume and functional residual capacity (FRC) are increased, but the total lung capacity may remain normal. The condition eventually leads to hypercapnic respiratory failure, with pCO_2 of > 45 mm Hg. The four types of obstructive lung disease discussed below are emphysema, asthma, chronic bronchitis, and bronchiectasis.

EMPHYSEMA

Basic description: Disease process that is characterized by the loss of pulmonary parenchyma (i.e., loss of alveolar septae and walls of airways) and dilation of terminal airways.

Types of emphysema

▪ **Centriacinar emphysema,** which affects the respiratory bronchioles and involves the upper lobes. Centriacinar emphysema is associated with smoking.

▪ **Panacinar emphysema,** which affects the alveoli and alveolar ducts and eventually the respiratory bronchioles and involves the lower lobes. Panacinar emphysema is associated with α_1-antitrypsin deficiency.

Mechanism of emphysema: The loss of pulmonary parenchyma causes a loss of elastic recoil. When the patient breathes out, the airways collapse, trapping air because of reduced driving pressure.

Causes of emphysema

▪ Both centriacinar and panacinar emphysema are caused by an imbalance in protease-antiprotease and oxidant-antioxidant.

▪ Centriacinar emphysema is caused by cigarette smoking. The nicotine plays several roles.

  ○ Nicotine is a chemoattractant of neutrophils by induction of nuclear factor-$\kappa\beta$ and resultant production of tumor necrosis factor (TNF) and interleukin-8 (IL-8). TNF and IL-8 activate neutrophils, which release damaging proteases.

  ○ Nicotine causes inactivation of antiproteases.

  ○ Nicotine causes production of reactive oxygen species, which inactivate proteases and deplete antioxidants.

▪ Panacinar emphysema is caused by a deficiency in α_1-antitrypsin. The normal allele encoding α_1-antitrypsin is PiMM, but 0.012% of the population has a PiZZ allele, which is associated with a significant decrease in the amount of α_1-antitrypsin.

Complications of emphysema

▪ **Pulmonary hypertension** as a result of hypoxia-induced vasospasm and loss of vascular surface area (i.e., losing alveolar septae causes loss of alveolar capillaries).

▪ **Cor pulmonale** (right-sided heart failure secondary to pulmonary hypertension).

▪ **Mismatched ventilation-perfusion,** with shunting of blood to areas of poor ventilation.

Morphology of emphysema: Dilation of airspaces; bullae formation at the pleural surface (Figure 13-2 A–C).

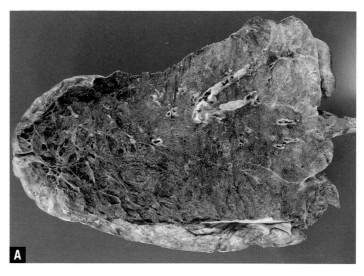

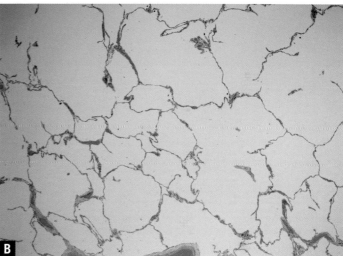

Figure 13-2. Emphysema. **A,** The lung is lying on its posterior surface, and the upper lobe is at the left side of the image. Note the loss of parenchyma and greatly increased size of the airspaces (imparting a spiderweb-like appearance). **B,** The microscopic appearance of emphysema correlates with the gross appearance in A. Once again, note the loss of pulmonary parenchyma and greatly increased size of the airspaces. Hematoxylin and eosin, 40×. (*Continued*).

CHRONIC BRONCHITIS

Basic description: Productive cough for at least 3 months in 2 consecutive years.

Pathogenesis: Related to cigarette smoking. Toxins in smoke irritate the airway, resulting in increased production of mucus, which, in turn, stimulates hyperplasia of mucous-secreting glands.

Types of chronic bronchitis: Simple, obstructive, and asthmatic.

Complications of chronic bronchitis

- Obstruction of the airway by mucus, leading to bronchiectasis or atelectasis.
- Pulmonary hypertension.

Morphology of chronic bronchitis

- **Gross:** Mucous plugging.
- **Microscopic:** Submucosal gland hypertrophy producing increased **Reid index.** The Reid index is the thickness of mucous glands in relation to thickness of the wall; in chronic bronchitis, it is > 0.40.

Clinical presentation of chronic bronchitis (see basic description of chronic bronchitis)

- **Signs and symptoms:** Chronic productive cough; hypercapnia (patients are referred to as "blue bloaters").
- **Important point:** Can have asthmatic component ("**asthmatic bronchitis**").

BRONCHIECTASIS

Basic description: Abnormal, permanent dilation of airways.

Pathogenesis: Requires two components, infection and obstruction, each one of which can occur first and start the disease process. The infection results in destruction of the smooth muscle and elastic fibers in the wall of the airway.

Causes of bronchiectasis: Allergic bronchopulmonary aspergillosis, cystic fibrosis, and **Kartagener syndrome** (see related condition below); necrotizing pulmonary infections leading to obstruction (e.g., *Staphylococcus*, *Klebsiella*); and other sources of obstruction including tumors, foreign bodies, and mucus in the airways (e.g., from asthma, chronic bronchitis, cystic fibrosis).

Complications of bronchiectasis

- Hemoptysis, with potentially life-threatening hemorrhage.
- Rarely, pulmonary hypertension, abscess formation, and amyloidosis.

Morphology of bronchiectasis

- **Gross:** Dilation of airways, usually involving lower lobes, right side more often than left, with airways almost extending to the pleural surface (Figure 13-4).
- **Microscopic:** Appearance depends upon stage, inflammatory infiltrate, and tissue destruction.

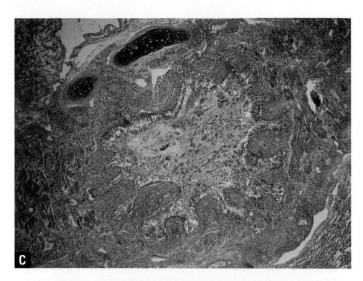

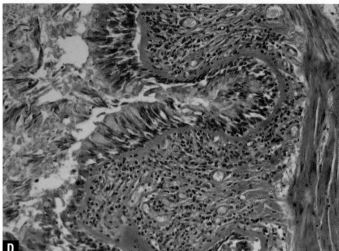

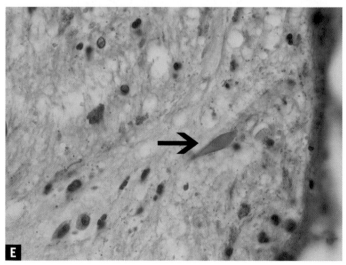

Figure 13-3. (*Continued*) **C,** Low-power histologic changes associated with asthma, mucous plug of the airway, prominent basement membrane, and smooth muscle hypertrophy. The smooth muscle hypertrophy is producing a vaguely polyp-like architecture to the airway lining, with projections into the lumen. **D,** The characteristic eosinophilic infiltrate associated with some forms of asthma. **E,** A Charcot-Leyden crystal (*arrow*), formed by major basic protein. Hematoxylin and eosin, C, 40×; D, 200x; E, 1000×.

Clinical presentation of bronchiectasis

- **Symptoms:** Dyspnea, chronic cough (dry, or with large amounts of purulent sputum production). Hemoptysis is common.

- **Signs:** Clubbing of the fingers (i.e., **pulmonary osteoarthropathy**), hypoxemia, and hypercapnia.

- **Chest radiograph:** Parallel lines in peripheral lung fields, which represent nontapering thickened bronchial walls.

Related condition: Primary ciliary dyskinesia

- **Genetic abnormality:** Hereditary condition associated with short dynein arms.

- **Subset of primary ciliary dyskinesia is Kartagener syndrome,** which includes bronchiectasis, sinusitis, situs inversus, and sterility.

CHRONIC OBSTRUCTIVE PULMONARY DISEASE

Overview: Chronic bronchitis is a clinical diagnosis, and emphysema is an anatomic diagnosis. Patients with symptoms of obstructive lung disease (except asthma and bronchiectasis) are often assigned the clinical diagnosis of chronic obstructive pulmonary disease (COPD). The cause of death in patients with COPD is respiratory acidosis, cor pulmonale, or potentially a pneumothorax.

Clinical presentation of COPD

- **Symptoms:** Earliest is chronic productive cough, followed by dyspnea on exertion.

- **Signs:** Increased anteroposterior chest diameter (i.e., barrel chest) due to chronic lung overinflation. Patients use accessory muscles to breath. Patients are often dependent on supplemental oxygen, and pulmonary function tests are consistent with a diagnosis of obstructive lung disease with decreased FEV_1/FVC ratio.

RESTRICTIVE LUNG DISEASE

Overview: There are two categories of restrictive lung disease, **extrapulmonary and intrapulmonary.** Extrapulmonary sources include obesity and kyphoscoliosis, and cause a restrictive lung disease by externally impairing filling of the lung. There are two subcategories of intrapulmonary restrictive lung disease, **acute and chronic.** Acute restrictive lung disease is primarily confined to the diagnosis of acute respiratory distress syndrome (ARDS). Chronic restrictive lung disease is a broad group, which includes many distinct entities. Chronic restrictive lung disease will be discussed following acute restrictive lung disease.

ACUTE RESTRICTIVE LUNG DISEASE

Basic description: Disease developing over a short time period (minutes to days), usually secondary to a major systemic insult (e.g., sepsis, shock), which causes an acute restrictive lung disease, hypoxemic respiratory failure (pO_2 is < 60 mm Hg), and diffuse pulmonary infiltrates, and is not attributable to left-sided heart failure. The clinical term for acute restrictive lung disease is **acute respiratory distress syndrome** (ARDS), and the pathologic term is **diffuse alveolar damage.**

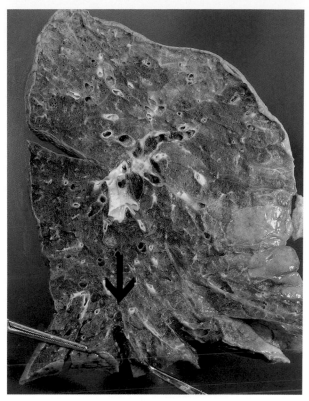

Figure 13-4. Bronchiectasis. In the lower lobe of this lung, the bronchi can be traced to the pleural surface (*arrow*).

Pathogenesis of diffuse alveolar damage: Damage to the epithelium or endothelium causes the alveolar septae to become leaky (i.e., increased vascular permeability and loss of diffusion capacity), allowing protein to enter the alveoli. The epithelial cells undergo necrosis and slough into the alveoli. There are three stages of diffuse alveolar damage: exudative, proliferative, and fibrosis.

Stages of diffuse alveolar damage (in order of appearance)

- **Exudative stage:** The protein and necrotic cells layer out on the alveolar septae, forming **hyaline membranes.**
- **Proliferative stage:** Occurs in response to the damage. Type II pneumocytes undergo hyperplasia.
- **Fibrosis.**

Causes of diffuse alveolar damage

- **Four main causes:** Severe pulmonary infection, aspiration, sepsis, and severe trauma with shock.
- **Other causes:** Acute pancreatitis, cardiopulmonary bypass, fat emboli, viral infection (e.g., Hantavirus, severe acute respiratory syndrome [SARS]).
- **Acute interstitial pneumonitis** (see idiopathic pulmonary fibrosis below) is diffuse alveolar damage of undetermined etiology.

Complications of diffuse alveolar damage: High mortality rate. With survival, patients may develop fibrosis, causing development of a chronic restrictive lung disease, which can lead to pulmonary hypertension.

Morphology of diffuse alveolar damage

- **Gross:** Firm lungs.
- **Microscopic:** Hyaline membranes in the exudative stage (Figure 13-5); type II pneumocyte hyperplasia in the proliferative stage; and fibrosis.

Clinical presentation of diffuse alveolar damage

- **Symptoms:** Severe dyspnea and pink frothy sputum within 72 hours of exposure to an inciting agent.
- **Signs:** Diffuse crackles, hypoxemia, and diffuse alveolar infiltrates seen on chest radiograph.

CHRONIC RESTRICTIVE LUNG DISEASE

Basic description: Chronic restrictive lung disease, also referred to as interstitial lung disease, is characterized by chronic diffuse lung injury with inflammation and fibrosis, impaired gas exchange (low diffusing capacity of lung for carbon monoxide [DLCO]), decreased FEV_1 and FVC, and normal FEV_1/FVC ratio.

Causes of interstitial lung disease, by etiology: There are four general categories of causes of interstitial lung disease, which are drug-related, occupational, autoimmune, and idiopathic (Table 13-2).

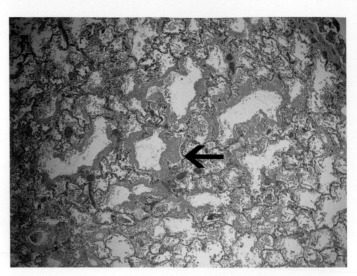

Figure 13-5. Diffuse alveolar damage. Diffuse alveolar damage (the histologic correlate of the clinical condition, acute respiratory distress syndrome) is characterized by the formation of hyaline membranes (*arrow*) on the alveolar septae. These hyaline membranes impair oxygen exchanged between the alveoli and alveolar capillaries, producing an acute restrictive lung disease. Hematoxylin and eosin, 40×.

TABLE 13-2. Causes of Chronic Restrictive Lung Disease

General Category	Specific Causes
Autoimmune	Systemic lupus erythematosus Wegener granulomatosis Rheumatoid arthritis
Idiopathic	Idiopathic pneumonias (e.g., UIP, DIP) Sarcoidosis
Work related	Asbestosis Silica-induced lung disease Coal-induced lung disease
Drug related	Bleomycin Busulfan Amiodarone Methotrexate

UIP, usual interstitial pneumonia; DIP, desquamative interstitial pneumonia.

- **Drug-related causes:** Bleomycin, busulfan, methotrexate, amiodarone, oxygen therapy.
- **Occupational causes:** Asbestosis, silicosis.
- **Autoimmune causes:** Systemic lupus erythematosus (SLE), Wegener granulomatosis, rheumatoid arthritis.
- **Idiopathic causes:** Idiopathic pneumonias, sarcoidosis.

Pathogenesis of interstitial lung disease: Exposure to the inciting agent eventually causes alveolitis that leads to the release of cellular mediators, causing injury and eventually fibrosis of the alveolar septae. The resultant appearance of the fibrotic lung parenchyma is referred to as **honeycomb lung** (Figure 13-6 *A* and *B*).

Clinical presentation of interstitial lung disease

- **Symptoms:** Insidious onset of dyspnea on exertion and dry nonproductive cough; tachypnea.
- **Signs:** Fine bibasilar end-inspiratory crackles; clubbing of fingers. Signs and symptoms of right-sided heart failure may be present.
- **Chest radiograph:** Reticular or reticulonodular pattern with diminished lung volumes.
- **Diagnosis:** Lung biopsy.

CAUSES OF CHRONIC RESTRICTIVE LUNG DISEASE

Overview: As described above, the causes of chronic restrictive lung disease (i.e., interstitial lung disease) can be divided into four categories: drug-related, occupational, autoimmune, and idiopathic. The term **pneumoconiosis** describes lung disease, including chronic restrictive lung disease arising due to exposure to inorganic or organic dust or to chemical fumes or vapors. Discussed below are asbestosis, other pneumoconioses, sarcoidosis, idiopathic pulmonary fibrosis, and hypersensitivity pneumonitis, which represent some of the more common forms of chronic restrictive lung disease (see Table 13-2).

ASBESTOSIS (FIGURE 13-7 *A-C*)

Basic description: Chronic restrictive lung disease occurring with evidence of exposure to asbestos.

Other features of asbestos exposure

- Pleural plaques or pleural effusions.
- Increased risk for development of bronchogenic carcinoma: If the patient has asbestosis and a bronchogenic carcinoma, the bronchogenic carcinoma may be considered to have been caused by the asbestos exposure and not by another source such as smoking. However, it is also important to understand that smoking and asbestos exposure are synergistic risk factors for bronchogenic carcinoma; that is, the risk for development of a bronchogenic lung carcinoma in a patient with exposure to both toxins is markedly increased over the simple additive risk of exposure to both toxins.

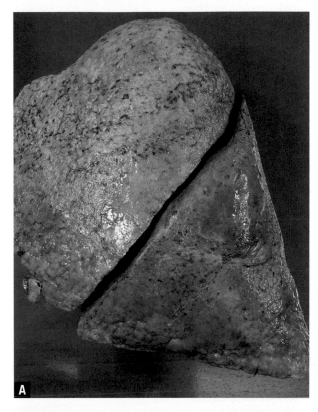

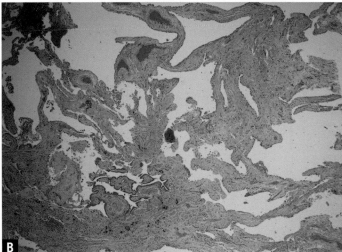

Figure 13-6. Chronic restrictive lung disease due to amiodarone exposure. **A,** Note the cobblestone appearance of the pleural surface (from fibrosis retracting the pleura). **B,** Note the prominent fibrosis of the alveolar septae. This fibrosis produces the honeycomb lung that is associated with chronic restrictive lung disease. In the lower left corner is type II pneumocyte hyperplasia, a reactive change. Hematoxylin and eosin, 40×.

- **Mesothelioma:** Only seen due to exposure to amphibole fibers (see types of asbestos fibers below). Smoking does not increase the risk for development of mesothelioma in patients with asbestos exposure.
- **Ferruginous bodies:** Asbestos particles coated with iron by macrophages.

Types of asbestos fibers

- **Amphibole fibers:** Straight and less soluble; therefore, they penetrate deeper into the lungs and are more damaging.
- **Chrysotile fibers:** Curvy and more soluble; the curved nature does not allow them to penetrate as deeply into the lungs, and thus they are cleared by the mucociliary escalator.

OTHER PNEUMOCONIOSES

Basic description: Lung disease (not including asthma, emphysema or chronic bronchitis) arising due to exposure to inorganic or organic dust or to chemical fumes or vapors. Although there are many pneumoconioses other than asbestosis, only coal, silica, and beryllium-induced lung disease will be discussed below.

Coal-induced lung disease: three forms of the disease

- **Anthracosis:** Collections of anthracotic pigment-laden macrophages in the lymphatics.
- **Simple coal workers' pneumoconiosis:** Coalescence of pigment-laden macrophages into 1–2 mm macules and slightly larger nodules.
- **Complicated coal workers' pneumoconiosis** (also referred to as **progressive massive fibrosis,** a general term for the end stage of many work-related pneumoconioses): Development of large scars (2–10 cm or larger) in the pulmonary parenchyma.

Silica-induced lung disease

- **Forms: Acute and chronic silicosis.**
- **Morphology of silica-induced lung disease**
  - **Acute silicosis:** Appears similar to **pulmonary alveolar proteinosis** (i.e., alveoli are filled with eosinophilic, fine, proteinaceous-like material).
  - **Chronic silicosis:** Nodular fibrosis (Figure 13-8), progressing to progressive massive fibrosis.
- **Important points**
  - Classic radiologic appearance of chronic silicosis: Involvement of upper lobe with nodules and "eggshell-like" calcification of hilar nodes.
  - Silicosis predisposes to infection with mycobacteria (**silicotuberculosis**).

Beryllium-induced lung disease

- **Acute berylliosis:** Intense inflammatory reaction resembles a chemical pneumonia.
- **Chronic berylliosis:** Granulomas in the alveolar septae.

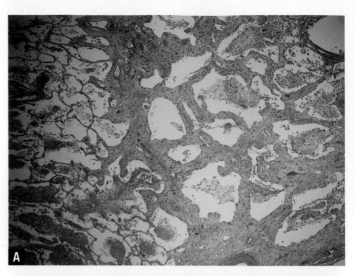

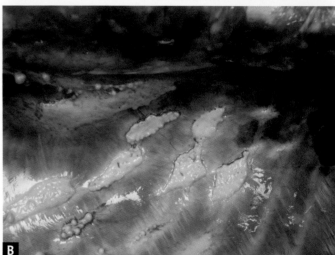

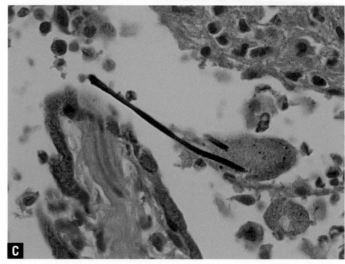

Figure 13-7. Asbestos exposure. **A,** Asbestosis, a chronic restrictive lung disease, is due to asbestos exposure. Note the thick and fibrotic alveolar septae. **B,** Multiple flat yellow-tan plaques line the parietal pleura. Pleural plaques are seen in patients with asbestos exposure, but are not specific to the condition. **C,** A ferruginous body. Macrophages engulf the asbestos fibers but cannot degrade them and, therefore, coat them with iron. Hematoxylin and eosin, A, 40×; C, 1000×.

SARCOIDOSIS

Basic description: Multisystem disease of uncertain (possibly autoimmune) etiology that produces noncaseating granulomas.

Organ involvement

- Lungs: 90% of cases; can lead to diffuse interstitial fibrosis and pulmonary hypertension.

- Lymph nodes: 75–90% of cases.

- Eye: 20% of cases; uveitis, iritis, and iridocyclitis, leading to glaucoma, cataracts, and possible visual loss.

- Heart: 30% of cases; leading to arrhythmias.

- Skin: 25% of cases; **erythema nodosum** (i.e., raised tender red nodules on the anterior surface of the legs).

- Spleen, liver, and bone marrow.

Epidemiology: Younger than 40 years of age; African Americans have a 10 to 15 times higher incidence of being diagnosed with the disease than do whites; increased incidence in nonsmokers.

Microscopic morphology of sarcoidosis: Noncaseating granulomas, **asteroid bodies** (eosinophilic, star-shaped inclusions), and **Schaumann bodies** (concentrically calcified bodies). Sarcoidosis can lead to alveolar septal fibrosis (Figure 13-9 A–C).

Clinical presentation: There are three manners by which sarcoidosis can present clinically.

- **Asymptomatic patients** with abnormal chest radiograph (hilar lymphadenopathy).

- Patients with **pulmonary symptoms** (e.g., nonproductive cough and dyspnea).

- Patients with **extrapulmonary manifestations** (e.g., uveitis, lupus pernio, erythema nodosum).

Important points

- Sarcoidosis is a diagnosis of exclusion; thus all other causes of the granulomas should be excluded.

- The mononuclear cells can produce the active form of vitamin D, causing hypercalcemia.

- **Laboratory studies:** Patients may have an elevated level of angiotensin-converting enzyme (ACE).

- Circulating CD4$^+$ lymphocytes are decreased.

- Sarcoidosis is associated with pure thymic hyperplasia.

IDIOPATHIC PULMONARY FIBROSIS

Basic description: Chronic restrictive lung disease occurring with no identifiable etiology, such as exposure to asbestos or drugs (e.g., amiodarone).

Pathogenesis of idiopathic pulmonary fibrosis: Idiopathic pulmonary fibrosis is usually an end stage of a form of idiopathic pneumonia, most commonly the end stage of **usual interstitial pneumonia**. The likely pathogenesis for the idiopathic pneumonias is repeated cycles of alveolitis by an unknown agent.

Five types of idiopathic pneumonia

- Usual interstitial pneumonia (UIP)

- Desquamative interstitial pneumonia (DIP)

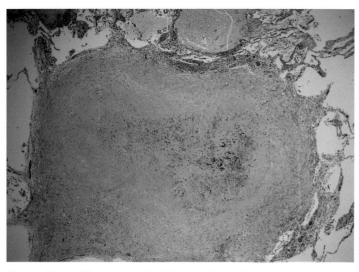

Figure 13-8. Silicotic nodule. The acellular fibrotic nodule in this image is due to exposure to silica. Large nodules can merge, leading to progressive massive fibrosis. Hematoxylin and eosin, 40×.

Microscopic morphology: Interstitial lymphocytic infiltrate (Figure 13-14); may have diffuse alveolar damage.

Clinical presentation of community-acquired atypical pneumonia

- **Signs and symptoms:** Insidious onset of low-grade fever, nonproductive cough, headache, and myalgias. Symptoms may vary depending on the causative organism. Chest radiograph usually shows diffuse interstitial or alveolar infiltrates, and consolidation is less commonly observed than in typical pneumonia.

- **Important point:** SARS is caused by a coronavirus, and the course of the infection first affects the lower respiratory tract and then spreads throughout the body.

NOSOCOMIAL PNEUMONIA

Basic description: Pulmonary infection acquired while hospitalized; usually bacterial, but sometimes fungal.

Causative organisms: Gram-negative bacilli, *Pseudomonas*, and, less commonly, *Staphylococcus aureus*.

Important point regarding nosocomial pneumonia: Organisms can be difficult to treat because they are often multidrug-resistant to antibiotics.

ASPIRATION PNEUMONIA

Basic description: Pneumonia that occurs as a result of aspiration, usually in intoxicated or neuromuscularly impaired individuals.

Causative organisms: Mixed aerobic and anaerobic (oral flora) organisms, including aerobic and anaerobic streptococcus; *Staphylococcus aureus*, gram-negative organisms, and anaerobic organisms including *Bacteroides* species. Chemical injury also plays a role.

Complication of aspiration pneumonia: Lung abscess (Figure 13-15).

Microscopic morphology of aspiration pneumonia: Food material (e.g., skeletal muscle, vegetable matter) surrounded by neutrophils (Figure 13-16).

NECROTIZING PNEUMONIA

Basic description: Pneumonia with prominent necrosis of the parenchyma and abscess formation.

Causative organisms: *Streptococcus pneumoniae*, *Staphylococcus aureus*, *Klebsiella*, *Pseudomonas aeruginosa*, *Nocardia*.

Morphology of necrotizing pneumonia: Abscesses and focal destruction of parenchyma.

CHRONIC PNEUMONIA

Basic description: Pneumonia of long duration.

Causative organisms: *Mycobacterium tuberculosis* and dimorphic fungi.

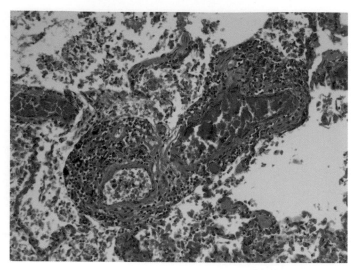

Figure 13-14. Interstitial pneumonia. Note the lymphocytic infiltrate within the tissue surrounding this vessel. Interstitial pneumonia is consistent with a viral or mycoplasmal etiology. Hematoxylin and eosin, 200×.

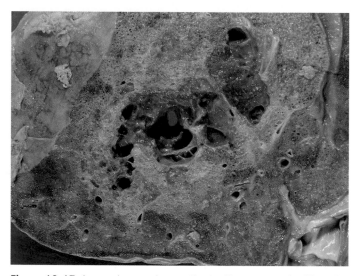

Figure 13-15. Lung abscess in a patient with pneumonia. Note the loss of parenchyma in the center of the image. This area represents an abscess.

Pulmonary tuberculosis (TB)

Forms of TB: include primary TB, secondary TB, primary progressive TB, and miliary TB

▨ **Primary TB:** Patients have **Ghon complex**, which is **Ghon focus** (i.e., granuloma at the periphery of the lung near the interlobar groove), plus enlarged and involved hilar lymph nodes. Primary TB is common. Lesions usually heal on their own and the granulomas become calcified; however, the organism is still present and held in check by the immune system. If the patient becomes immunocompromised, secondary TB can occur (Figure 13-17 A and B).

▨ **Secondary TB** (or **reactivation TB**): Granulomas occur at apices of the lung, because TB is aerophilic.

▨ **Primary progressive TB:** Morphologically, has the appearance of bronchopneumonia; usually due to primary TB infection occurring in a patient who is already immunocompromised.

▨ **Miliary TB:** Hematogenous dissemination of the organism to the lungs, liver, and spleen produces "millet seed" appearance.

Complications of pulmonary tuberculosis

▨ Exsanguination, due to erosion of granulomas into the blood vessels.

▨ Basilar meningitis.

▨ **Pott disease:** Involvement of the vertebral column.

▨ Spread to other organs.

Clinical presentation of pulmonary tuberculosis

▨ **Signs and symptoms:** Persistent productive cough, fever, chills, loss of appetite, night sweats, and weight loss. With blood vessel invasion, patients may have hemoptysis. With extensive involvement of the lung, patients may have dyspnea on exertion.

▨ **Testing:** Tuberculin skin test; culture of sputum.

Dimorphic fungi: *Histoplasmosis capsulatum*, *Blastomyces dermatitidis*, and *Coccidioides immitis*.

Geographic distribution of dimorphic fungi

▨ *Histoplasmosis capsulatum*: Ohio and Mississippi River Valleys. Usually associated with exposure to and subsequent inhalation of bird or bat droppings.

▨ *Blastomyces dermatitidis*: Distribution overlaps with *Histoplasmosis capsulatum* in central and southeastern United States.

▨ *Coccidioides immitis*: San Joaquin Valley in California and Arizona.

Morphology of infection with dimorphic fungi

▨ **Gross:** Can appear similar to tuberculosis.

▨ **Microscopic**

   ○ *Histoplasmosis capsulatum:* 2–5 μm organisms, in macrophages.

   ○ *Blastomyces dermatitidis:* Broad-based budding yeasts.

   ○ *Coccidioides immitis:* Spherules containing endospores.

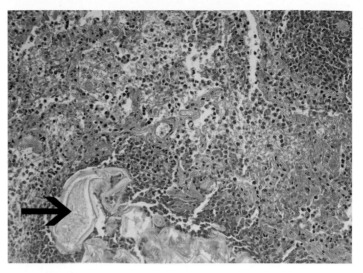

Figure 13-16. Aspiration pneumonia. The arrow indicates foreign material within the pulmonary parenchyma. The neutrophilic infiltrate that dominates the remainder of the image is in response to the aspiration of this material. Hematoxylin and eosin, 200×.

PNEUMONIA IN THE IMMUNOCOMPROMISED PATIENT

In HIV patients

- If CD4 count is > 200 cells/ μL, pneumonia is likely bacterial.

- If CD4 count < 200 cells/ μL, pneumonia is likely *Pneumocystis* pneumonia.

- If CD4 count is < 50 cells/ μL, pneumonia is likely cytomegalovirus (CMV) or *Mycobacterium avium-intracellulare*.

PULMONARY ABSCESS

Overview: Pulmonary abscesses are a complication of several of the seven categories of pulmonary infections, including community-acquired typical and atypical pneumonias, aspiration pneumonia, and necrotizing pneumonia. Other causes of a pulmonary abscess include bronchial obstruction, neoplasms, and septic emboli due to hematogenous dissemination from another source (e.g., endocarditis).

Location of abscess: Usually lower lobes (right side more frequently than left side). The right main stem bronchus has a less acute angle than the left main stem bronchus; therefore, aspirated material enters the right bronchus more easily.

Complications of lung abscess

- Pneumothorax, due to rupture into pleural cavity.

- Empyema, due to rupture into pleural cavity with subsequent extension of infection into the pleural cavity.

PULMONARY NEOPLASMS

Overview: There are only two general categories of pulmonary neoplasms of clinical importance: small cell and non–small cell carcinoma. The importance of the small cell versus non–small cell designation is that small cell lung carcinoma is considered to have already metastasized at the time of diagnosis; therefore, it is treated with radiation and chemotherapy, and no further surgery. About 85–90% of lung tumors arise in active smokers or those who have recently stopped smoking, and the favored sites of metastases for pulmonary neoplasms are, in descending order, liver, brain, and bone. The three types of non–small cell carcinoma (squamous cell carcinoma, adenocarcinoma, and large cell carcinoma) as well as small cell carcinoma will be discussed below.

SQUAMOUS CELL CARCINOMA

Epidemiology: Age 55–60 years or older; more common in males.

Location: Central or at or near the hilum of the lung (Figure 13-18).

Risk factors for squamous cell carcinoma of the lung: Cigarette smoking leads to squamous metaplasia, which can lead to squamous dysplasia, and then to carcinoma.

Mutations: Squamous cell carcinoma has the highest rate of *p53* mutations among lung tumors.

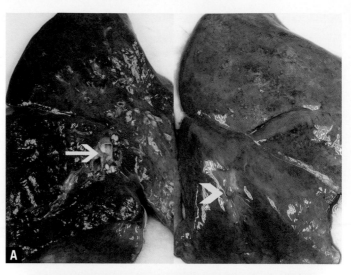

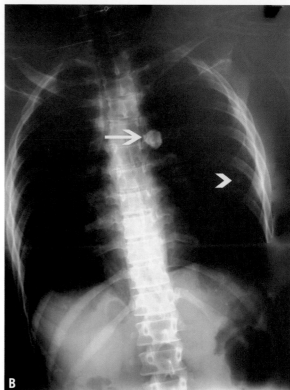

Figure 13-17. Healed primary pulmonary tuberculosis. **A,** A lung sectioned from superior to inferior, with the halves placed side-by-side on the table. The pleural surface has a contracted nodule, which represents the Ghon focus (*arrowhead*), and the hilum has multiple lymph nodes with calcified caseous necrosis (*arrow*). Together, the Ghon focus and the hilar lymphadenopathy are referred to as the Ghon complex. **B,** A chest radiograph of a patient with healed primary pulmonary tuberculosis. The hilar lymphadenopathy (*arrow*) and Ghon focus (*arrowhead*) will calcify, allowing them to be visualized by chest radiograph.

Associated conditions: Squamous cell carcinoma can produce parathormone-like protein, which can result in hypercalcemia.

Morphology of squamous cell carcinoma

▨ **Gross:** Lung mass, which often cavitates due to necrosis.

▨ **Microscopic:** Keratin pearls and intercellular bridges.

ADENOCARCINOMA

Epidemiology: Age younger than 45 years; female predominance.

Location: Peripheral or at or near the pleural surface (Figure 13-19).

Risk factors for pulmonary adenocarcinoma: Weakly linked to cigarette smoking.

Pathogenesis of adenocarcinoma

▨ **Atypical adenomatous hyperplasia** can lead to bronchioalveolar carcinoma, which can lead to invasive adenocarcinoma.

▨ **Important points regarding bronchioalveolar carcinoma**

  ○ Grows along the alveolar septae (referred to as **lepidic growth**) (Figure 13-20).

  ○ No invasive component.

  ○ Can present in patchy distribution similar to pneumonia.

  ○ Classic symptom is bronchorrhea.

Microscopic morphology of invasive adenocarcinoma: Infiltrative glandular formations; architecture includes papillary and solid forms.

LARGE CELL CARCINOMA

Basic description: Most likely a poorly differentiated squamous cell carcinoma or adenocarcinoma. Anaplasia inhibits determination of epithelial-type origin of tumor (Figure 13-21).

SMALL CELL LUNG CARCINOMA

Epidemiology: Older males.

Location: Central, along bronchi.

Risk factors for small cell lung carcinoma: Smoking (only 1% of cases occurs in nonsmokers).

Mutations: *c-MYC, RB*.

Associated paraneoplastic syndromes

▨ Small cell lung carcinoma can produce adrenocorticotropic hormone (ACTH), antidiuretic hormone (ADH), and calcitonin-like substances.

▨ Clubbing of fingers.

▨ **Lambert-Eaton syndrome,** due to autoantibodies to neuronal calcium channels.

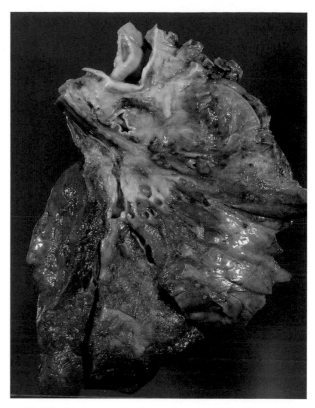

Figure 13-18. Squamous cell carcinoma of the lung. Note the white-tan contracted mass centered at the hilum of this lung. Characteristically, squamous cell carcinoma has a central location.

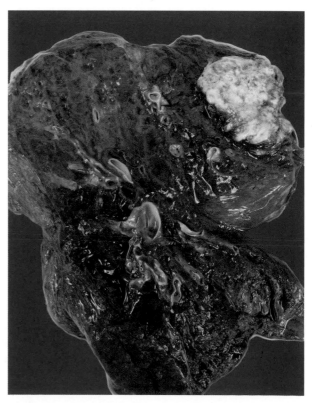

Figure 13-19. Adenocarcinoma of the lung. Note the white-tan nodule at the periphery of this lung. Characteristically, adenocarcinoma has a peripheral location.

Two types of pneumothorax (by etiology)

- **Spontaneous:** May be primary (no underlying lung disease) or secondary (patient has underlying lung disease). The classic spontaneous pneumothorax occurs in a tall, thin, young male patient.
- **Traumatic.**

Clinical presentation of pneumothorax

- **Symptoms:** Sudden onset of sharp chest pain, worsened by inspiration; tachypnea. With a tension pneumothorax, patients also have hypotension and cyanosis.
- **Signs:** Hyperresonance to percussion, decreased tactile fremitus, and decreased breath sounds over the affected area. With a tension pneumothorax, patients will have elevated jugular venous pressure.

MESOTHELIOMA

Basic description: Malignant tumor of the pleural cavity derived from mesothelial cells.

Important point: Almost always due to exposure to asbestos.

Morphology of mesothelioma

- **Gross:** Tumor encases the lung.
- **Microscopic:** Epithelioid or sarcomatoid components.

UPPER RESPIRATORY TRACT PATHOLOGY

Overview: Briefly discussed below are vocal cord nodules and squamous cell carcinoma of the larynx. The final entry of this section discusses the **field effect,** an important concept when considering the effects and treatment of smokers with a malignancy of the upper or lower respiratory tract.

Vocal cord nodules: Seen in singers and smokers.

Squamous cell carcinoma of the larynx: The type is based upon location of tumor and includes glottic, supraglottic, and subglottic (Figure 13-23).

- **Glottic:** Patients present earlier because the tumor produces symptoms earlier. There are fewer lymphatics on the true vocal cords, so these tumors are less likely to have metastasized. It is the most common location for squamous cell carcinoma of the larynx.
- **Supraglottic:** Area is rich in lymphatics; therefore, tumors in this site will metastasize sooner than those in other areas.
- **Subglottic:** Patients present late in the course of disease, because the tumor must cause significant obstruction of the upper airway to produce symptoms and thus to be diagnosed.

FIELD EFFECT

Basic description: Cigarette smoke exposes multiple areas of the body to carcinogens; therefore, development of carcinoma in one area of the body may precede development in another area. For example, patients with squamous cell carcinoma of the larynx often develop squamous cell carcinoma of the lung at a later time. Patients can also have synchronous tumors (i.e., occurring at the same time) in different locations.

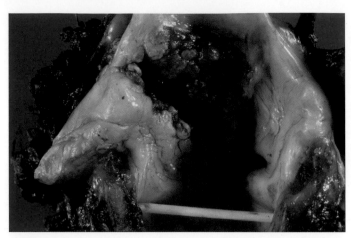

Figure 13-23. Laryngeal squamous cell carcinoma. Centered above the left true vocal cord is an ulcerated polypoid mass. The presentation of laryngeal squamous cell carcinoma depends upon its location. Tumors growing on the vocal cords present the earliest, due to changes in the voice induced by the growth of the neoplasm.

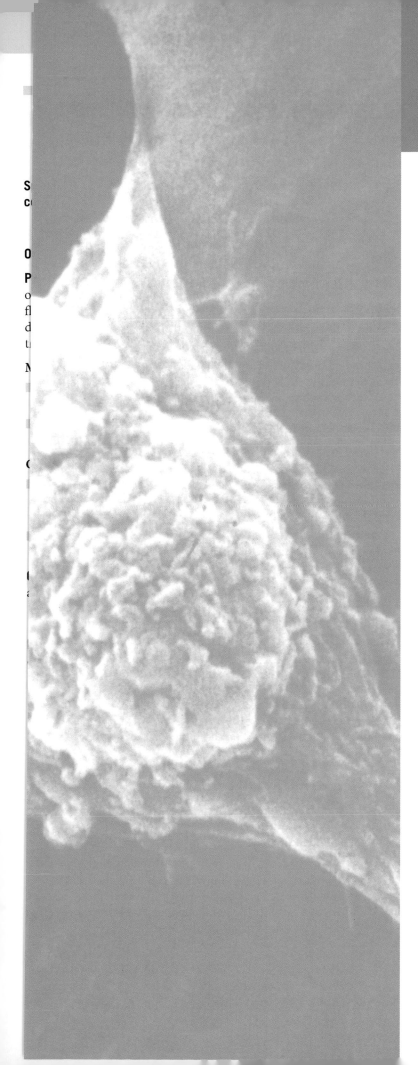

CHAPTER 14

GASTROINTESTINAL PATHOLOGY

OVERVIEW

The main purpose of the gastrointestinal tract is the transport of food and the absorption of nutrients. Many pathologic conditions of the gastrointestinal tract impair either or both of these functions. The gastrointestinal tract, and especially the colon, is a common site of malignancy. The two main symptoms related to pathology of the gastrointestinal tract are abdominal pain and gastrointestinal hemorrhage.

The differential diagnosis for abdominal pain can be classified as either acute or chronic, based upon the length of time of the pain (Table 14-1). The four categories of the causes of acute abdominal pain are (1) inflammation, including appendicitis, cholecystitis, pancreatitis, and diverticulitis; (2) perforation; (3) obstruction; and (4) vascular disease, including acute ischemia and ruptured abdominal aortic aneurysm. The five categories of causes of chronic abdominal pain are (1) inflammation, including peptic ulcer disease, esophagitis, inflammatory bowel disease, and chronic pancreatitis; (2) vascular disease, including chronic ischemia; (3) metabolic disease, including porphyria; (4) abdominal wall pain; and (5) functional causes, including irritable bowel syndrome. The most frequent causes of chronic abdominal pain are functional.

The second main symptom of gastrointestinal pathology is bleeding (Table 14-2). The character of the blood can help identify the source: **hematemesis** (i.e., vomiting of bright red blood), if the source is gastrointestinal, is most likely due to a source proximal to the ligament of Treitz. **Melena** (i.e., black, tarry stool) is most often due to upper gastrointestinal bleeding. **Hematochezia** (i.e., bright red blood per rectum) usually indicates a lower gastrointestinal bleed (or very rapid upper gastrointestinal bleed). The differential diagnosis of upper gastrointestinal bleeding includes gastritis, esophageal varices, and peptic ulcer disease (as a result of erosion into a blood vessel). The diagnosis of the source of an upper gastrointestinal bleed is often made by endoscopy. The differential diagnosis of lower gastrointestinal bleeding includes a rapid upper gastrointestinal bleed, diverticulosis, infections (e.g., *Salmonella*, *Shigella*), cancer, inflammatory bowel disease, and anal fissures or hemorrhoids. The diagnosis of a lower gastrointestinal bleed is often determined by flexible sigmoidoscopy or colonoscopy.

Clinical presentation of disaccharidase deficiency

■ **Symptoms:** Bloating, flatus, abdominal discomfort.

■ **Diagnosis:** Confirmed by the presence of high hydrogen gas levels after the patient is given a test dose of lactose. The hydrogen is a byproduct of bacterial breakdown of the lactose.

INFLAMMATORY BOWEL DISEASE

Basic description: Conditions characterized by mucosal (and deeper) damage to the gastrointestinal tract, the etiology of which is uncertain.

Epidemiology: Bimodal, two age peaks; one in the second to fourth decades and one about the sixth decade; occurs equally in males and females; whites from northern climates in the United States and Europe.

Pathogenesis: Possible dysfunction of immune response toward normal intestinal flora. *NOD2* gene on chromosome 16 plays a role in the development of inflammatory bowel disease.

Two types of inflammatory bowel disease: ulcerative colitis and **Crohn disease.** Ulcerative colitis is confined to the colon, and the inflammation affects only the mucosa. Crohn disease can affect any portion of the gastrointestinal tract, and the inflammation is transmural (Table 14-5).

TABLE 14-5.   Comparison and Contrast of Crohn Disease and Ulcerative Colitis

Feature	Crohn Disease	Ulcerative Colitis
Region affected	From mouth to colon	Colon
Location of inflammation	Transmural	Mucosal
Extraintestinal manifestations	Migratory polyarthritis, iritis, uveitis, sclerosing cholangitis	Migratory polyarthritis, iritis, uveitis, sclerosing cholangitis
p-ANCA	11% of cases	75% of cases
Anti-*Saccharomyces cerevisiae*	Common	Rare
Increased risk of colonic adenocarcinoma (above normal)	5–6x	10–20x
Anatomic features	Fistula formation, skip lesions, creeping fat, cobblestoning of mucosa	Pseudopolyps, crypt abscesses
Submucosal granulomas	Yes	No
Rectal involvement	No	Yes

CROHN DISEASE

Location: Can affect any region of the gastrointestinal tract from mouth to anus. The forms of Crohn disease are based upon the location and include ileocecal (most common form), terminal ileum, colon only, and other sites (rare).

Theories of pathogenesis of Crohn disease

1. Crohn disease may be an immune response to normal gastrointestinal flora, and there is epithelial barrier malfunction.

2. The NOD2 protein is an intracellular receptor for microbes and triggers NF-κβ. The NOD2 protein has decreased function in Crohn disease.

3. T-cell hyperreactivity.

Extraintestinal associations of Crohn disease: Migratory polyarthritis (most common), iritis, uveitis, erythema nodosum, primary sclerosing cholangitis, and obstructive uropathy.

Important points regarding Crohn disease

■ p-ANCA is positive in 11% of cases; anti-*Saccharomyces cerevisiae* antibody is common (rare in ulcerative colitis).

■ Approximately 30–50% concordance among monozygotic twins.

■ Differential diagnosis of lower right quadrant pain and fever: Crohn disease, acute appendicitis, and *Yersinia enterocolitica* infection.

Complications of Crohn disease

■ Risk of colonic adenocarcinoma: 5–6 times higher versus the normal population, which is not as much of an increase as seen in patients with ulcerative colitis.

■ Fistula formation.

■ Abdominal abscesses, intestinal stricture, and toxic megacolon.

■ Extensive ileal mucosal damage, leading to vitamin B_{12} deficiency and malabsorption of bile salts.

■ Urinary calcium oxalate stones from chronic fat malabsorption, leading to binding of free fatty acids to calcium and allowing oxalate to be absorbed (normally oxalate is excreted bound to the calcium).

Gross morphology of Crohn disease

■ Long, linear, serpentine ulcers and fissures with no rectal involvement.

■ Skip lesions: Unaffected bowel mucosa between lesions, with sharp demarcation between normal and abnormal mucosa.

■ Fistula formation.

■ Mesenteric fat wraps around the bowel (i.e., "**creeping fat**").

■ Thick wall with stenotic lumen, which is responsible for the "string sign" on barium enema.

Microscopic morphology of Crohn disease: Has transmural inflammation, submucosal granulomas, and mural thickening (Figure 14-16 *A* and *B*).

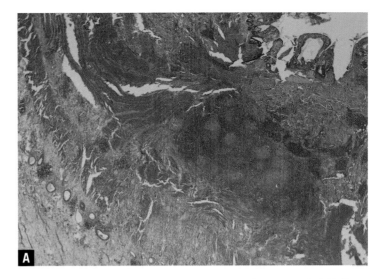

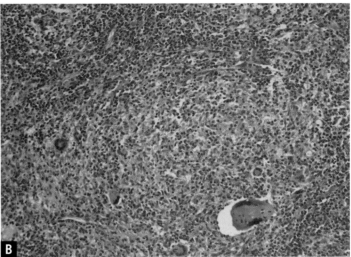

Figure 14-16. Crohn disease. **A**, Note the transmural nature of the inflammatory infiltrate. Within the muscularis propria and submucosa is a large cluster of lymphocytes associated with multiple granulomas. **B**, A high-power view of one of the granulomas. Hematoxylin and eosin, A, 40×; B, 400×.

obstructive liver disease pattern, also called **cholestasis**, which has an elevated ALP and bilirubin (Table 15-1).

Ascites is often associated with cirrhosis; however, both transudative ascites (seen in patients with cirrhosis, alcoholic hepatitis, or congestive heart failure) and exudative ascites (seen in patients with peritoneal carcinomatosis or tuberculosis) may occur. Differentiating between the two types requires a determination of gradient (i.e., difference between serum albumin and ascitic fluid albumin). Transudative ascites has a high gradient ($>$ 1.1 g/dL), and exudative ascites has a low gradient ($<$ 1.1 g/dL).

This chapter discusses liver pathology, including jaundice and cholestasis, hepatic failure, cirrhosis, vascular and circulatory disorders, alcoholic liver disease, metabolic diseases, obstructive biliary tract disorders, and hepatic tumors; gallbladder pathology, including gallstones and acute and chronic cholecystitis; and pancreatic pathology, including pancreatitis and pancreatic adenocarcinoma.

GENERAL RESPONSES OF THE LIVER TO INJURY

Overview: Although many different toxins, infections, and other conditions affect the liver, the liver only has five general responses to injury: inflammation, cellular accumulations, cell death, fibrosis, and regeneration. **Cirrhosis** results from a combination of fibrosis and regeneration after cell death. Of the five general responses of the liver, only cellular accumulations and cell death will be discussed here.

Cellular accumulations

Macrovesicular steatosis: One large fat vacuole in hepatocytes; associated with alcohol use, obesity, and diabetes mellitus.

Microvesicular steatosis: Many small vacuoles in hepatocytes; associated with acute fatty liver of pregnancy, Reye syndrome (occurs in children with viral illness when given aspirin), alcohol, and certain drugs (e.g., tetracycline).

Cell death (i.e., necrosis and apoptosis): Several patterns of necrosis are specific to the liver.

Spotty necrosis: Focal areas of necrosis in the lobular parenchyma.

Interface hepatitis: Necrosis at the edge of the limiting plate.

Bridging necrosis: Necrosis spanning between the portal tracts and from the portal tracts to the centrilobular hepatocytes.

Submassive necrosis: Necrosis of entire lobules.

Massive necrosis: Necrosis of almost the entire liver.

JAUNDICE AND CHOLESTASIS

Overview: Jaundice is an accumulation of unconjugated or conjugated bilirubin in skin that produces a golden yellow color. Jaundice is evident in skin when the serum bilirubin level is 2.5–3 mg/dL or higher. Yellow discoloration of the sclerae is referred to as **icterus** (Figure 15-1). **Cholestasis** is an accumulation of bile. Bile contains much more than just bilirubin, including bile salts and cholesterol.

TABLE 15-1. Laboratory Studies and Patterns of Liver Disease

Patterns of Liver Disease	Laboratory Studies
Acute hepatitis pattern	↑ AST, ALT
Cirrhosis pattern	↓ albumin, ↑ gamma globulins
Chronic liver disease pattern	↑ AST, ALT ↓ albumin, ↑ gamma globulins
Obstructive liver disease pattern	↑ ALP, bilirubin

AST, aspartate aminotransferase; ALT, alanine aminotransferase; ALP, alkaline phosphatase.

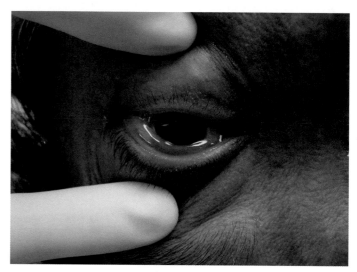

Figure 15-1. Scleral icterus. Note the yellow discoloration of this patient's conjunctivae. Scleral icterus is a manifestation of jaundice, and can be seen in patients with elevated levels of bilirubin.

TABLE 15-2. Mechanisms of Jaundice and Cholestasis and Their Causes

Mechanism of Jaundice and Cholestasis	Form of Hyperbilirubinemia	Causes
Increased bilirubin production	Unconjugated	Hemolytic anemia, ineffective hematopoiesis
Decreased hepatic uptake	Unconjugated	Gilbert syndrome, rifampin use
Impaired conjugation	Unconjugated	Physiologic jaundice of newborn, Crigler-Najjar syndrome, diffuse hepatocellular disease
Decreased hepatic excretion	Conjugated	Dubin-Johnson syndrome, diffuse hepatocellular disease
Impaired intrahepatic bile flow	Conjugated	Primary biliary cirrhosis, primary sclerosing cholangitis
Impaired extrahepatic bile flow	Conjugated	Gallstone, pancreatic carcinoma

Mechanisms of jaundice and cholestasis (Table 15-2)

Excessive production of bilirubin results in unconjugated hyperbilirubinemia (causes: hemolytic anemias and ineffective erythropoiesis, such as in megaloblastic anemia).

Reduced hepatic uptake results in unconjugated hyperbilirubinemia (causes: rifampin, which competes for bilirubin uptake; Gilbert syndrome).

Impaired conjugation results in unconjugated hyperbilirubinemia (causes: physiologic jaundice of the newborn, Crigler-Najjar syndrome, diffuse hepatocellular damage).

Decreased hepatocellular excretion causes conjugated hyperbilirubinemia (causes: Dubin-Johnson syndrome, diffuse hepatocellular damage).

Impaired bile flow (from intrahepatic or extrahepatic obstruction) results in conjugated hyperbilirubinemia.

○ Causes of intrahepatic obstruction: primary biliary cirrhosis, primary sclerosing cholangitis.

○ Causes of extrahepatic obstruction: gallstones, carcinoma of the pancreas, extrahepatic biliary atresia or biliary strictures, and extrahepatic primary sclerosing cholangitis.

SPECIFIC CONDITIONS CAUSING JAUNDICE AND CHOLESTASIS

Overview: Although there are many causes of jaundice and cholestasis, the five conditions that will be discussed in this section are hereditary conditions or conditions associated with the neonate. These conditions are physiologic jaundice of the newborn, Gilbert syndrome, Crigler-Najjar syndrome, Dubin-Johnson syndrome, and neonatal cholestasis.

PHYSIOLOGIC JAUNDICE OF THE NEWBORN

Basic description: The enzymes that conjugate bilirubin do not mature for a few weeks after birth; therefore, neonates are prone to development of unconjugated hyperbilirubinemia.

GILBERT SYNDROME

Epidemiology: Common (> 5% of the population); male predominance.

Mechanism: Mutations of the *UGT* gene lead to decreased levels of uridine diphosphate-glucuronyl transferase (at 30% of normal level), which causes decreased ability to conjugate bilirubin with glucuronic acid.

Clinical presentation of Gilbert syndrome: Patients become jaundiced when stressed (e.g., illness, exercise).

CRIGLER-NAJJAR SYNDROME (TYPES I AND II)

Inheritance pattern: Both types I and II are autosomal recessive.

Mechanism: Type I has a complete lack of enzyme needed for the conjugation of glucuronic acid to bilirubin; type II has partial lack of the enzyme.

DUBIN-JOHNSON SYNDROME

Mechanism: Absence of canalicular protein multidrug-resistant protein 2 (MRP2), which transports bilirubinglucuronides.

Gross morphology: Black liver.

NEONATAL CHOLESTASIS

Causes: Bile duct obstruction, infections (e.g., caused by cytomegalovirus, sepsis), toxins, metabolic (e.g., α_1-antitrypsin deficiency), and idiopathic (50% of cases).

Microscopic morphology of neonatal cholestasis: Giant cells, cholestasis, mononuclear cells in portal tracts, and extramedullary hematopoiesis.

Gross morphology of jaundice and cholestasis: Scleral icterus; skin xanthomas due to impaired excretion of cholesterol.

Microscopic morphology of jaundice and cholestasis (Figures 15-2 and 15-3)

   Bile plugs within canaliculi (seen in cholestasis).

   Foamy degeneration of hepatocytes (due to intracellular accumulation of bile).

   If cholestasis is due to intra- or extrahepatic bile duct obstruction:

   ○ Distension of upstream bile ducts; proliferation and edema of bile ducts.

   ○ Bile lakes (i.e., focal destruction of parenchyma with accumulation of bile).

   ○ Cirrhosis due to portal tract fibrosis.

Clinical presentation of jaundice and cholestasis

Symptoms: Patients with cholestasis have pruritus as a result of deposition of bile salts in tissue, and may have clay-colored stools resulting from failure of bile to reach the intestines.

Signs: Elevated bilirubin (unconjugated or conjugated, depending upon the cause of jaundice); also increased concentration of ALP in cholestasis. ALP is produced by bile duct epithelium and canalicular hepatocytes and is released by detergent action of bile. ALP is increased to three to four times the normal level, and the AST and ALT are increased more than five to ten times the normal levels.

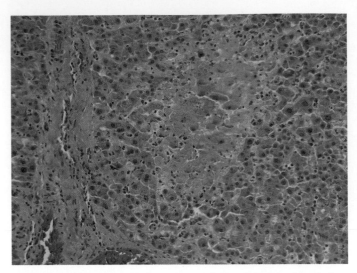

Figure 15-2. Bile lake. In the center of the photomicrograph is a yellow-green pool of bile, which has displaced the surrounding hepatocytes. Bile lakes can be seen in patients with obstruction of the bile ducts. Hematoxylin and eosin, 200×.

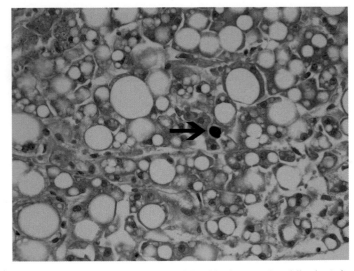

Figure 15-3. Bile plug. At the tip of the black arrow is a bile ductule plugged with bile. This histologic feature is indicative of cholestasis. Hematoxylin and eosin, 400×.

Laboratory studies to differentiate causes of jaundice and cholestasis

  Hemolytic causes: No urine bilirubin, elevated urine urobilinogen, and elevated unconjugated bilirubin.

  Hepatocellular cause: Increased urine bilirubin, normal urine urobilinogen, and elevated unconjugated and conjugated bilirubin.

  Obstructive causes: Increased urine bilirubin, decreased urine urobilinogen, and elevated conjugated bilirubin.

Diagnosis of cause of jaundice and cholestasis: Biopsy of liver; radiographic imaging to determine location and source of obstruction.

HEPATIC FAILURE

Overview: For liver failure to occur, there must be a loss of 80–90% of hepatic parenchyma. Hepatic failure occurs in one of three situations: massive hepatic necrosis, chronic liver disease, or widespread but nonfatal injury to the hepatocytes. Hepatic failure as a result of chronic liver disease is most often due to the end stage of cirrhosis. Widespread damage to hepatocytes, which maintain viability, has several causes, including acute fatty liver of pregnancy. Massive hepatic necrosis as a cause of hepatic failure will be discussed below.

MASSIVE HEPATIC NECROSIS

Basic description: Massive hepatic necrosis is often the result of fulminant hepatitis or toxic injury. The definition of fulminant hepatic failure is the onset of **encephalopathy** within 8 weeks of the onset of jaundice in a patient with hepatic injury and no history of prior liver disease.

Causes of massive hepatic necrosis

  Acetaminophen toxicity (35–40% of cases).

  Other toxins: Halothane, isoniazid.

  Acute hepatitis A (4% of cases).

  Acute hepatitis B (8% of cases).

  Others causes: Acute fatty liver of pregnancy, Wilson disease, hepatic ischemia, *Amanita* mushroom poisoning.

  Specific cause: Reye syndrome (clinical presentation in children: Reye syndrome presents as vomiting a few days after treatment of a viral infection with aspirin; patients progress to seizures, cloudy sensorium, and coma).

COMPLICATIONS OF HEPATIC FAILURE

Overview: Include hepatic encephalopathy, hepatorenal syndrome, jaundice, hyperammonemia, coagulopathy, hypoglycemia, and infections. Several of these complications are simply due to loss of normal liver functions. Coagulopathy is a result of deficiency of vitamin K–dependent factors II, VII, IX, and X. Hypoglycemia is a result of impaired gluconeogenesis. Infections are one of the leading causes of death in patients with fulminant hepatic failure. Hepatic encephalopathy and hepatorenal syndrome are discussed below.

HEPATIC ENCEPHALOPATHY

Basic description: Complex neuropsychiatric syndrome that complicates advanced liver disease.

Forms: acute and chronic

- **Acute hepatic encephalopathy:** Occurs in the setting of fulminant hepatic failure. Cerebral edema is more prominent in acute hepatic encephalopathy than in the chronic form.
- **Chronic hepatic encephalopathy:** Occurs with chronic liver disease; is reversible.

Pathogenesis of hepatic encephalopathy: Inadequate removal of nitrogenous compounds or other toxins that are ingested or formed in the gastrointestinal tract. Common precipitants include gastrointestinal bleeding and gastrointestinal protein loading, portosystemic shunting, and infections.

Microscopic morphology: Characterized by Alzheimer type II astrocytes in the central nervous system (CNS).

Clinical presentation of hepatic encephalopathy

- Disturbance of sleep is often the earliest sign of hepatic encephalopathy.
- **Asterixis** and hyperreflexia.
- **Fetor hepaticus** (musty odor of breath).
- Alterations in personality and cognitive function.

HEPATORENAL SYNDROME

Pathogenesis: Severe cortical vasoconstriction.

Clinical presentation of hepatorenal syndrome

- **Signs and symptoms:** Decreased glomerular filtration rate (GFR), oliguria, low urine sodium and disproportionately high ratio of blood urea nitrogen (BUN) to creatinine (i.e., prerenal pattern of acute renal failure).
- **Clinical course:** Often progressive and fatal, with mortality rate of 95%.

Important point: Kidneys are histologically normal.

CIRRHOSIS OF THE LIVER

Basic description: Diffuse scarring of the liver with nodular regeneration of hepatocytes, resulting in severe disruption of hepatic architecture (Figure 15-4).

Causes of cirrhosis in the Western world (Table 15-3)

- Viral hepatitis; hepatitis C (about 50% of patients with hepatitis C infection develop cirrhosis). Hepatitis C has now surpassed alcoholism as the leading cause of cirrhosis in the United States. Hepatitis B is less likely to progress to cirrhosis.
- Alcohol abuse (6–15% of chronic alcoholics develop cirrhosis).
- Nonalcoholic fatty liver disease (NAFLD) or nonalcoholic steatohepatitis (NASH). Incidence is rising dramatically. Up to 10% of patients with NAFLD/NASH will go on to develop cirrhosis.

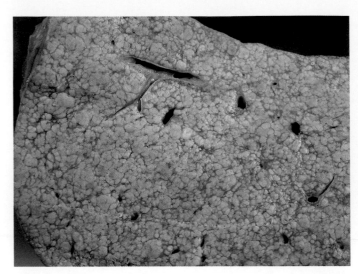

Figure 15-4. Cirrhosis. This cross-section of the liver reveals parenchyma that is effaced by innumerable nodules, most of which are > 3 mm in size.

TABLE 15-3. Causes of Cirrhosis

Source of Cirrhosis	Causes
Infectious	Viral (hepatitis B, C, D)
Toxins	Ethanol
Metabolic	Hereditary hemochromatosis, Wilson disease, α_1-antitrypsin deficiency
Biliary disease	Primary biliary cirrhosis, primary sclerosing cholangitis
Other	Autoimmune, cryptogenic

Sclerosing cholangitis, primary biliary cirrhosis, biliary atresia, autoimmune hepatitis, hereditary hemochromatosis, Wilson disease, and α_1-antitrypsin deficiency are less common causes of cirrhosis.

Cryptogenic cirrhosis: Term used when there is no recognizable cause for the cirrhosis.

Mechanism of cirrhosis: Chronic inflammation causes the release of transforming growth factor-β (TGF-β), which promotes collagen synthesis by stellate cells, leading to fibrosis. Cycles of cell death, fibrosis, and regeneration result in cirrhosis of the liver; reorganization of vascular microarchitecture plays a role.

Complications of cirrhosis include portal hypertension, ascites, hepatocellular dysfunction, portal vein thrombosis, and hepatocellular carcinoma (Figure 15-5 A–D).

Portal hypertension: The portal vein normally drains into the liver. If the liver is scarred, intrahepatic vascular tone increases, causing an increased resistance to portal venous flow and thus an increase in portal venous pressure. Portal hypertension forces blood returning to the heart to take alternate routes such as esophageal varices, hemorrhoids, and **caput medusae** (i.e., dilated veins in abdominal wall). Portal hypertension contributes to the development of ascites and splenomegaly. Splenomegaly also traps red blood cells and platelets. *Note: The cause of portal hypertension can be prehepatic, intrahepatic, or posthepatic, depending upon the site of the pathology.* Cirrhosis is an intrahepatic cause of portal hypertension.

Rupture of esophageal varices can lead to massive gastrointestinal hemorrhage.

Ascites: Occurs as a result of portal hypertension (increased hydrostatic pressure) and hypoalbuminemia (decreased osmotic pressure).

○ **Important points**

   Ascites is detectable on physical examination (shifting dullness and fluid wave) at amounts of > 500 mL.

   Serum-ascites albumin gradient (SAAG) > 1.1 is diagnostic of portal hypertension.

○ **Spontaneous bacterial peritonitis**

   Basic description: Infection of ascitic fluid, usually by *Enterobacteriaceae* or *Pneumococcus.*

   Symptoms and signs: Fever, abdominal pain, and tenderness; rebound tenderness and guarding; and leukocytosis.

   Outcomes: Can precipitate hepatic encephalopathy or renal insufficiency.

Hepatocellular dysfunction, leading to impaired protein synthesis (e.g., decreased albumin and clotting factors), which causes bleeding tendencies and contributes to ascites. Hepatocellular dysfunction also leads to low BUN levels and elevated ammonia levels.

Other complications of cirrhosis: Portal vein thrombosis, hepatocellular carcinoma, hyperestrinism leading to testicular atrophy and gynecomastia.

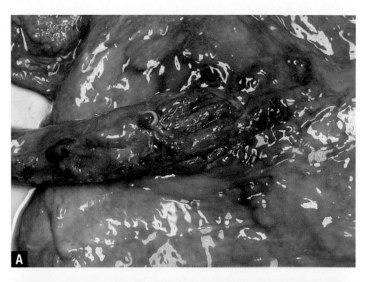

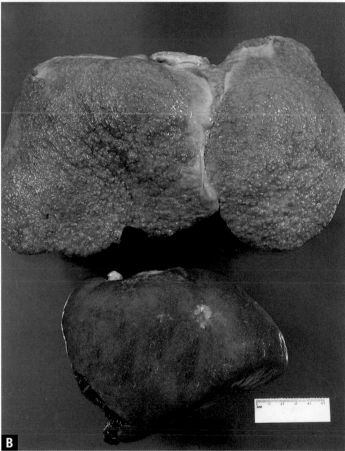

Figure 15-5. Complications of cirrhosis. **A**, Esophageal varices. The blue ring is attempted ligation of the varices by the patient's physician. **B**, Congestive splenomegaly. With portal hypertension, blood return through the splenic vein is impaired. Normally, the spleen is about one tenth the size of the liver; in the photograph, the spleen is about one third the size of the cirrhotic liver.

Note: Remember, cirrhosis is one of the main causes of hepatic failure.

Morphology of cirrhosis

Gross: Diffusely nodular liver, with a micronodular (< 3 mm nodules) or macronodular (> 3 mm nodules) architecture. Macronodular cirrhosis is associated with hepatitis, autoimmune diseases, and end-stage cirrhosis of all etiologies. Micronodular cirrhosis is associated with alcohol use and with other causes such as α_1-antitrypsin deficiency and hemochromatosis.

Microscopic: Bridging fibrosis between the portal tracts and central veins, which divide residual and regenerating hepatocytes into nodules. Other features depend upon the cause of cirrhosis.

ACUTE AND CHRONIC HEPATITIS

Overview: Acute and chronic hepatitis are nonspecific terms relating to the time course of the disease within the liver. The basic description of acute and chronic hepatitis, causes, clinical presentation, and important distinguishing points are discussed below.

ACUTE HEPATITIS (FIGURE 15-6)

Basic description: Inflammation of the liver lasting < 6 months.

Causes of acute hepatitis

Viral: Hepatitis A, B, C, D, and E, Epstein-Barr virus (EBV), and cytomegalovirus (CMV).

Toxins: Alcohol, acetaminophen, isoniazid, halothane, and phenytoin.

Clinical presentation

Signs and symptoms: Enlarged and tender liver; AST and ALT increased 20–100 times normal levels.

Results of acute hepatitis: Vary from complete resolution to rapid progression, with extensive necrosis and fatal outcome.

CHRONIC HEPATITIS (FIGURE 15-7)

Basic description: Sustained inflammation of the liver lasting > 6 months.

Important points

It is difficult to distinguish acute from chronic hepatitis on a histologic basis. The diagnosis of chronic hepatitis requires histologic evidence of progression toward cirrhosis.

Classification of chronic hepatitis is based upon the etiologic agent; the grade of injury, which depends upon numbers and locations of inflammatory cells; the stage of disease, which depends upon the degree, location, and extent of fibrosis; and the distortion of normal architecture.

Alcohol abuse and chronic viral hepatitis are rarely associated with AST or ALT values > 1000 U/L. Values > 1000 U/L are suggestive of acute viral, toxic, or ischemic causes of liver damage.

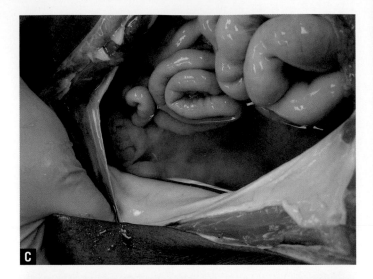

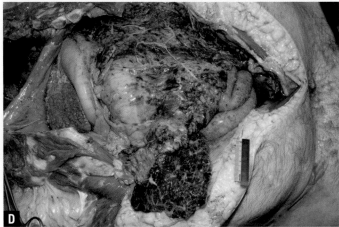

Figure 15-5. (*Continued*) **C**, Ascites. Ascites occurs in patients with cirrhosis because of increased vascular pressure caused by portal hypertension, and also because of decreased plasma osmotic pressure caused by hypoalbuminemia. **D**, Spontaneous bacterial peritonitis. Patients with cirrhosis are prone to development of peritonitis, with no other underlying risk factors identified (e.g., perforated gastric ulcer, diverticulitis).

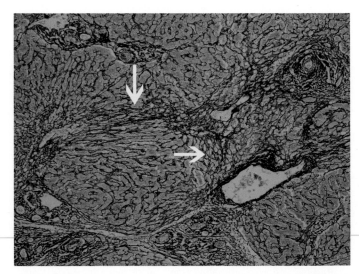

Figure 15-6. Acute hepatitis. This photomicrograph exhibits collapse of the hepatic parenchyma (bridging necrosis indicated by the arrows). Bridging necrosis is a histologic feature of acute hepatitis. Elastin, 100×.

Complicati

Microscop

chronic hep

Overview:

lar damage

Important

Acetami
tocytes.
reduce (
of toxic
relative
farther
the poss

Vinyl ch

Oral co

Chlorpr

Halotha

Phenyt(

Methot

Sulfona

Overview:

include he
tures of h
below.

Overview:

exposure (

Morphol(

Gross:
patchy
15-8).

Micros
ure 15

Clinical p

Sympt(
sense (

Signs:

Import

Microsco

Balloo

Neutr(

Sinusc

VIRAL HEPATITIS

Important clinical points

Hepatitis A (HAV) and hepatitis E (HEV): Have no chronic carrier state so there is no risk of cirrhosis; rarely can HAV cause fulminant hepatic failure. When HEV causes fulminant hepatic failure, it is most commonly associated with Southeast Asian pregnant females.

Of the forms of viral hepatitis, acute hepatitis B (HBV) is most likely to cause fulminant hepatic failure, especially if the patient is co-infected with hepatitis D (HDV).

Immune response is critical in the pathogenesis of acute hepatitis. A vigorous immune response on exposure to HBV increases the risk of acute hepatitis and fulminant hepatic failure but decreases the risk of subsequent development of the chronic carrier state.

The immune response to chronic viral hepatitis (e.g., TGF-β) is responsible for most of the damage to the liver.

HAV is transmitted by the fecal-oral route. HBV is transmitted by exposure to blood or body fluid, sexual contact, or congenital transmission. Transmission of hepatitis C (HCV) requires exposure to blood, and conclusive evidence of routine sexual or congenital transmission is lacking.

Serologic testing in HBV: In the acute phase of HBV infection, HBV surface antigen (HBsAg) and antibodies to HBV core antigen (anti-HBc) are detected in the serum. HBsAg disappears within 3–5 months, and antibodies to HBV surface antigen (HbsAb) do not appear until 6 months after infection. During this variable length "window period," anti-HBc antibody is the only serologic marker of infection. Immunity to HBV is conferred by anti-HBV surface antibodies (HBsAb) and is seen in resolved acute infection (Table 15-4).

Outcomes of viral hepatitis

Carrier state: Patients have *no* symptoms but can transmit the disease; a carrier state is not seen with HAV. HBe antigen is associated with a highly infectious state.

Asymptomatic infection: No symptoms.

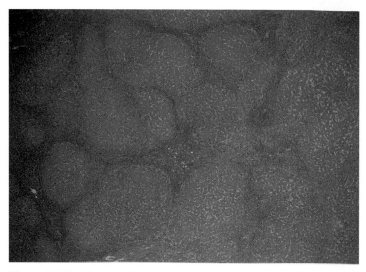

Figure 15-7. Chronic hepatitis. Acute and chronic hepatitis can often appear similar histologically. Chronic hepatitis can be separated from acute hepatitis by demonstration of scarring. In the photomicrograph, the hepatic parenchyma is vaguely divided into nodules, due to early bridging fibrosis. The early bridging fibrosis is associated with a prominent lymphocytic infiltrate. Hematoxylin and eosin, 40×.

TABLE 15-4. Serologic Diagnosis of Viral Hepatitis

Stage of Infection	HBsAg	HBsAb	Anti-HBc	HBe Antigen
Acute infection	+	−	+	+
Acute infection, window period	−	−	+	+
Chronic infection	+	−	+	+/−
Resolved infection	−	+	+	−
Immunized	−	+	−	−

HBsAg, hepatitis B surface antigen; HBsAb, hepatitis surface antigen antibody; anti-HBc, antibody versus hepatitis B core antigen; HBe, hepatitis B envelope antigen.

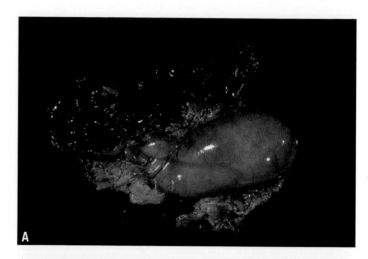

PATHOLOGY OF THE PANCREAS

Overview: Although there are other diseases of the pancreas, the three most important conditions affecting the pancreas are acute and chronic pancreatitis and pancreatic neoplasms (most importantly pancreatic adenocarcinoma and islet cell tumors), which are discussed here. Pancreatic cysts will also be discussed briefly in this section.

ACUTE PANCREATITIS (FIGURE 15-20 *A* and *B*)

Causes

The two most common causes of acute pancreatitis are alcohol use and gallstones.

Other causes: Hypercalcemia, hypertriglyceridemia, drugs (e.g., thiazide diuretics, estrogen), trauma, steroids, and autoimmune disease.

Mechanism of acute pancreatitis: Uncontrolled activation of pancreatic enzymes.

Complications: Chronic pancreatitis, pseudocysts.

Clinical presentation of acute pancreatitis

Signs and symptoms: Acute epigastric abdominal pain, radiating to the back; anorexia and nausea.

Laboratory findings: Elevated amylase and lipase levels (lipase is more sensitive than amylase). Amylase remains elevated for 4–7 days, whereas lipase remains elevated for a longer time period. Hypocalcemia and leukocytosis are common.

Ranson criteria are used to predict severity of acute pancreatitis and include two general categories: those at presentation, and those within 48 hours of presentation. The presence of three or more criteria indicates severe pancreatitis.

At presentation

- Age: Older than 55 years.
- Blood glucose level of > 200 mg/dL.
- White cell count of > 16,000/mm³.
- Lactate dehydrogenase of > 350 IU/L.
- Alanine aminotransferase of > 250 IU/L.

Within 48 hours of presentation

- Hematocrit: > 10% decrease.
- Serum calcium < 8 mg/dL.
- Base deficit of > 4 mEq/L.
- BUN of > 5 mg/dL.
- Fluid sequestration of > 6 L.
- Partial pressure of arterial oxygen of < 60 mm Hg.

Important point: Acute pancreatitis is a severe systemic disorder; it causes diffuse alveolar damage and disseminated intravascular coagulation (DIC).

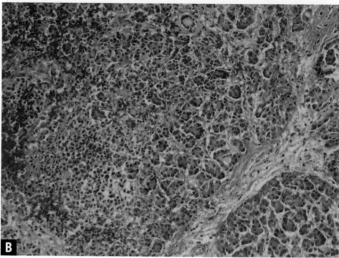

Figure 15-20. Acute hemorrhagic pancreatitis. In this block of organs (**A**), the esophagus and stomach are present as well as the pancreas (the pancreas is the hemorrhagic mass above the stomach). Acute pancreatitis is most commonly due to gallstones or alcohol use, and is a potentially life-threatening condition that causes widespread systemic changes, including diffuse alveolar damage and disseminated intravascular coagulation. In (**B**), note the neutrophilic infiltrate and hemorrhage within the pancreatic parenchyma. Hematoxylin and eosin, 200×.

CHRONIC PANCREATITIS (FIGURE 15-21 *A* and *B*)

Causes: In many patients, chronic pancreatitis is the result of recurring bouts of acute pancreatitis due to causes such as alcohol abuse and gallstones.

Complications: Diabetes mellitus and malabsorption

Clinical presentation of chronic pancreatitis: Weight loss, abdominal pain, and symptoms associated with malabsorption, such as diarrhea.

PANCREATIC CYSTS

True cysts: True cysts of the pancreas (i.e., those with epithelial lining) are seen in patients with polycystic kidney disease.

Pseudocysts: No epithelial lining; seen as a result of acute pancreatitis; most commonly in alcoholics.

Pancreatic neoplasms: Features of pancreatic adenocarcinoma and islet cell tumors, the two most common pancreatic neoplasms, are discussed below.

PANCREATIC ADENOCARCINOMA

Epidemiology: 60–80 years of age.

Risk factor: Smoking.

Prognosis: Poor; most patients do not survive more than 5 years after diagnosis.

Location of tumor: Most are in the head of the pancreas.

Clinical presentation of pancreatic adenocarcinoma

Symptoms: Abdominal pain radiating to the back; weight loss as a result of malabsorption and anorexia.

Signs: Obstructive jaundice with palpable gallbladder (i.e., **Courvoisier sign**). Dilated proximal pancreatic duct on CT and MRI. Elevated CA19-9.

Important points

Trousseau syndrome: Migratory thrombophlebitis.

Pancreatic adenocarcinoma is known for perineural invasion (painful).

If pancreatic adenocarcinoma occurs in the ampulla, patients can present with jaundice. Because of the early production of symptoms, the tumor can be resected at an early stage (i.e., when it is small), and patients then have a better prognosis. In contrast, a tumor in the tail can grow large before it presents with symptoms, and patients have a poor prognosis.

ISLET CELL TUMOR

Important points: Most islet cell tumors are benign (i.e., do not invade or metastasize), but they can produce insulin or glucagon and have systemic effects. Insulinomas (i.e., a type of islet cell tumor that produces insulin) usually cause hypoglycemia with an elevated C-peptide level. About 5% of cases are associated with MEN 1.

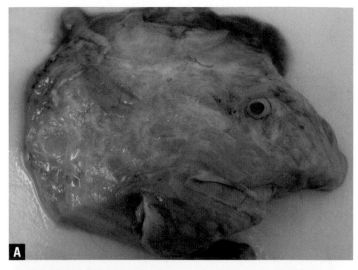

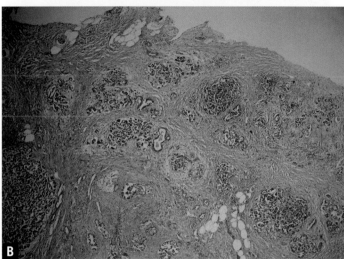

Figure 15-21. Chronic pancreatitis. **A**, Note the loss of pancreatic parenchyma and its replacement with fibrosis. Chronic pancreatitis is not an immediately life-threatening condition as is acute pancreatitis; however, it can lead to secondary diabetes mellitus and malabsorption, depending upon its extent. **B**, Note the loss of pancreatic glandular parenchyma and its replacement with fibrosis (the glandular parenchyma should be back to back). The islets are resistant to the changes and, in cases of chronic pancreatitis, only clusters of pancreatic islets may be present among the fibrosis. Hematoxylin and eosin, 40×.

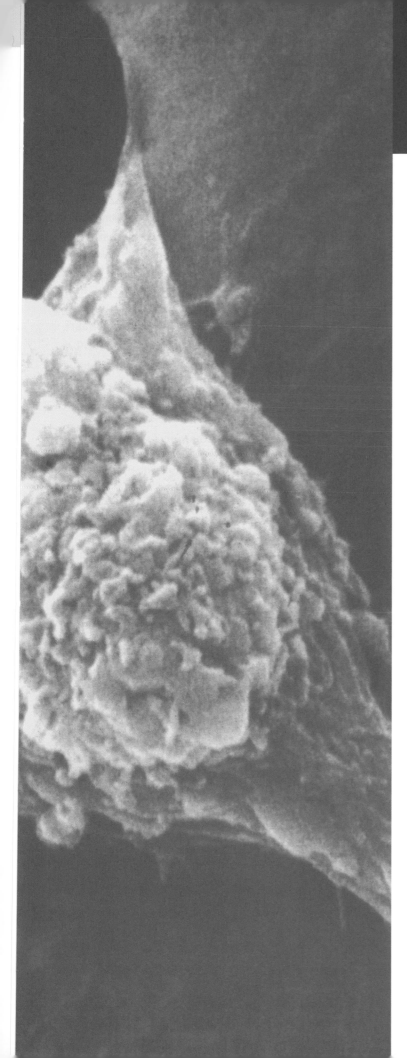

CHAPTER 16

PATHOLOGY OF THE KIDNEY AND BLADDER

OVERVIEW

In this chapter, the pathology of the kidney is organized into four anatomic categories: diseases of the glomeruli, tubules, interstitium, and vessels. Diseases that affect the glomeruli often have an immunologic etiology, whereas those that affect the tubules and interstitium usually have an infectious or toxic etiology. Early in the disease process, most disorders predominantly affect one of the anatomic structures listed above. Over time, however, the entire kidney usually becomes diseased. Because of the large physiologic reserve of the kidneys, many diseases do not become clinically apparent until the majority of the organ is affected, making subtle abnormalities in laboratory findings the only early indication of renal disease. Recognition of these patterns of abnormalities, pathologic findings, and clinical presentation is perhaps more important to renal pathology than in any other organ system. This chapter describes acute and chronic renal failure, disorders of volume regulation, glomerular diseases, tubulointerstitial diseases, nephrolithiasis, cystic diseases of the kidney, renal tumors, pathology of the bladder, acid-base disorders, and electrolyte disorders.

ACUTE RENAL FAILURE

Overview: Acute renal failure is rapid onset of **azotemia** (i.e., elevated blood urea nitrogen [BUN] and creatinine [Cr]) combined with oliguria or anuria. Azotemia can occur by itself, in which case a patient has an elevated BUN and creatinine but normal urine output. Therefore, the difference between azotemia and acute renal failure is the amount of urine output (normal with azotemia; decreased or absent with acute renal failure). There are three types of acute renal failure and azotemia: **prerenal, intrinsic** (i.e., **renal**), and **postrenal,** which are based upon the location of the source of the azotemia or acute renal failure. To simplify the following discussion, the three forms will be listed as prerenal azotemia, intrinsic azotemia, and postrenal azotemia; however, remember that azotemia and acute renal failure are technically on a spectrum defined by urine output. For example, the listed causes of prerenal azotemia can also lead to acute renal failure.

Type I RPGN

- **Distinguishing feature:** Linear pattern of immunofluorescence due to causative IgG binding directly to glomerular basement membrane antigens.
- **Causes:** Goodpasture syndrome; idiopathic.

Type II RPGN

- **Distinguishing feature:** Immune complex mediated.
- **Causes:** Postinfectious glomerulonephritis, IgA nephropathy and Henoch-Schönlein purpura, SLE, idiopathic.

Type III RPGN

- **Distinguishing feature:** Type III RPGN is referred to as pauci-immune (i.e., no immune complexes). ANCA is positive (e.g., Wegener granulomatosis) in up to 80% of cases.
- **Causes:** Wegener granulomatosis, microscopic polyarteritis, idiopathic.

MEMBRANOPROLIFERATIVE GLOMERULONEPHRITIS (MPGN)

Presentation: About 50% of patients present with nephrotic syndrome, 30% with asymptomatic hematuria, and 20% with acute nephritic syndrome.

Epidemiology: Most patients are diagnosed between the ages of 5 and 30 years.

Important point: About 50% of patients develop chronic renal failure within 10 years.

Histologic evaluation of membranoproliferative glomerulonephritis (see Table 16-2)

- **Light microscope:** Lobular appearance of glomeruli, thickening of basement membrane, and an increase in the number of cells in the glomerulus. Glomerular basement membranes have "**tram-track**" appearance (like railroad tracks) on silver stain, due to splitting of the basement membrane by extensions of mesangial and inflammatory cell processes. There is a proliferation of glomerular cells combined with leukocyte infiltrate. The proliferation of cells is commonly in a mesangial location, hence the alternative name "**mesangiocapillary glomerulonephritis**" (Figure 16-7).
- **Immunofluorescence:** See types of MPGN.
- **Electron microscopy:** See types of MPGN.

Types of MPGN (I and II): There are two types of MPGN based upon the immunofluorescence and electron microscopic findings.

Type I MPGN

- **Immunofluorescence:** Granular pattern; positive for C_3 and IgG.
- **Electron microscopy:** Subendothelial immune complex deposits.
- **Important point:** Associated with hepatitis B and C and SLE.

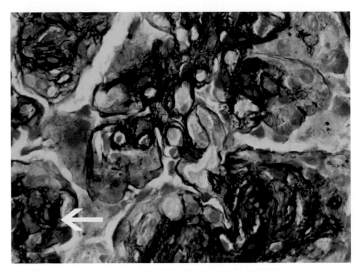

Figure 16-7. Membranoproliferative glomerulonephritis. Note the redundancy of the basement membrane ("tram-track" appearance) at the arrow. Jones silver stain, 1000×.

Type II MPGN

■ **Immunofluorescence:** Positive for C_3 (on either side of dense deposit); no IgG.

■ **Electron microscopy:** Long dense band of unknown composition in lamina densa and subendothelial region.

■ **Important point:** Associated with C_3 nephritic factor, which stabilizes C_3 convertase; thus, patients have hypocomplementemia.

CHRONIC GLOMERULONEPHRITIS

Overview: Chronic glomerulonephritis is a condition resulting from long-term damage to the glomeruli. In addition, other compartments of the kidney begin to show damage. For example, glomerular failure due to global sclerosis of the glomeruli leads to decreased blood flow to the kidney, and decreased blood flow to the kidney triggers release of renin, which results in hypertension. Hypertension causes hyaline arteriolosclerosis, which damages the vessels, resulting in a thinned renal cortex and atrophy of tubules (Figure 16-8).

Causes of chronic glomerulonephritis

■ **Common causes:** Diabetes mellitus, lupus nephritis, RPGN, FSGS, and membranoproliferative glomerulonephritis.

■ **Less common causes:** IgA nephropathy and membranous glomerulonephropathy.

■ **Rare causes:** Postinfectious glomerulonephritis.

■ **Important point:** In most cases, the original condition that resulted in the chronic damage cannot be identified because the glomeruli are too sclerotic.

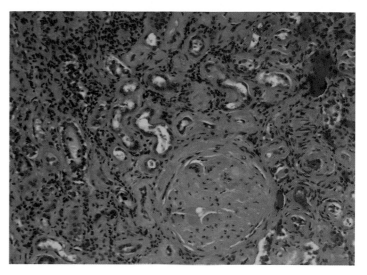

Figure 16-8. Chronic glomerulonephritis. Over time, with many renal diseases, all four components of the renal cortex (i.e., glomeruli, tubules, interstitium, and vessels) are damaged. In this section, there is one globally sclerotic glomerulus and many atrophic tubules. Diabetes mellitus and hypertension are common etiologies of chronic renal failure; however, at the end stage of the disease, histologic examination of the kidney often will not reveal changes to identify the underlying cause. Hematoxylin and eosin, 400×.

ASYMPTOMATIC HEMATURIA

Overview: Asymptomatic hematuria is hematuria without other associated symptoms. For example, nephritic syndrome is associated with hematuria, but hypertension, oliguria, and other symptoms are usually present.

Important laboratory finding: Red cell casts.

General pathogenesis: Most forms of asymptomatic hematuria caused by glomerular disease are due to abnormalities in the basement membrane; however, the most common glomerular cause of asymptomatic hematuria is IgA nephropathy, which is caused by immune complex deposition.

Specific causes of asymptomatic hematuria: The four most common conditions causing asymptomatic hematuria are IgA nephropathy, Henoch-Schönlein purpura, Alport syndrome, and thin basement membrane disease.

IGA NEPHROPATHY (BERGER DISEASE)

Epidemiology: Accounts for 40–50% of patients with asymptomatic hematuria. IgA nephropathy is the most common primary cause of glomerulonephritis. Most patients are between the ages of 15 and 35 years. It has a male to female ratio of 2–3:1, and is more common in whites than African Americans. IgA nephropathy is associated with celiac disease and Henoch-Schönlein purpura.

Causes of chronic tubulointerstitial nephritis

- Urinary tract obstruction (most important cause).
- Chronic pyelonephritis and reflux nephropathy.
- **Drugs:** NSAIDs (analgesic nephropathy), cisplatin, cyclosporine.
- **Vascular disease:** Hypertension, atherosclerosis.
- **Heavy metals:** Lead, cadmium.
- **Malignancies:** Multiple myeloma.

ACUTE TUBULAR NECROSIS

Basic description: Rapid onset of necrosis of tubular epithelium with subsequent acute loss of renal function. Acute tubular necrosis is the most common cause of acute renal failure.

Causes of acute tubular necrosis

- **Ischemic category:** Trauma with blood loss; sepsis.
- **Toxic category:** Aminoglycosides, intravenous contrast, mercury, oxalic acid (due to ethylene glycol poisoning), myoglobinuria, hemoglobinuria; hyperuricemia (associated with rapid cellular turnover with certain malignancies).

Pathogenesis: Tubular injury and decreased GFR leads to acute tubular necrosis.

Stages of acute tubular necrosis

- **Initiating:** The initiating stage is the event that causes the acute tubular necrosis; no change in renal output.
- **Maintenance:** Oliguria; urine flow decreases to < 400 mL/day within 24 hours of initiating event.
- **Recovery:** Increased urine output (up to 3 L); electrolyte disturbances at this time increase the risk of death.

Microscopic morphology of acute tubular necrosis: Tubulorrhexis; coagulative necrosis of epithelial cells, protein casts (composed of **Tamm-Horsfall protein**), and dilation of proximal convoluted tubules (Figure 16-10 A and B).

Clinical presentation of acute tubular necrosis: Acute renal failure with granular or "muddy brown" epithelial casts in urine.

INFECTIONS OF THE KIDNEY AND URINARY TRACT

Overview: The three most important infections of the kidneys and urinary tract are classified as cystitis and acute and chronic pyelonephritis. Although each is a separate entity, they all are also interrelated. These three infections and xanthogranulomatous pyelonephritis are all discussed in this section.

CYSTITIS

Basic description: Infection of the bladder.

Clinical presentation of cystitis

- **Symptoms:** Dysuria, urinary frequency, urgency.
- **Signs:** Suprapubic discomfort.
- **Laboratory testing:** Urine is positive for leukocyte esterase and has elevated pH and elevated nitrates.

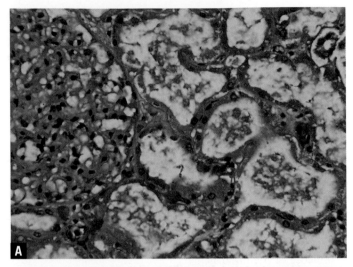

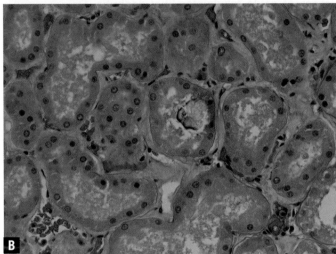

Figure 16-10. Acute tubular necrosis. **A,** The tubules are dilated and lined with flattened epithelial cells, some of which are necrotic (eosinophilic, with loss of nuclear basophilia). Acute tubular necrosis is due to an ischemic or toxic insult. One toxin that affects the kidney is ethylene glycol. Ethylene glycol is, by itself, harmless to the kidney; however, metabolism of the toxin converts it to oxalic acid, which damages the kidney. **B,** An oxalic acid crystal is in the center of the photomicrograph. Hematoxylin and eosin, **A** and **B,** 400×.

Complications of cystitis: Acute pyelonephritis.

ACUTE PYELONEPHRITIS (FIGURE 16-11 *A–C*)

Basic description: Inflammation (usually bacterial in origin) of the kidney (primarily tubules and interstitium). The glomeruli are fairly resistant, but eventually can become involved.

Pathogenesis of acute pyelonephritis

- **Two sources of infection:** Ascending infections from the bladder (most common), or hematogenous spread from another site of infection.

- **Causative organisms:** *Escherichia coli*, *Proteus*, *Enterobacter*, and *Staphylococcus*. *Staphylococcus* is more common from hematogenous sources.

- **Mechanism of ascending infections:** Bacteria adhere to the mucosa of the lower urinary tract (i.e., colonization of urethra) and enter into the bladder following instrumentation or other trauma (e.g., from sexual intercourse). From the bladder, bacteria ascend to the pelvis of the kidney because of vesicoureteral reflux (i.e., incompetent valves between the ureter and bladder).

- **Risk factors for ascending infections**
  - **Obstruction** (e.g., benign prostatic hyperplasia, uterine prolapse) impairs voiding. Voiding is a mechanism the bladder has for remaining sterile by washing the bacteria out frequently.
  - **Vesicoureteral reflux** (see Figure 16-11 *A*).
  - **Diabetes mellitus:** Patients have increased risk of infection and can have bladder dysfunction due to nerve damage.
  - **Gender:** Females have shorter urethra.
  - **Other risk factors:** Presence of renal lesion, immunosuppression, and trauma, including sexual intercourse and pregnancy.

Morphology of acute pyelonephritis: Abscesses in cortex.

Clinical presentation of acute pyelonephritis: Acute onset of fevers, chills, rigors, and back pain with costovertebral angle tenderness. Leukocytosis is almost always present. Hematuria, dysuria, and frank pyuria may occur. White blood cells, white cell casts, and positive leukocyte esterase in urine.

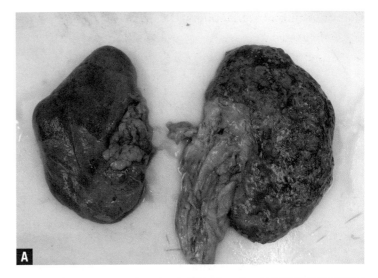

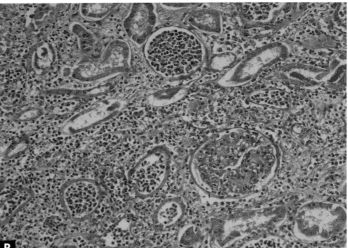

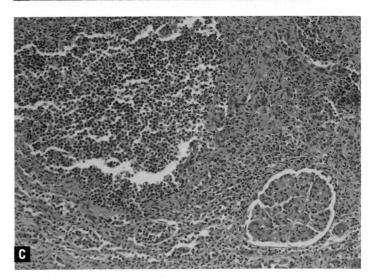

Figure 16-11. Acute pyelonephritis. **A**, Both kidneys are from the same patient. The right kidney has a friable cortex, and the ureter is dilated. The left kidney is essentially normal. The fact that only one kidney is affected supports the concept that a urinary tract infection alone is not enough to result in pyelonephritis. This patient most likely had vesicoureteral reflux on the right side, but none on the left. **B**, Note the infiltrate of neutrophils in the interstitium and filling the tubules. **C**, The neutrophilic infiltrate can result in abscess formation (left upper corner), which contributed to the degeneration and subsequent friable nature of the cortex in (**A**). Hematoxylin and eosin, **B** and **C**, 200×.

SIMPLE CYSTS

Basic description: Fluid-filled cyst, usually in the cortex of the kidney.

Important points

- Simple cysts are common and benign.
- Patients on chronic dialysis can develop many cysts, and have an increased risk of developing renal cell carcinoma.

CYSTIC RENAL DYSPLASIA

Location: Can be bilateral or unilateral.

Microscopic morphology: Undifferentiated mesenchyme surrounding immature collecting ducts; can also have cartilage.

Pathogenesis: Abnormality in metanephric differentiation.

AUTOSOMAL DOMINANT POLYCYSTIC KIDNEY DISEASE (ADPCKD)

Basic description: Hereditary condition that usually has its clinical onset (i.e., symptoms) during adulthood.

Mutations

- Chromosome 16p13.3 involves *PKD1* gene, which encodes polycystin.
- Chromosome 4q21 involves *PKD2* gene, which encodes polycystin 2.

Complications of ADPCKD

- **Renal failure:** Most common cause of death. ADPCKD causes 5–10% of all cases of chronic renal failure. About 50% of patients progress to chronic renal failure by 60 years of age.
- Hypertension.
- Chronic urinary tract infections.

Important points regarding ADPCKD

- Associated with berry aneurysms, which can be a source of subarachnoid hemorrhage.
- Associated with cysts of liver and pancreas.
- Can see a myxomatous mitral valve in 20% of patients.

Gross morphology: Multiple cysts (up to 4 cm in size), which usually distort the normal architecture of the kidney to a point where it is no longer identifiable as a kidney (Figure 16-16).

Clinical presentation of ADPCKD

- **Symptoms:** Abdominal flank pain, back pain, hematuria.
- **Signs:** Abdominal mass, microscopic hematuria, hypertension.

AUTOSOMAL RECESSIVE POLYCYSTIC KIDNEY DISEASE

Basic description: Hereditary condition that usually has its clinical onset (i.e., symptoms) during infancy or childhood.

Mutation: 6p21-23 involves *PKHD1* gene, which encodes fibrocystin.

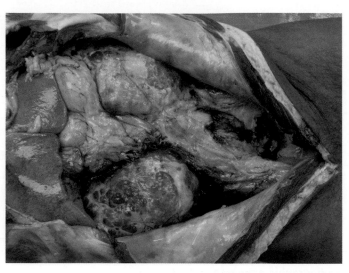

Figure 16-16. Adult polycystic kidney disease. Both kidneys are enlarged and multicystic. Adult polycystic kidney disease is responsible for a portion of cases of chronic renal failure. The condition is associated with cerebral berry aneurysms, which may be responsible for the sudden death of the patient.

Morphology

- **Gross:** Multiple cysts in cortex and medulla; normal kidney architecture (i.e., the general shape of the kidney) is preserved.
- **Microscopic:** Dilation of collecting tubules.

RENAL NEOPLASMS

Overview: Although there are many different renal neoplasms, the most common tumor in adults is a renal cell carcinoma, and the most common tumor in children is Wilms tumor.

RENAL CELL CARCINOMA

Epidemiology: Occurs in sixth and seventh decades of life; predominance of male to female, with a ratio of 2:1.

Risk factors: Smoking, cadmium, chronic dialysis.

Types of renal cell carcinoma: Although there are several histologic variants of renal cell carcinoma, the most common is the clear cell type, which, along with the chromophobe and papillary types, will be discussed below.

CLEAR CELL RENAL CELL CARCINOMA

Incidence: About 85% of all renal cell carcinomas.

Morphology (Figure 16-17 *A* and *B*)

- **Gross:** Yellow (from glycogen) and hemorrhagic.
- **Microscopic:** Clear cells with variably pleomorphic nuclei (graded I–IV, based upon pleomorphism of nuclei); well vascularized.

Mutations: Deletion or unbalanced translocations involving 3p. *VHL* gene is on chromosome 3p25 and produces a protein that is a component of ubiquitin-ligase complex, which targets proteins for degradation.

CHROMOPHOBE RENAL CELL CARCINOMA

Incidence: About 5% of all renal cell carcinomas.

Morphology

- **Gross:** Brown mass.
- **Microscopic:** Neoplastic cells with abundant eosinophilic cytoplasm.

Important point: Unique among tumors in that they usually have multiple losses of entire chromosomes.

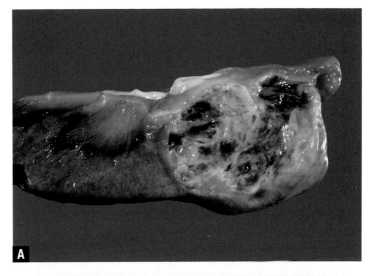

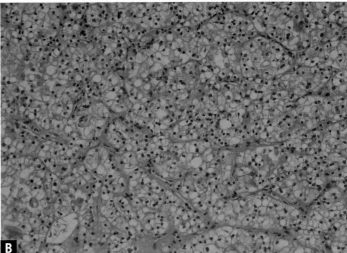

Figure 16-17. Renal cell carcinoma, clear cell type. Clear cell renal cell carcinoma has a very characteristic gross appearance, yellow coloration from the glycogen in the tumor cells and hemorrhage due to the prominent vascularity of the tumor (**A**). Histologically, the neoplasm is composed of clear cells with a background of prominent vascularity (**B**). Although the tumor cells appear bland (i.e., no pleomorphism, few mitotic figures), renal cell carcinoma is a highly malignant tumor and known for its propensity to metastasize to unusual locations. Hematoxylin and eosin, 200×.

neoplasms metastasize sooner, are radioresistant, and tend to metastasize via hematogenous routes. The classic presentation of testicular cancer is a painless testicular mass.

Sites of metastases from testicular neoplasms

- **Lymph nodes:** Para-aortic, mediastinal, and supraclavicular lymph nodes.
- **Hematogenous dissemination:** Lungs, liver, brain, bone.

Two categories of testicular neoplasms

- Germ cell (most common type of testicular neoplasm).
- Non–germ cell (including sex cord–stromal tumors and Leydig cell tumors).

Risk factors for development of testicular neoplasms

- **Cryptorchidism** (i.e., undescended testicle).
- Syndromes with testicular dysgenesis (e.g., Klinefelter syndrome).
- Family history and history of a tumor in the contralateral testis.

World Health Organization (WHO) classification of testicular neoplasms

- Tumors with one histologic pattern.
- Tumors with more than one histologic pattern (also referred to as mixed germ cell tumor), which account for 60% of testicular tumors.

Mutations: Isochromosome (12p) is found in virtually all germ cell tumors. It encodes the *DAD-R* gene, which produces a protein that prevents apoptosis.

TYPES OF GERM CELL TUMORS AND THEIR PRECURSORS

Overview: Intratubular germ cell neoplasia and five common types of germ cell tumors (seminoma, embryonal carcinoma, yolk sac tumor, choriocarcinoma, and teratoma) are discussed below. Remember, although the germ cell tumors are being discussed under testicular tumors, they also occur in the ovary. For clinical purposes, the important distinction is seminoma versus non–seminomatous germ cell tumor, because seminomas are radiosensitive and the other germ cell tumors are radioresistant (Table 17-1).

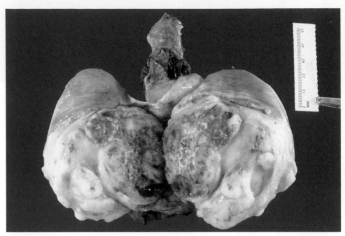

Figure 17-1. Mixed germ cell tumor of testis. This testicle has been bisected (the spermatic cord is at the 12-o'clock position), revealing an expansive mass in the parenchyma. The mass has a variegated appearance, consistent with a mixed germ cell tumor.

TABLE 17-1. Comparison of Germ Cell Neoplasms

Neoplasm	Radiosensitive?	Protein Secreted	Age Range
Seminoma	Yes	hCG (15% of tumors)	15–35 years
Embryonal carcinoma	No	hCG and AFP	20–30 years
Yolk sac tumor	No	AFP	If pure, 3 years
Choriocarcinoma	No	hCG	20–30 years
Teratoma	No	None	18 years

hCG, human chorionic gonadotropin; AFP, α-fetoprotein.

INTRATUBULAR GERM CELL NEOPLASIA

Basic description: Preneoplastic proliferation of germ cells within seminiferous tubules.

Important points: Approximately 50% of cases progress to a germ cell tumor within 5 years. The main risk factor for intratubular germ cell neoplasia is cryptorchidism.

SEMINOMA

Epidemiology: Most arise between 15 and 35 years of age.

Important points

- Seminomas are radiosensitive.
- A dysgerminoma is the ovarian correlate of the seminoma (i.e., the tumors have the same features but different names).

Morphology of seminoma

- **Gross:** Homogenous tan mass.
- **Microscopic:** Large mononuclear cells with clear cytoplasm and fibrous septae with lymphocytes (Figure 17-2). Approximately 10–15% of seminomas can have giant cells (syncytiotrophoblasts), in which case human chorionic gonadotropin (hCG) can be detected in the blood.

Clinical presentation of seminoma: Painless testicular mass. Approximately 15% have metastasized to local lymph nodes at the time of diagnosis. Prognosis is excellent, with cure rates close to 100% for stage I and stage II disease.

EMBRYONAL CARCINOMA

Epidemiology: Many occur between 20 and 30 years of age.

Important points

- Approximately 90% of patients have elevated β-hCG or α-fetoprotein (AFP).
- An embryonal carcinoma is only pure in 2–3% of cases. In most cases, an embryonal carcinoma occurs as part of a mixed tumor.

Morphology of embryonal carcinoma

- **Gross:** Hemorrhagic and necrotic mass.
- **Microscopic:** Alveolar or tubular architecture; pleomorphic, primitive looking "ugly" cells with abundant mitotic figures.

YOLK SAC TUMOR (FIGURE 17-3)

Epidemiology: Only occurs as a pure tumor in young males (at about 3 years of age). In adults, yolk sac tumors are part of mixed germ cell tumors.

Important point: Positive for AFP (see Figure 17-3).

Microscopic morphology of yolk sac tumor: May have a variety of histologic patterns. One characteristic feature is **Schiller-Duval bodies,** which resemble endodermal sinuses. Schiller-Duval bodies have a capillary at the core and are surrounded by a visceral and a parietal layer (i.e., resemble primitive glomerulus).

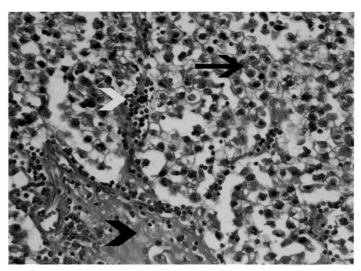

Figure 17-2. Seminoma. The three characteristic microscopic features of seminomas are large mononuclear cells (*arrow*), fibrous septae (*black arrowhead*), and lymphocytes (*white arrowhead*). Seminomas have a characteristic gross appearance (i.e., homogeneous and tan). Hematoxylin and eosin, 400×.

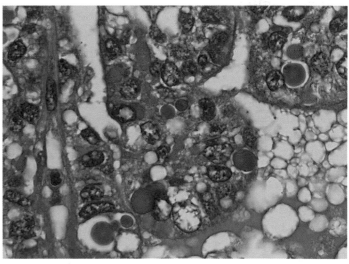

Figure 17-3. Yolk sac tumor. The eosinophilic globules are composed of α-fetoprotein (AFP). The production of AFP is characteristic of yolk sac tumors. Hematoxylin and eosin, 400×.

PATHOLOGY OF THE PROSTATE

Overview: The three main pathologic conditions affecting the prostate are acute prostatitis, benign prostatic hyperplasia, and prostatic adenocarcinoma.

ACUTE PROSTATITIS (FIGURE 17-5)

Associated conditions: Infection of the urinary bladder or urethra, obstruction (e.g., due to prostatic hyperplasia), and human immunodeficiency virus (HIV) infection.

Causative organisms: In men older than 35 years of age, *Escherichia coli*, *Enterobacter*, and other urinary tract pathogens are the most common cause of acute prostatitis. In men younger than age 35 years, *Neisseria gonorrhoeae* and *Chlamydia* are the causative agents until proven otherwise.

Complications of acute prostatitis: Chronic prostatitis, which can be source of recurring urinary tract infections in older males because antibiotics poorly penetrate the prostate.

Clinical presentation of acute prostatitis

- **Symptoms:** Dysuria, urinary frequency, lower back pain.

- **Signs:** Boggy, tender prostate on examination. Leukocytosis, fever, and elevated prostate-specific antigen (PSA) are common.

BENIGN PROSTATIC HYPERPLASIA

Basic description: Hyperplasia of glandular and stromal elements of prostate.

Epidemiology: More common with increasing age; usually males older than 50 years of age.

Location of benign prostatic hyperplasia: Usually involves the parenchyma around the urethra (i.e., transitional zone) first, and produces urinary obstruction.

Pathogenesis: Results from action of androgens. Testosterone is converted to dihydrotestosterone by 5α-reductase.

Complications of benign prostatic hyperplasia

- Urinary obstruction, which is subsequently risk for urinary tract infection; postrenal azotemia, hydronephrosis, renal failure, and kidney stones.

- Benign prostatic hyperplasia is *not* considered a premalignant condition.

Morphology of benign prostatic hyperplasia

- **Gross:** Well-circumscribed nodules in the center of the gland around the urethra (Figure 17-6).

- **Microscopic:** Nodules of glandular hyperplasia associated with stromal hyperplasia; can have squamous metaplasia surrounding infarcts.

Clinical presentation of benign prostatic hyperplasia

- **Symptoms:** Increased frequency of urination, nocturia, difficulty starting and stopping urine flow, and incomplete voiding.

- **Signs:** Enlarged gland on digital rectal examination, with no nodules; gland may be tender upon palpation.

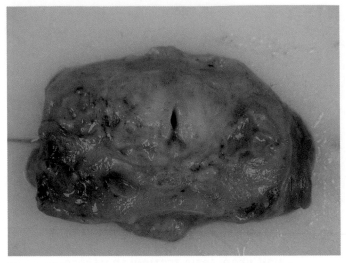

Figure 17-5. Acute prostatitis. Note the scattered yellow-green depressed regions, which are abscesses. Prostatitis can serve as the source of bacteria in patients with chronic urinary tract infections.

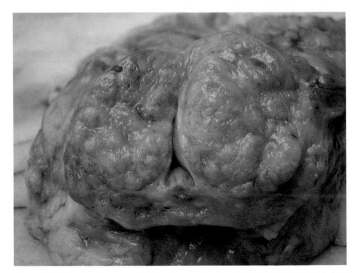

Figure 17-6. Benign prostatic hyperplasia. Note the large nodules of hyperplastic parenchyma compressing the urethra (center). The posterior aspect of the gland is at the 6-o'clock position and is uninvolved. Prostatic adenocarcinoma more commonly arises in this region and can be palpated upon digital rectal examination.

PROSTATIC ADENOCARCINOMA

Epidemiology: Males, age 60 years and older; second leading cause of cancer deaths in men.

Location: Peripheral portion of gland and, therefore, palpated by digital rectal examination.

Important point: Prostatic adenocarcinoma is known for osteoblastic metastases to lumbar spine, proximal femur, and pelvis, which can cause increased alkaline phosphatase.

Genetics: Prostatic adenocarcinoma commonly has hypermethylation of glutathione S-transferase gene promoter (GSTP1), which is found on chromosome 11q13.

Precursor: High-grade prostatic intraepithelial neoplasia (PIN).

Gleason grading system for prostatic adenocarcinoma: Final grade is two numbers (e.g., 3 + 3) representing the dominant (first number) and subdominant (second number) histologic appearance. The dominant and subdominant histologic appearances are each graded from 1 to 5, depending upon the fusion of tubules and the presence of single cells; the lower the number, the lower the grade of the tumor.

Morphology of prostatic adenocarcinoma (Figure 17-7 A and B)

- **Gross:** Yellow discoloration; usually involves periphery of the gland first.
- **Microscopic**
  - **Low power:** Small glands, back-to-back.
  - **High power:** Single cell layer (i.e., no basal cell layer as found in the normal prostate), prominent nucleoli, crystals, blue mucin; known for perineural invasion.

Clinical presentation of prostatic adenocarcinoma

- **Symptoms:** Decreased urinary stream, urinary frequency; back pain from osteoblastic metastases to lumbar spine.
- **Signs:** Nodules or induration (i.e., hardness) felt upon digital rectal examination.
- **PSA**
  - PSA level of 4–10 ng/mL is gray zone; < 4 ng/mL is rarely cancer; > 10 ng/mL is most likely cancer; and 4–10 ng/mL is of uncertain etiology.
  - **Important point regarding PSA testing:** Free PSA level is good for evaluation of patients in the 4–10 ng/mL range; normal free PSA level is < 24% of the total PSA
  - **Other causes of elevated PSA:** BPH, prostatitis, prostate massage, cystoscopy, transurethral resection of the prostate (TURP), prostate biopsy.
- **Other laboratory studies for evaluating PSA**
  - **PSA density:** Is calculated as PSA divided by weight of prostate gland (weight of prostate determined by transrectal ultrasound); a PSA density of > 0.15 suggests carcinoma.
  - **PSA velocity:** Rate of change in PSA; suspicious for carcinoma if > 0.75 ng/mL/year.

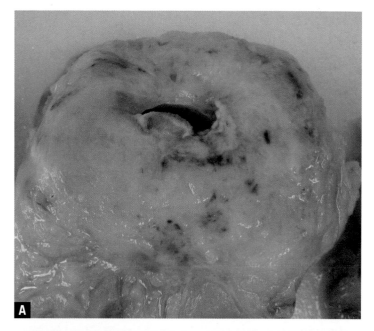

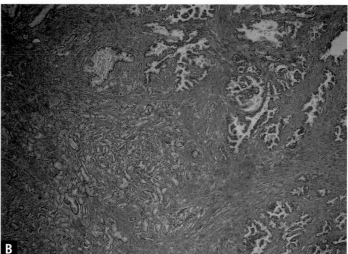

Figure 17-7. Prostatic adenocarcinoma. **A,** Note the blurring and obliteration of normal parenchyma from the 5-o'clock to the 9-o'clock position in this prostate. This tumor has arisen in the posterior portion of the gland. **B,** The initial diagnosis of prostatic adenocarcinoma is based upon the low power appearance. The small glands that are back-to-back in the left lower corner are characteristic of prostatic adenocarcinoma; compare these to the larger, more widely separated normal glands in the upper right corner. Hematoxylin and eosin, 40×.

Precursor lesion for endometrial adenocarcinoma: Endometrial hyperplasia.

Mutations: Approximately 35% of cases of endometrial adenocarcinoma have a mutation of *PTEN*. *PTEN* is located at 10q23, and is a tumor suppressor gene whose function is to cause arrest of the cell cycle at G_1, enabling apoptosis. Endometrial adenocarcinoma can also have a mutation of β-catenin.

Important points regarding endometrial adenocarcinoma

■ Higher-grade variants of endometrial adenocarcinoma such as clear cell adenocarcinoma and papillary serous adenocarcinoma are less commonly related to increased estrogen and hyperplasia. They have a poorer prognosis, and are associated with microsatellite instability or mutation of *p53*.

■ Endometrial adenocarcinoma metastases to lungs, liver, and bone.

Clinical presentation of endometrial adenocarcinoma

■ **Symptoms:** Vaginal bleeding.

■ **Important points**

  ○ Vaginal bleeding in a postmenopausal woman is endometrial hyperplasia or cancer until proven otherwise, and *always* necessitates biopsy. Because of this sentinel symptom, endometrial cancer is usually diagnosed at an early stage.

  ○ Granulosa cell tumors secrete estrogen, and thus are an uncommon cause of endometrial hyperplasia and endometrial adenocarcinoma.

LEIOMYOMA (UTERINE FIBROIDS)

Basic description: Benign tumor of smooth muscle.

Epidemiology: Very common during reproductive years; found in up to 75% of women of reproductive age. More common in African Americans.

Locations: Leiomyomas can occur in subserosal, intramural, or subendometrial locations. Leiomyomas are usually multiple in number.

Mutations: t(12;14) and del 7.

Complications of leiomyomas

■ Menorrhagia with severe anemia.

■ Infertility, abortion, and premature labor.

■ Compression of the bladder or ureter, causing hydroureter or hydronephrosis.

■ Development of leiomyosarcoma is extremely rare.

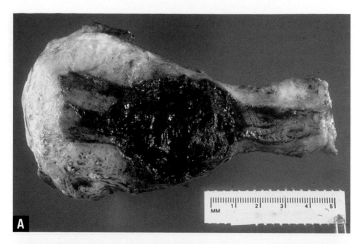

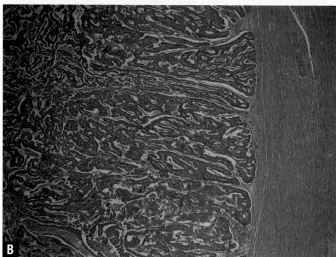

Figure 17-13. Endometrial adenocarcinoma. **A**, Bulging forth from the endometrial surface is a large, red-tan polypoid mass. Endometrial adenocarcinoma can be detected early in its course because of vaginal bleeding. **B**, This low-power view illustrates an invasive endometrial adenocarcinoma. Note the complexity of the glands (compare to Figure 17-12 **B**). One of the only histologic differences between complex hyperplasia with atypia and endometrial adenocarcinoma is the presence of invasion. Hematoxylin and eosin, 40×.

Morphology of leiomyomas

▣ **Gross:** Firm, tan, well-circumscribed mass (Figure 17-14).

▣ **Microscopic:** Interlocking fascicles of smooth muscle cells.

Clinical presentation of leiomyoma: Abnormal uterine bleeding (menorrhagia), anemia, enlarged irregular uterus, recurrent abortions, infertility.

Important points

▣ Leiomyomas are estrogen sensitive and increase in size with pregnancy and decrease in size with menopause.

▣ The most important risk factor for malignant degeneration to leiomyosarcoma is prior pelvic irradiation.

LEIOMYOSARCOMA

Basic description: Malignant tumor of smooth muscle.

Epidemiology: Females between ages 40 and 60 years.

Clinical presentation: Rapidly enlarging pelvic mass. May present in a woman with a history of leiomyomas. Metastases to lungs, bone, and brain.

OTHER NEOPLASMS

Endometrial stromal sarcoma: Malignant tumor of endometrial stroma; represent < 5% of endometrial tumors.

Combination tumors

▣ **Endometrial carcinoma with stromal differentiation** (called **carcinosarcoma** or **malignant mixed müllerian tumor**).

▣ **Adenosarcoma:** Stromal tumor associated with benign glands.

NON-NEOPLASTIC OVARIAN DISEASE

Overview: One of the most important conditions involving the ovaries is tumors, which will be discussed in the next section. Many ovaries have non-neoplastic conditions, most commonly cysts of various types, which are usually incidental findings during surgery and of little or no clinical importance. However, polycystic ovarian disease (formerly known as **Stein-Leventhal syndrome**) is a condition associated with multicystic ovaries and is discussed below.

Polycystic ovarian disease (PCOD)

▣ **Mechanism:** Multiple cysts in the ovary result in excessive production of estrogen and androgens, which are converted to estrone. Estrone then inhibits FSH.

▣ **Complications:** Increased risk for endometrial hyperplasia and cancer, diabetes mellitus, and metabolic syndrome. Infertility responds well to metformin, although the mechanism is poorly understood.

▣ **Clinical presentation of PCOD:** Include obesity, hirsutism and acne, and infertility. Patients have insulin resistance and may have signs of diabetes mellitus, including **acanthosis nigricans.** The LH/FSH ratio is > 2:1.

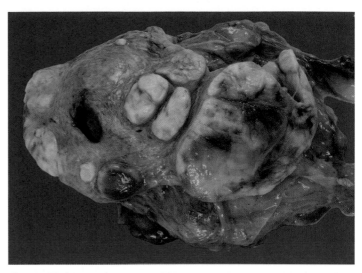

Figure 17-14. Leiomyomas. This uterus has been bisected (the lumen is present on the left side), revealing multiple well-circumscribed, tan-white masses (leiomyomas) that bulge from the cut surface. Often, more than one leiomyoma is present. These tumors can cause pelvic pain, infertility (preventing expansion of the uterus during pregnancy), and vaginal bleeding (if they project into the endometrial cavity).

Morphology of mature cystic teratoma

- **Gross:** Cyst containing hair, sebaceous material, and teeth (Figure 17-19).

- **Microscopic:** Usually contain a large component of epidermis and dermal appendages; however, the tumor can also contain tissue from the gastrointestinal system, liver, peripheral nervous system, and brain, among other organs.

DYSGERMINOMA

Epidemiology: About 75% occur during the second and third decades of life.

Important points: A dysgerminoma is the female counterpart of the male seminoma. All dysgerminomas are malignant.

FIBROTHECOMA

Incidence: A form of sex cord–stromal tumor. Fibrothecomas represent 4% of ovarian tumors.

Important points: Fibrothecomas are benign. Most are inactive, but some produce estrogen and some are associated with **Meigs syndrome** (i.e., ascites and hydrothorax).

GRANULOSA CELL TUMOR

Important points

- Most are benign; however, between 5 and 25% are malignant. Malignancy cannot absolutely be predicted by the histology, and requires the presence of invasion and/or metastases to confirm the diagnosis.

- The tumors can produce estrogen, thus leading to endometrial hyperplasia and cancer.

Microscopic morphology of granulosa cell tumor: Have **Call-Exner bodies** (appear similar to ovarian follicle), and produce inhibin, which can be identified in serum and by immunohistochemistry.

KRUKENBERG TUMOR

Basic description: Bilateral metastatic ovarian tumor composed of signet ring cells, usually gastrointestinal in origin (e.g., gastric carcinoma).

PLACENTAL AND PREGNANCY-RELATED PATHOLOGY

Overview: The major conditions associated with pregnancy, including abortion, infections (chorioamnionitis), gestational trophoblastic disease, placental abruption, abnormal placental implantation (ectopic pregnancy, placenta previa and placenta accreta), and toxemia of pregnancy, are discussed in this section.

ABORTION

Basic description: Pregnancy that fails before 20 weeks' gestation. The death of a fetus after this time (i.e., 20 weeks' gestational age) is referred to as a **stillbirth.**

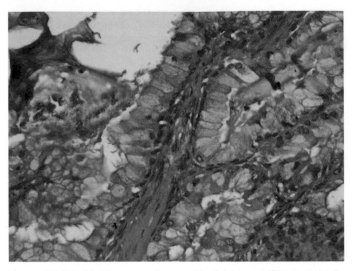

Figure 17-17. Mucinous surface epithelial tumor. The neoplastic cells produce mucin, as can be seen in the image. Similar to serous tumors, mucinous surface epithelial tumors occur in benign, borderline, and malignant forms. Hematoxylin and eosin, 400×.

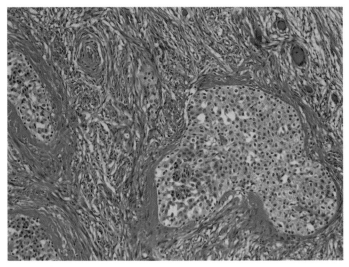

Figure 17-18. Brenner tumor. This neoplasm has a characteristic histologic appearance of nests of transitional epithelium-like cells admixed with a fibrous stroma. Most Brenner tumors are benign. Hematoxylin and eosin, 200×.

Types of abortion

- **Threatened abortion:** Patients have uterine bleeding, and the cervical os is closed. About 50% of threatened abortions will eventually result in miscarriage.
- **Inevitable abortion:** Patients have uterine bleeding, and the cervical os is open.
- **Incomplete abortion:** Fetus is not passed.
- **Complete abortion:** All tissue is passed. Cervical os is closed.

Complications of abortion: Hemorrhage with resultant hypovolemic shock, sepsis, and psychological distress.

Important point: Chromosomal abnormalities are the most common identifiable cause of spontaneous abortion.

Clinical presentation of abortion

- **Symptoms:** Vaginal bleeding, cramping abdominal pain.
- **Signs:** Open or closed cervical os, depending upon the form of abortion. Passage of clots or tissue.
- **Laboratory evaluation:** Failure of serial serum hCG to double in 48 hours and serum progesterone < 5 ng/mL are indicative of a nonviable pregnancy.

CHORIOAMNIONITIS

Basic description: Infection of the fetal membranes.

Mechanism

- Ascending infection from the uterus, often associated with premature rupture of membranes. Most common causative organisms include group B *Streptococcus* and *Escherichia coli*.
- Hematogenous (less common).

Risk factors for chorioamnionitis: Premature and prolonged rupture of membranes, multiple vaginal examinations during labor, and colonization of vagina and perineum with group B *Streptococcus*.

Complications: Premature labor, endometritis, fetal and newborn sepsis, and stillbirth.

Clinical presentation of chorioamnionitis: Fever, maternal and fetal tachycardia, leukocytosis, uterine tenderness, and foul-smelling vaginal discharge.

GESTATIONAL TROPHOBLASTIC DISEASE (HYDATIDIFORM MOLE)

Incidence: Occurs in 1 in 1500 pregnancies.

Three main types of hydatidiform moles: Complete, partial, and invasive (Table 17-3). Uterine choriocarcinoma is directly related to gestational trophoblastic disease, and will be discussed below as a fourth entry.

1. Complete hydatidiform mole

Mechanism of development: Approximately 90% of cases are due to an empty egg fertilized by one sperm (with subsequent duplication of DNA); 10% of cases are due to an empty egg fertilized by two sperm.

Karyotype: Most are 46,XX.

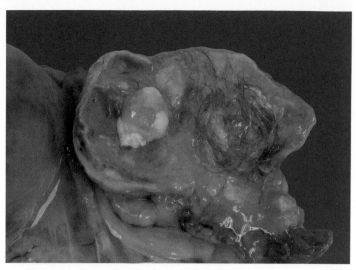

Figure 17-19. Mature cystic teratoma. A frequently occurring benign ovarian tumor; the gross appearance of a mature cystic teratoma is characteristic, with a cyst containing hair, sebaceous fluid (the thick green liquid), and occasionally teeth. The components of a mature cystic teratoma can, rarely, undergo malignant change (resulting in a squamous cell carcinoma or adenocarcinoma).

TABLE 17-3. Comparison and Contrast of Complete and Partial Moles

Feature	Complete Mole	Partial Mole
Mechanism of formation	Empty egg fertilized by one or two sperm	Normal egg fertilized by two sperm
Karyotype	46, XX	69, XXY
Risk for choriocarcinoma	2%	Rare
Presence of fetal parts	No	Yes
Morphology	All villi are hydropic and have trophoblastic proliferation	Some villi are hydropic and have trophoblastic proliferation

Risk of choriocarcinoma: 2%

Important point: Approximately 20% of women will have recurrence in subsequent pregnancies.

Morphology of complete hydatidiform mole

- **Gross:** Markedly hydropic villi, which resemble cluster of grapes. No fetal parts.
- **Microscopic:** All villi are edematous and have prominent trophoblast proliferation (Figure 17-20).

2. **Partial hydatidiform mole**

Mechanism of development: Normal egg fertilized by two sperm.

Karyotype: Triploid (69,XXY).

Risk of choriocarcinoma: Patients rarely develop choriocarcinoma.

Morphology of partial hydatidiform mole

- **Gross:** Difficult to distinguish from spontaneous abortion; some hydropic villi; fetal parts are present.
- **Microscopic:** Some edematous villi; some trophoblast proliferation.

3. **Invasive mole**

Basic description: Molar pregnancy that penetrates the uterine wall.

Important points

- Locally destructive.
- May embolize.
- Approximately 10% of complete moles become an invasive mole.

4. **Uterine choriocarcinoma**

Precursor conditions to choriocarcinoma

- Approximately 50% arise in molar pregnancies; 25% from previous abortion and 25% from normal pregnancies.
- Complicate about 1 in 100,000 normal pregnancies.

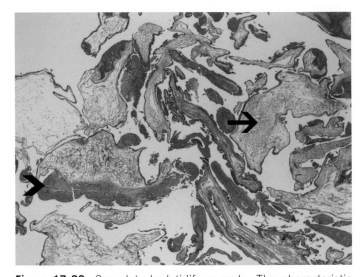

Figure 17-20. Complete hydatidiform mole. The characteristic gross appearance of this condition is described as "grape-like clusters." The grape-like clusters are produced by edematous villi (*arrow*). In a complete mole, all villi are edematous and have prominent trophoblastic proliferation (*arrowhead*). Hematoxylin and eosin, 40×.

Important points

▨ Metastases: Lungs (50%), vagina (30%), then brain, liver, and kidney.

▨ Produce β-hCG.

▨ Responds to methotrexate.

Clinical presentation of gestational trophoblastic disease

▨ **Signs and symptoms:** The clinical hallmarks of trophoblastic disease are uterine enlargement and elevated hCG in excess of what is expected for gestational age. Hyperemesis and bleeding are common, and new onset of hypertension in the first trimester should raise suspicion of molar pregnancy.

▨ **Radiologic finding:** The classic sonographic finding is the "snowstorm pattern."

▨ **Important point:** The two main risk factors for molar pregnancy are extreme maternal age (either very young or old) and prior molar pregnancy.

PLACENTAL ABRUPTION

Basic description: Premature separation of the placenta from the uterus due to hemorrhage between the placenta and uterine wall.

Incidence: Occur in 1 in 150 pregnancies; usually during the third trimester.

Complications of placental abruption: Hemorrhage between the uterus and the placenta results in decreased oxygen and nutrients delivered to the fetus, with 20% chance of fetal mortality. The mother can develop hypovolemic shock. Maternal coagulopathy and disseminated intravascular coagulation (DIC) are common.

Risk factors: Increasing age, multiparity, hypertension, trauma, cocaine use.

Clinical presentation of placental abruption

▨ **Symptoms:** Painful vaginal bleeding, uterine tenderness, back pain.

▨ **Diagnosis:** Because blood has a similar echotexture to placenta, ultrasound cannot be used to rule out placental abruption; thus diagnosis is clinical and confirmed at delivery.

ECTOPIC PREGNANCY

Basic description: Pregnancy occurring when the fetus implants in a location other than the uterine cavity.

Location: Fallopian tubes (90% of cases), ovaries, and abdominal cavity.

Risk factors for ectopic pregnancy

▨ Scarring of the fallopian tube due to PID.

▨ Tumors, endometriosis.

▨ Intrauterine devices (IUD).

▨ Adhesions (e.g., from previous surgery).

Complications of ectopic pregnancy: Hemorrhage from rupture of pregnancy.

Clinical presentation of ectopic pregnancy

- ◼ Triad (seen in 15% of patients): Unilateral abdominal or adnexal pain, abnormal vaginal bleeding, and adnexal mass.

- ◼ With rupture, patients have severe abdominal pain, peritoneal signs, tachycardia, and shock.

PLACENTA PREVIA

Basic description: Abnormal insertion of placenta, in which placenta partially or completely covers the cervical os (Figure 17-21).

Incidence: 1 in 200 pregnancies.

Complications of placenta previa: Hemorrhage.

Risk factors: Previous caesarean section; multiple gestation pregnancies.

Clinical presentation of placenta previa

- ◼ **Symptoms:** Painless vaginal bleeding; postcoital spotting at > 30 weeks' gestation.

- ◼ **Diagnosis:** Ultrasound is diagnostic and should be performed prior to vaginal examination in any third trimester bleed to avoid tearing the placenta and causing hemorrhage.

PLACENTA ACCRETA

Basic description: Placental villi in direct contact with myometrium, due to partial or complete loss of decidua (Figure 17-21).

Risk factors: Low lying placenta or placenta previa; prior cesarean section.

Complications of placenta accreta: Postpartum bleeding as a result of failure of placental separation; perforation of uterus.

TOXEMIA OF PREGNANCY

Basic description: Hypertension, proteinuria, and edema occurring during pregnancy. This constellation of symptoms is referred to as **preeclampsia.** If the patient develops seizures, the condition is referred to as **eclampsia.**

Incidence: About 7% of pregnancies.

Epidemiology: Occurs from 20 weeks' gestation to 6 weeks' postpartum; primigravidas are more commonly affected than multigravidas.

Pathogenesis of toxemia of pregnancy: Possibly the result of abnormal placentation leading to ischemia. A shallow implantation results in incomplete conversion of decidual vessels to vessels adequate for pregnancy. The incomplete conversion of decidual vessels may be due to a defect in trophoblasts.

Risk factors for toxemia of pregnancy: Hypertension, diabetes mellitus, and chronic renal disease.

Morphology of toxemia of pregnancy

- ◼ Placental infarcts.

- ◼ Retroplacental hemorrhage.

- ◼ **Specific microscopic finding: Atherosis,** which is fibrinoid necrosis and lipid deposition in walls of vessels.

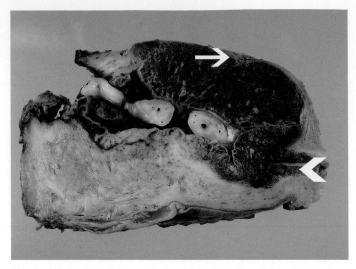

Figure 17-21. Placenta accreta and placenta previa. This cross section of a uterus, with the placenta still within the uterine cavity, reveals placental previa (at the *arrowhead,* note the placenta completely covers the cervical os) and placenta accreta (at the *arrow,* note the placenta has invaded the wall of the uterus, extending almost to the serosal surface; compare to the opposite uterine wall).

TABLE 17-4. Risk for Future Development of Breast Carcinoma Associated with Certain Conditions

Condition	No or Minimal Risk	Slight Risk	Moderate Risk	Great Risk
Fibrocystic disease with no proliferative activity	X			
Ductal hyperplasia, fibroadenoma, sclerosing adenosis		X		
Atypical ductal hyperplasia			X	
Carcinoma in situ				X

Clinical presentation of toxemia of pregnancy

■ **Symptoms:** Headache, visual disturbances, weight gain, and nausea and vomiting.

■ **Signs:** Hypertension, oliguria; right upper quadrant tenderness resulting from subcapsular liver hemorrhage.

Associated condition: HELLP syndrome (features are *h*emolysis, *e*levated *l*iver function tests, *l*ow *p*latelets).

NON-NEOPLASTIC DISEASES OF THE BREAST

Overview: The three most clinically important categories of breast disease are non-neoplastic diseases, carcinoma in situ, and breast neoplasms (Table 17-4). Because of their importance, both carcinoma in situ of the breast and breast neoplasms will be discussed separately, following this section covering non-neoplastic lesions of the breast. After a brief discussion of acute mastitis, fibrocystic change, sclerosing adenosis, fibroadenoma, phyllodes tumor, and intraductal papilloma and their risk for future development of carcinoma will be discussed.

ACUTE MASTITIS

Basic description: Bacterial infection of the breast occurring during lactation.

Causative organism: Most commonly *Staphylococcus aureus*.

Mechanism: Bacteria enter the breast through cracks in the nipple.

Clinical presentation of acute mastitis: Erythematous and painful breast.

FIBROCYSTIC CHANGE

Epidemiology: Females older than 35 years of age.

Two forms of fibrocystic change: nonproliferative and proliferative

■ **Nonproliferative form:** No epithelial hyperplasia in ducts; no increased risk for development of breast cancer.

HYPOADRENALISM

Overview: Hypoadrenalism is due to an adrenal gland that produces an insufficient amount of cortisol. Primary hypoadrenalism occurs in two major forms: acute and chronic. Secondary hypoadrenalism, and its relation to cortisol therapy, is discussed below, following acute and chronic primary adrenocortical insufficiency.

Causes of acute primary adrenocortical insufficiency

■ Rapid withdrawal of exogenous steroids in patients on chronic corticosteroid therapy: Exogenous steroids feed back on the pituitary gland to reduce the level of ACTH. Thus, the adrenal glands have no stimulus for growth and, therefore, undergo atrophy during treatment with steroids. Steroids must be withdrawn slowly to allow regeneration of glucocorticoid-producing cells in the zona fasciculata of the adrenal cortex (Figure 18-14 *A* and *B*).

■ Acute exacerbation of chronic adrenal insufficiency.

■ Anticoagulant therapy, postoperative patients with DIC, and pregnancy.

■ **Waterhouse-Friderichsen syndrome:** Overwhelming sepsis due to *Neisseria meningitidis* and *Pseudomonas* associated with hemorrhagic necrosis of the adrenal glands (Figure 18-15).

Clinical presentation of acute adrenocortical insufficiency

■ **Symptoms:** Severe abdominal pain, nausea and vomiting, and somnolence.

■ **Signs:** Hypotension.

Causes of chronic adrenocortical insufficiency

ADDISON DISEASE

Overview: Addison disease, an autoimmune disorder, is the most common cause of chronic primary adrenal insufficiency in developed nations.

Important point: Patients have increased pigmentation of pressure points and buccal mucosa due to increased levels of melanocyte-stimulating hormone. Melanocyte-stimulating hormone is produced along with ACTH in the form of pro-opiomelanocortin, which is cleaved to its respective segments. Note that patients with adrenal insufficiency due to pituitary disorders (secondary adrenal insufficiency) do not have hyperpigmentation, since these conditions are characterized by low ACTH levels.

Pathogenesis of Addison disease: Autoantibody to 21-hydroxylase and 17-hydroxylase.

Other causes of chronic adrenal insufficiency: Metastatic tumor (Figure 18-16), infections (e.g., tuberculosis, *Histoplasma*, *Coccidioides immitis*), amyloidosis, and hemochromatosis.

Clinical presentation of chronic adrenocortical insufficiency

■ **Symptoms:** Weakness, gastrointestinal disturbances, weight loss, salt craving.

■ **Signs:** Hyponatremia, hyperkalemia, hypoglycemia, hypotension, decreased aldosterone.

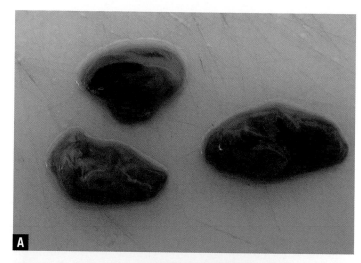

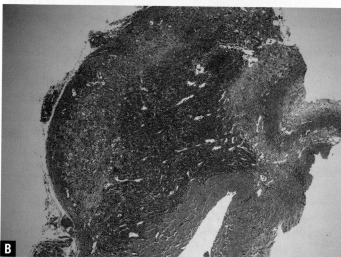

Figure 18-14. Adrenal atrophy due to corticosteroid therapy. **A,** The adrenal gland is markedly atrophic, with little if any normal cortex identified grossly. **B,** Microscopically, the medulla (central basophilic cells) is much more prominent than the cortex. Slow withdrawal of steroids is mandatory to allow the regrowth of the cortex. Hematoxylin and eosin, 40×.

SECONDARY HYPOADRENALISM

Basic description: Condition due to pituitary gland destruction (see hypopituitarism) or due to suppression of adrenal gland (due to exogenous steroids).

Important points

▪ Hyperpigmentation does not occur in secondary hypoadrenalism, since ACTH levels (and, thus, MSH production) are decreased.

▪ Mineralocorticoid levels are normal, so hyperkalemia and salt craving do not occur. Hyponatremia can still occur because of increased ADH, which occurs in response to volume depletion.

Clinical presentation of secondary hypoadrenalism

▪ **Symptoms:** Weakness, weight loss, anorexia, and nausea and vomiting.

▪ **Laboratory finding:** Patients do *not* have decreased levels of aldosterone.

Distinguishing primary hypoadrenalism from secondary hypoadrenalism

▪ In primary hypoadrenalism, ACTH is increased. In secondary hypoadrenalism, ACTH is decreased. Aldosterone levels are normal or decreased in primary hypoadrenalism and normal in secondary hypoadrenalism.

▪ **ACTH stimulation test:** Give ACTH and measure plasma cortisol level; in secondary hypoadrenalism, the cortisol level should increase.

CONGENITAL ADRENAL HYPERPLASIA

Basic description: Condition due to a deficiency of an enzyme in the pathway of cortisol synthesis. Lack of cortisol stimulates production of ACTH, which stimulates adrenal glands, causing hyperplasia.

Types: Five types; most common type is due to 21-hydroxylase deficiency (95% of cases).

Pathogenesis: Failure of 21-hydroxylation of 17-hydroxyprogesterone and progesterone to 11-deoxycortisol and 11-deoxycortisone results in deficient cortisol and aldosterone production. ACTH secretion is increased, resulting in increased production of androstenedione and dehydroepiandrosterone (DHEA).

Forms of congenital adrenal hyperplasia: classic and late onset

1. Classic congenital adrenal hyperplasia

Epidemiology: Diagnosed at birth. Two thirds of patients are salt wasting.

2. Late onset congenital adrenal hyperplasia

Epidemiology: Diagnosed at or after puberty.

Clinical presentation: Virilization (e.g., hirsutism, acne), amenorrhea, or oligomenorrhea.

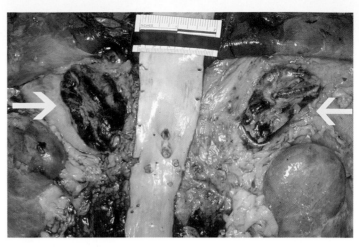

Figure 18-15. Waterhouse-Friderichsen syndrome. The adrenal glands are in situ. The aorta has been opened, and the perirenal adipose tissue removed from the kidneys. Both adrenal glands are hemorrhagic (*arrows*). Waterhouse-Friderichsen syndrome is a cause of acute adrenal insufficiency due to overwhelming sepsis caused by *Neisseria meningitidis*, *Pseudomonas*, and other organisms. Courtesy of Dr. Gary Dale, Forensic Science Division, Montana State Department of Justice, Missoula, MT.

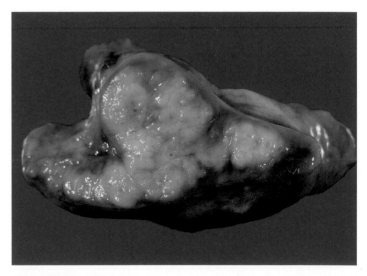

Figure 18-16. Metastatic squamous cell carcinoma of the adrenal gland. The normal architecture of this adrenal gland is nearly obliterated by this focus of metastatic squamous cell carcinoma in a patient with squamous cell carcinoma of the lung. This condition would lead to chronic adrenocortical insufficiency.

HYPERALDOSTERONISM

PRIMARY HYPERALDOSTERONISM (CONN SYNDROME)

Causes

- Neoplasm (usually adrenal adenoma).
- Adrenocortical hyperplasia.

Laboratory findings: Hypernatremia and hypokalemia. The two most common causes of hypokalemia are primary hyperaldosteronism and diuretic therapy. Patients with primary hyperaldosteronism also have increased aldosterone and decreased renin levels.

SECONDARY HYPERALDOSTERONISM

Causes: Decreased renal perfusion (e.g., due to renal artery stenosis or atherosclerosis), hypovolemia and edema, and pregnancy.

Laboratory findings: Increased aldosterone and increased renin.

ADRENAL NEOPLASMS

Overview: Adrenal adenomas, Conn syndrome, adrenocortical carcinoma, and pheochromocytomas represent the majority of adrenal neoplasms.

Adrenal adenoma

- **Important point:** Most adrenal adenomas are nonfunctioning, and if plasma ACTH is detected, a primary adrenal adenoma as a source for Cushing syndrome is unlikely. A functioning adrenal adenoma would produce cortisol, which will feed back on the pituitary gland and inhibit ACTH production.
- **Morphology:** Yellow nodule in adrenal cortex.

Conn syndrome

- **Basic description:** Adenoma of the glomerulosa cells that produces aldosterone, which results in secondary hypertension. Conn syndrome can also be due to hyperplasia of the adrenal glands, but is most commonly associated with an adrenal adenoma.
- **Laboratory findings:** Include hypokalemia and low plasma renin level.

Adrenocortical carcinoma: Size (weight) is important in differentiating an adrenocortical carcinoma from an adenoma. A tumor weighing > 100 grams is more likely to be a carcinoma than an adenoma.

Pheochromocytoma

- **Basic description:** A tumor of the adrenal medulla that secretes epinephrine and norepinephrine, causing episodic hypertension.
- **Associated conditions** (i.e., conditions that often manifest with a pheochromocytoma): MEN 2A and 2B, von-Hippel Lindau syndrome, von Recklinghausen disease of bone, and Sturge-Weber syndrome.

■ **Important points regarding pheochromocytoma**

  ○ 10% are familial.

  ○ 10% are extra-adrenal (e.g., in the carotid body or sympathetic chain).

  ○ 10% are bilateral.

  ○ 10% are malignant (require metastases to determine malignancy).

  ○ 10% occur during childhood.

■ **Morphology of pheochromocytoma** (Figure 18-17 *A* and *B*)

  ○ **Gross:** Yellow-tan; can be hemorrhagic.

  ○ **Microscopic:** Bland, monomorphous cells in nests (referred to as **Zellballen pattern**); nuclei have salt and pepper chromatin.

■ **Clinical presentation of pheochromocytoma**

  ○ **Signs and symptoms:** Precipitous tachycardia, palpitations, pounding headache, sweating, and weight loss. Symptoms can be precipitated by stress (e.g., surgery, acute infections) and hypertension (episodic in classic cases, but in other cases may be more sustained).

■ **Laboratory diagnosis of pheochromocytoma**

  ○ **Plasma:** Free metanephrine level > 0.61 nmol/L and normetanephrine level > 0.31 nmol/L. A 24-hour metanephrine test is almost 100% sensitive.

  ○ **Urine:** Free catecholamines; vanillylmandelic acid (VMA).

  ○ **Important point:** Plasma testing is performed first; urine testing if needed.

MULTIPLE ENDOCRINE NEOPLASIA (MEN) 1

Name: Wermer syndrome.

Mutation: *MEN1* gene at 11q13 (protein is menin, a tumor suppressor gene).

Organs affected

■ **Parathyroid gland:** Hyperplasia or adenoma.

■ **Pancreas:** Endocrine tumors, which are usually aggressive and multifocal and may secrete gastrin or insulin.

■ **Pituitary gland:** Prolactinoma, most common form of pituitary adenoma in MEN 1.

MEN 2A

Name: Sipple syndrome.

Mutation: *RET* proto-oncogene (10q11.2); mutation causes activation of receptor producing "gain of function."

Organs affected

■ **Thyroid gland:** Medullary thyroid carcinoma.

■ **Adrenal medulla:** Pheochromocytoma.

■ **Parathyroid gland:** Hyperplasia.

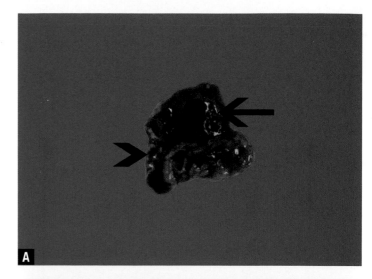

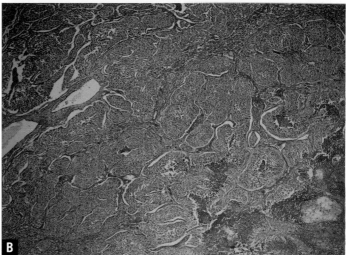

Figure 18-17. Pheochromocytoma. **A**, The mass in the adrenal medulla (*arrow*) is a pheochromocytoma. The arrowhead indicates the adrenal cortex. **B**, Histologically, pheochromocytomas appear as bland monomorphic cells in nests (the "zellballen" pattern. Hematoxylin and eosin, 40×.

MEN 2B

Mutation: *RET* proto-oncogene; different mutation than in MEN 2a.

Organs affected

- **Thyroid gland:** Medullary thyroid carcinoma.
- **Adrenal medulla:** Pheochromocytoma.

Difference from MEN 2a

- MEN 2b does *not* develop parathyroid gland hyperplasia.
- MEN 2b has ganglioneuromas and marfanoid habitus.

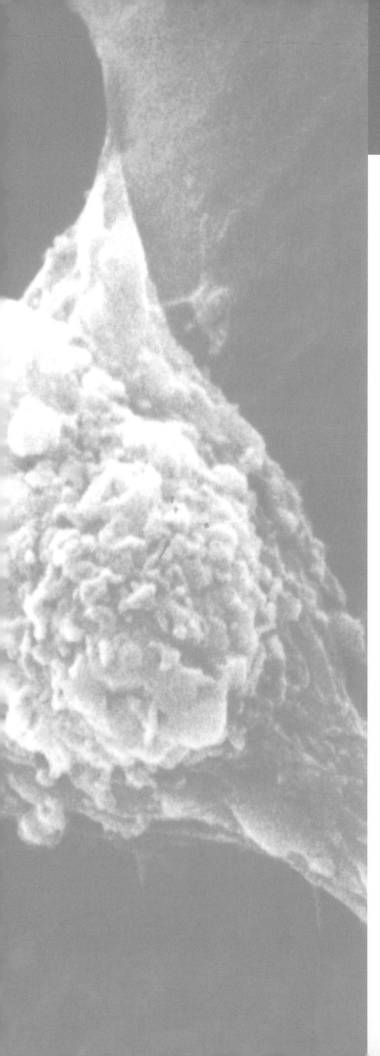

CHAPTER 19

PATHOLOGY OF THE BONES AND JOINTS

OVERVIEW

Diseases of the bone include non-neoplastic disorders such as genetic defects (e.g., achondroplasia), osteoporosis, infections of the bone (i.e., osteomyelitis), and Paget disease. The age of the patient and the location of the tumor are very important considerations in the diagnosis of bone tumors. For example, most chondrosarcomas occur in older adults and almost never occur in the bones of the hands, whereas most Ewing sarcomas occur in the diaphysis of long bones of children.

Diseases of the joints include inflammatory and noninflammatory arthritides. The two major types of arthritis are osteoarthritis and rheumatoid arthritis. Wear and tear is one of the major etiologic agents for the development of osteoarthritis, whereas rheumatoid arthritis is considered to be an autoimmune condition. An important molecular topic regarding bone pathology is the receptor for nuclear factor-$\kappa\beta$ (RANK), which is expressed on macrophages, monocytes, and preosteoclasts. The binding of RANK ligand (RANKL) to RANK stimulates osteoclastogenesis. RANKL is produced by osteoblasts and marrow stromal cells. Osteoprotegerin binds to RANK and blocks the binding of RANKL; therefore, it is inhibitory.

This chapter will discuss non-neoplastic bone diseases (including those caused by genetic defects, osteoporosis, osteonecrosis, osteomyelitis, Paget disease, renal osteodystrophy, and fractures), bone neoplasms, and joint disorders, primarily osteoarthritis, rheumatoid arthritis, and gout.

INHERITED DEFECTS IN BONE STRUCTURE

Overview: There are many inherited conditions that result in abnormalities of bone structure. Three of the more common types, achondroplasia, osteogenesis imperfecta, and osteopetrosis, will be discussed below.

ACHONDROPLASIA

Inheritance pattern: Autosomal dominant; 80% of new cases are the result of spontaneous mutations.

Mutation: Gene for FGF receptor 3 (*FGFR3*) on the p arm of chromosome 4.

Effect of mutation: FGF receptor 3 (FGFR3) is an inhibitor of cartilage proliferation. The mutation places the receptor in a constant state of activation.

Manifestations of achondroplasia

■ **Gross:** Disproportionate dwarfism with normal trunk length and short extremities, varus and valgus deformities of legs, short fingers and toes, and large head with prominent forehead.

■ **Microscopic:** Narrow and disorganized zones of proliferation and hypertrophy.

Important points: Achondroplasia accounts for 70% of cases of **dwarfism.** Less commonly, dwarfism may be due to pituitary dysfunction or secondary to a mutation in the growth hormone receptor (**Laron dwarfism**).

OSTEOGENESIS IMPERFECTA

Overview: There are several different types of osteogenesis imperfecta, each one caused by one of several different mutations. Some of the mutations have an autosomal dominant inheritance pattern. Only type I and type II osteogenesis imperfecta, two of the more common forms of the disease, will be discussed in detail here.

Mutations: Gene for α1 and α2 chains of type I collagen.

Effect of mutation: Varies, depending upon mutation. The results vary from phenotypically normal collagen produced in decreased amounts to absence of collagen production.

Two types of osteogenesis imperfecta

1. Type I osteogenesis imperfecta

Mutation: Decreased synthesis of pro-α1(1) collagen chain, which is compatible with normal life span or abnormal pro-α1(1) or pro-α2(1) collagen chains, which produce the complications discussed below.

Manifestations: Increased number of fractures; blue sclerae because of thin layer of collagen, causing choroid to be visible; hearing loss; and defective dentition. Patients can have a normal life span.

Microscopic morphology: Osteoporosis (i.e., decreased bone mass; bones have thin trabeculae).

2. Type II osteogenesis imperfecta

Mutation: Can involve gene for pro-α1(1) collagen chain in autosomal recessive form of the disease or produce an unstable triple helix in autosomal dominant form of the disease.

Manifestations: Death in utero or early perinatal period. Patients have multiple fractures.

OSTEOPETROSIS

Effect of mutation: Decreased resorption of bone by osteoclasts results in increased amount of bone, but the bone is structurally weak.

Types of osteopetrosis

1. **Infantile malignant osteopetrosis**
   - **Inheritance pattern:** Autosomal recessive.
   - **Manifestations:** Fractures, hydrocephaly, anemia, and infections due to decreased hematopoiesis, and hepato-splenomegaly due to extramedullary hematopoiesis.

2. **and** 3. **Autosomal dominant type I and type II**
   - **Manifestations of both type I and type II autosomal dominant osteopetrosis:** Fractures, anemia, and mild cranial nerve defects due to impingement.

4. **Carbonic anhydrase II deficiency**
   - **Effect of mutation:** Inability to excrete hydrogen ions.

Morphology of osteopetrosis

- **Gross:** No medullary canal; bulbous ends of long bones (i.e., **Erlenmeyer flask deformity**).

- **Microscopic:** Woven bone, with obliteration of marrow cavity.

Treatment of osteopetrosis: Bone marrow transplantation, since osteoclasts are derived from monocyte precursors.

OSTEOPOROSIS

Overview: Osteoporosis is due to a decrease in bone mass with a subsequent increase in the risk for fractures. Osteoporosis can be localized to one or a few bones (because of disuse) or generalized (involving a majority of the skeletal system). Osteoporosis can be a primary disorder, or it may be secondary to many other disorders.

Epidemiology: Incidence of osteoporosis increases with increasing age.

Forms of primary osteoporosis: Most common forms are type I (postmenopausal osteoporosis) and type II (senile osteoporosis).

Causes of secondary osteoporosis

- **Endocrine causes:** Increased levels of parathyroid hormone (PTH) due to an adenoma, or hyperplasia of the parathyroid glands; diabetes mellitus; Addison disease.

- **Gastrointestinal cause:** Malnutrition.

- **Drug causes:** Steroids, heparin.

Risk factors for primary osteoporosis

- Increasing age and family history.

- Smoking and alcoholism.

- Decreased estrogen; early or surgical menopause.

- Low body mass index, low calcium diet, and lack of weight-bearing exercise.

Pathogenesis of primary osteoporosis

- Decreased ability of cells to make bone, which occurs with senility of the bone.
- Decreased physical activity.
- Decreased estrogen, which results in increased level of interleukin-1 (IL-1) and IL-6. IL-1 and IL-6 increase the level of RANK and RANKL and decrease the level of osteoprotegerin.

Microscopic morphology: Thin cortex and thin trabeculae.

Clinical presentation of osteoporosis: Vertebral compression fractures with acute back pain and kyphosis; hip fracture. Most compression fractures are asymptomatic.

Diagnosis of osteoporosis: Bone density measurements (DEXA scan).

OSTEONECROSIS

Causes of osteonecrosis (avascular necrosis): Fractures and trauma, corticosteroids, sickle cell anemia and other hematologic diseases, and idiopathic.

Morphology of osteonecrosis

- **Gross:** If subchondral in location, the area of tissue death is wedge shaped.
- **Microscopic:** Empty lacunae.

Clinical presentation of osteonecrosis: Most commonly affects the epiphysis of the femur. Osteonecrosis of the jaw has been associated recently with bisphosphonate use. Patients present with pain and, as the lesion evolves, joint collapse may occur.

OSTEOMYELITIS

Overview: Osteomyelitis is infection of the bone. Two of the major forms of osteomyelitis are pyogenic and tuberculous.

PYOGENIC OSTEOMYELITIS

Causative organisms: *Staphylococcus aureus* causes 80–90% of cases. *S aureus* has a receptor for collagen, which contributes to its pathogenicity. Other organisms that cause osteomyelitis include:

- *Escherichia coli* and *Pseudomonas* in intravenous drug users and patients with urinary tract infections.
- *Haemophilus influenzae* and Group B *Streptococcus* in neonates.
- *Salmonella* in patients with sickle cell disease.

Routes of infection: Hematogenous, direct extension from infection in adjacent site, or traumatic implantation.

Bones affected by osteomyelitis: Long bones, vertebral bodies.

Location of infection within the bone

- **Neonates:** Metaphysis or epiphysis.
- **Child:** Metaphysis.
- **Adults:** Epiphysis.

Gross morphology of pyogenic osteomyelitis: The infection can lift the periosteum, which impairs blood flow and can lead to ischemia of the bone. In children, periosteal lifting can lead to abscess formation. The dead bone fragment is called a **sequestrum.** New bone growth around the sequestrum is called the **involucrum.** A **Brodie abscess** is a residual abscess surrounded by rim of new bone growth.

Clinical presentation of pyogenic osteomyelitis

- **Signs and symptoms:** Malaise, fever, chills, pain, warmth, swelling, erythema; range of motion may be limited by pain.
- **Laboratory findings:** Leukocytosis with or without a left shift; elevated erythrocyte sedimentation rate. Reactive thrombocytosis may be seen; platelet count can be extremely high.
- **Radiographic findings:** Destruction of bone; can have radiolucent or radiodense areas in chronic osteomyelitis.
- **Diagnosis:** Blood cultures are positive in 50% of acute cases. An aspirate with culture is more sensitive and should be performed if possible. Plain radiographs are the first test in the evaluation of suspected osteomyelitis and may reveal soft tissue swelling, periosteal elevation, and subperiosteal resorption and erosion. MRI is the test of choice for evaluating suspected osteomyelitis in diabetic patients. In nondiabetic patients with normal radiographs, a bone scan is indicated to rule out osteomyelitis.

Complications of pyogenic osteomyelitis

- Ruptured periosteum, leading to soft tissue abscess and fistula formation (e.g., draining sinuses to the skin) (Figure 19-1 A and B).
- Pathologic fractures.
- Squamous cell carcinoma in the fistulous tract; sarcomas.
- Suppurative arthritis, which is more common in children and less common in adults.
- Approximately 5–25% of cases of acute osteomyelitis progress to chronic osteomyelitis.

TUBERCULOUS OSTEOMYELITIS

Routes of infection: Usually hematogenous.

Bones affected: Most commonly the spine (i.e., **Pott disease**), followed by knee and hip.

PAGET DISEASE (OSTEITIS DEFORMANS)

Overview: Paget disease is a non-neoplastic disorder of bone characterized by disorganized growth of bony trabeculae, resulting in a thick, but fragile bone.

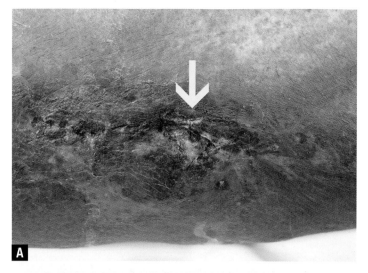

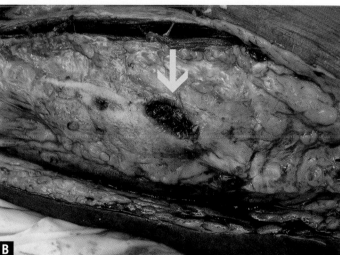

Figure 19-1. Osteomyelitis with draining fistula. **A**, The surface of the skin exhibits a draining fistula (*arrow*). The fistula developed due to underlying osteomyelitis. **B**, The arrow indicates the defect in the involucrum, through which the fistula connects with the overlying skin.

Three phases of Paget disease: Osteoclastic activity with hypervascularity; then mixed osteoclastic and osteoblastic stage; and finally, the osteosclerotic stage. The resultant bone is thick, but structurally weak.

Epidemiology: Prevalence in whites more than African Americans or Asians. Occurs in 1–10% of whites and commonly affects middle-aged adults.

Cause of Paget disease: Unknown, but may be viral. May be caused by paramyxovirus, which induces IL-6, which in turn stimulates osteoclasts.

Bones affected: Axillary skeleton (e.g., skull, ribs, vertebrae, pelvic bones) and proximal femur. The disease may be monostotic (15% of cases) or polyostotic (85% of cases).

Clinical presentation and complications of Paget disease

■ Most cases are diagnosed incidentally by radiography.

■ The classic presentation is a patient who complains that his hat size is enlarging. Increased thickness of the skull can cause headaches.

■ Pain caused by microfractures and bony overgrowth impinging the nerves. Patient may also have symptoms caused by impingement of the cranial nerves.

■ Pathologic fractures, especially **chalkstick-type fractures**.

■ High-output cardiac failure in initial hypervascular stage. The hypervascularity warms the skin and increases blood flow, functioning as an arteriovenous malformation.

■ Sarcoma (1%), usually osteosarcoma or chondrosarcoma. Patients can also develop giant cell tumors.

Morphology of Paget disease (Figure 19-2 *A* and *B*)

■ **Gross:** Thick bone.

■ **Radiographic finding:** Thick, coarse cortex.

■ **Microscopic:** Mosaic pattern of lamellar bone.

Laboratory findings: Elevated serum alkaline phosphatase and urinary excretion of hydroxyproline.

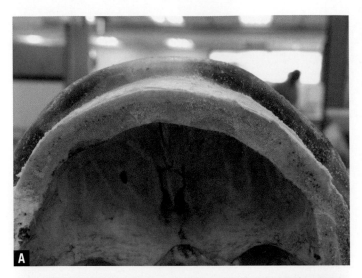

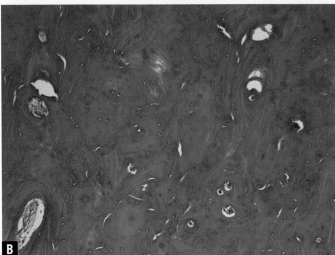

Figure 19-2. Paget disease of bone. **A,** The skull is markedly thick, and is a typical location for Paget disease. **B,** The bony trabeculae are thick and meshed together, creating the characteristic mosaic pattern of Paget disease and obliterating the marrow space. Hematoxylin and eosin, 200×.

RENAL OSTEODYSTROPHY

Basic description: Bony changes caused by renal disease.

Pathogenesis: Phosphate retention in renal failure leads to hypocalcemia and hyperparathyroidism. The inability of the failing kidneys to convert 25-OH-vitamin D to the active form, 1,25-OH-vitamin D, causes further stimulation of PTH secretion.

Clinical presentation of renal osteodystrophy: The presentation of renal osteodystrophy is essentially the same presentation as hyperparathyroidism (see Chapter 18). Bone pain and arthralgias are common and may be severe. Pathologic fractures are not uncommon. Spontaneous tendon rupture, which is classic for hyperparathyroidism, is less commonly seen in renal osteodystrophy. The characteristic radiographic finding is subperiosteal bone resorption, most easily demonstrated in the bones of the hands.

Radiographic findings of renal osteodystrophy: Two radiographic findings are classic for renal osteodystrophy and hyperparathyroidism: subperiosteal bone resorption (most easily demonstrated in the bones of the hands) and "rugger jersey spine," in which the upper and lower portions of the vertebral body have a higher bone density than the middle portion.

FRACTURES

Types of fractures

- Complete (extends through bone causing total separation at the site of the fracture), or incomplete.
- Closed (i.e., intact overlying skin), or compound (i.e., lacerated overlying skin, exposing bone).
- Comminuted (i.e., bone broken into many smaller fragments at the site of fracture).
- Displaced fracture: Edges of bone at fracture site are no longer aligned.
- Pathologic fracture: Fracture occurring at the site of another form of pathology (e.g., at the site of a tumor metastasis) (Figure 19-3).
- Spiral fracture: Caused when torque is directed along the axis of the shaft of a bone. In children, spiral fractures are often an indication of physical abuse.

Stages of repair

1. Formation of hematoma, which seals off fracture site and provides framework for repair.
2. Inflammatory cells release platelet-derived growth factor (PDGF), fibroblast growth factor (FGF), and other mediators, and activate osteoprogenitor cells.
3. Together, the hematoma and inflammatory cells (and the effects of their mediators) form a soft tissue callus.
4. Deposition of woven bone.

Important point regarding fractures: If the fracture is not immobilized, the callus can undergo cystic degeneration and a pseudoarthrosis is formed.

BONE TUMORS

Overview: The most common tumor arising within bone is multiple myeloma (see Chapter 12). The most common tumor of bone is a metastasis. With bone tumors, age and location are very important factors in the diagnosis (Table 19-1). Of primary bone tumors, > 40% are hematopoietic (most commonly multiple myeloma), > 20% chondrogenic, > 20% osteogenic, and 10% are of unknown origin. Not including multiple myeloma and metastases, the three most common malignant tumors of bone are osteosarcoma, chondrosarcoma, and Ewing sarcoma. Benign bone tumors are 100-fold more common than malignant tumors.

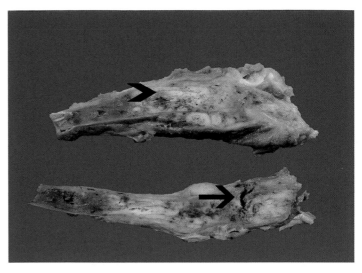

Figure 19-3. Pathologic fracture due to metastatic small cell carcinoma. This cross-section of a rib shows a metastasis (*arrowhead*) and the associated fracture of the rib (*arrow*). A pathologic fracture is a fracture due to another underlying disease of the bone. Metastatic and primary tumors are not the only cause of pathologic fractures.

OSTEOCHONDROMA (EXOSTOSIS)

Epidemiology: All ages are affected, but the tumor usually presents in late adolescence and in early adulthood. Prevalence of males to females is 5:1.

Location: Metaphysis near the growth plate of tubular bones; can be solitary or multiple.

Mutation: Inactivation of both *EXT* genes in sporadic and hereditary tumors.

Important points regarding osteochondroma

▪ Osteochondroma may be a malformation and not a neoplasm.

▪ Rarely result in development of sarcoma (< 1%).

Morphology of osteochondroma: Bony protuberance that communicates with bone marrow and has a cartilage cap (Figure 19-5).

CHONDROMA

Epidemiology: 20–50 years of age.

Location: Metaphysis of tubular bones (e.g., hands and feet).

Pathogenesis: Represent rests of growth plate cartilage that later enlarge.

Related conditions

▪ **Ollier syndrome:** Multiple enchondromas.

▪ **Maffucci syndrome:** Multiple enchondromas and hemangiomas.

Morphology of chondroma

▪ **Microscopic:** Nodules of cartilage.

▪ **Radiographic finding:** Well-circumscribed, oval lucency surrounded by a thin rim of radiodense bone.

▪ **Important point:** Chondromas are called **enchondromas** if they are subperiosteal in location.

Clinical presentation of chondroma: Pain; pathologic fracture.

CHONDROSARCOMA

Epidemiology: 40–60 years of age; predominance of males to females is 2:1.

Types of chondrosarcomas: Conventional, clear cell, dedifferentiated, and mesenchymal.

Location: Shoulder (e.g., scapula and humerus), spine, pelvis, proximal femur, and ribs. Clear cell variant of chondrosarcoma occurs in the epiphysis of tubular long bones.

Classification of chondrosarcoma (based upon two categories)

1. **Location:** Intramedullary or juxtacortical.

2. **Histology**

   • **Conventional chondrosarcoma** (grades I to III): Varying from grade I (which has increased cellularity and sparse binucleate cells) to grade III (which has much increased cellularity and extreme pleomorphism).

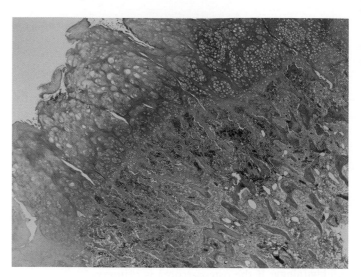

Figure 19-5. Osteochondroma. A bony protuberance (right lower half of image) capped with cartilage (left upper half of image), an osteochondroma is a benign mass, possibly of developmental origin. The cartilage cap may undergo malignant degeneration, developing into a chondrosarcoma. Hematoxylin and eosin, 40×.

- **Clear cell chondrosarcoma:** Clear cytoplasm, giant cells.
- **Dedifferentiated chondrosarcoma:** Conventional low-grade chondrosarcoma plus component of high-grade sarcoma (e.g., malignant fibrous histiocytoma, fibrosarcoma, or osteosarcoma).
- **Mesenchymal chondrosarcoma:** Well-differentiated hyaline cartilage plus small round cells.

Morphology of conventional chondrosarcoma

- **Gross:** Arise in medullary cavity and erode bone.
- **Microscopic:** Cartilage; multinucleated chondrocytes (Figure 19-6 *A* and *B*).

FIBROUS CORTICAL DEFECT

Epidemiology: Older than 2 years of age.

Locations: Metaphysis of distal femur or proximal tibia.

Morphology of fibrous cortical defect

- **Radiographic finding:** Well-defined radiolucency with a rim of sclerosis.
- **Microscopic:** Fibroblasts and histiocytes.

Important point: If size is > 5–6 cm, referred to as **nonossifying fibroma.**

FIBROUS DYSPLASIA

Overview: Fibrous dysplasia is not a neoplastic process, but instead is a development disorder that produces mass lesions within the skeletal system.

Types of fibrous dysplasia

1. **Monostotic (70% of cases); location:** Ribs, femur, and tibia.
2. **Polyostotic (27% of cases)**
   - **Epidemiology:** Occur in adolescents.
   - **Location:** Femur, skull, and tibia.
3. **Polyostotic with café au lait spots (McCune-Albright syndrome).**
   - **Mutation:** Gene for G protein, leading to activation and excessive production of cyclic adenosine monophosphate (cAMP).
   - **Other features:** Endocrine dysfunction (e.g., precocious puberty, hyperthyroidism).

Morphology of fibrous dysplasia

- **Gross:** Fibrous dysplasia is a tan-white, well-circumscribed, expansive lesion, which has an intramedullary location.
- **Microscopic:** Curvilinear trabeculae of woven bone surrounded by a fibroblastic proliferation.

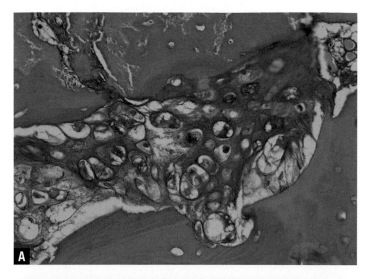

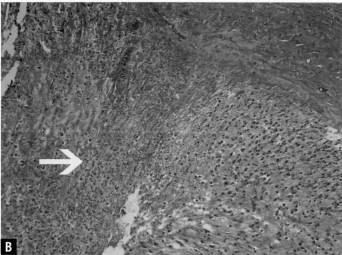

Figure 19-6. Chondrosarcoma. **A,** This chondrosarcoma is well differentiated. Note some of the chondrocyte lacunae have more than one nucleus, which is a feature of malignancy. **B,** This well-differentiated chondrosarcoma has outgrown its blood supply and become focally necrotic (*arrow*). Hematoxylin and eosin, **A,** 400×; **B,** 200×.

GIANT CELL TUMOR OF THE BONE

Epidemiology: 20–40 years of age; prevalent in females. Most occur after closure of the epiphyseal plate.

Location: In adults, epiphysis or metaphysis of long bones (e.g., distal femur, proximal tibia, proximal humerus, and distal radius); metaphysis in adolescents.

Important point: Histologically benign, but can recur. Only about 5% metastasize, usually to the lung, and can be locally aggressive.

Morphology of giant cell tumor

- **Gross:** Red-brown mass; may have cystic degeneration.
- **Microscopic:** Composed of giant cells and mononuclear cells. The mononuclear cells are neoplastic, and the giant cells are reactive (Figure 19-7).

Clinical presentation of giant cell tumor: Arthritis; pathologic fractures.

EWING SARCOMA AND PRIMITIVE NEUROECTODERMAL TUMOR (PNET)

Basic description: Ewing sarcomas are undifferentiated; PNETs have some neural differentiation. Ewing sarcomas and PNETs should be viewed as the same tumor.

Epidemiology: 10–20 years old.

Location: Diaphysis and metaphysis of femur, tibia, and pelvis.

Important point: Approximately 95% of Ewing sarcomas have translocation t(11;22) or t(21;22), which results in fusion of *EWS* (Ewing sarcoma gene) to *FLI* (chr 11) or *ERG* (chr 21). *FL1* and *ERG* are transcription factors.

Morphology of Ewing sarcoma

- **Gross:** Tan-white mass with hemorrhage and/or necrosis.
- **Radiographic findings:** Lytic tumor with permeative margins and extension into the surrounding soft tissue. Codman triangle may be present; however, the classic radiographic lesion of Ewing sarcoma is the "onion skin" periosteal reaction.
- **Microscopic** (Figure 19-8): **Small round cell tumor;** positive for CD 99; forms **Homer-Wright rosettes** (circle of neoplastic cells around a central fibrillary core).

Clinical presentation of Ewing sarcoma and PNET: Pain, tenderness, warmth, swelling, and fever. The tumor can masquerade as an infection.

METASTASES TO THE BONE

Important point: Overall, metastases are the most common tumor of bones.

Source of metastases

- **Adults:** Approximately 75% of metastases to the bone are derived from prostate, breast, kidney, and lung carcinomas.
- **Children:** Neuroblastoma, Wilms tumor, osteosarcoma, and Ewing sarcoma.

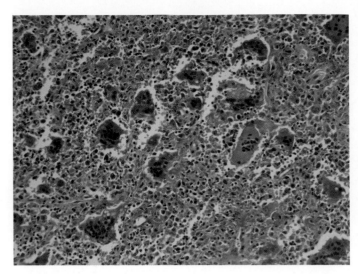

Figure 19-7. Giant cell tumor of bone. The photomicrograph depicts the two components of a giant cell tumor of bone, multinucleated giant cells, and mononuclear cells. The multinucleated giant cells are felt to be reactive in nature, and the mononuclear cells represent the neoplastic component of the tumor. Hematoxylin and eosin, 200×.

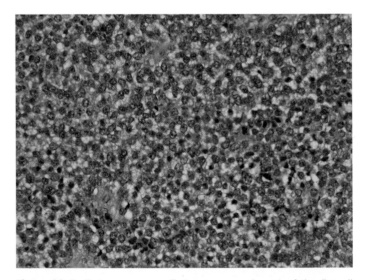

Figure 19-8. Ewing sarcoma. Ewing sarcoma is one of the "small round cell tumors" of childhood, as is evident by its histologic appearance. Immunohistochemical stains specific for CD99 help confirm its diagnosis. Hematoxylin and eosin, 200×.

TABLE 19-2. General Classification of Arthritis

Group	Descriptive Name of Group	Laboratory Findings	Common Cause
I	Noninflammatory arthritis	50–2000 WBC/mm^3; < 30% neutrophils	Osteoarthritis
II	Mildly inflammatory arthritis	0–9000 WBC/mm^3; < 20% neutrophils	Systemic lupus erythematosus
III	Severely inflammatory arthritis	100–160,000 WBC/mm^3; 70% neutrophils	Gout
IV	Purulent arthritis	150–250,000 WBC/mm^3; 90% neutrophils	Bacterial infections

WBC, white blood cells.

Important points regarding metastases to the bone

- Kidney and thyroid neoplasms are known for producing a solitary metastasis.

- Metastases to hand and foot bones are uncommon and, if present, the source is usually a lung, colon, or renal neoplasm.

ARTHRITIS

Overview: In general, arthritis is inflammation of the joint. Analysis of synovial fluid can help determine the cause of the arthritis. Arthritis is divided into four groups, based upon the number of white blood cells in the fluid and the percentage that are neutrophils (Table 19-2). This section will discuss only reactive arthritis. Two of the major forms of reactive arthritis are osteoarthritis and rheumatoid arthritis, each of which will be discussed in separate sections. The final section of this chapter will cover other joint diseases.

OSTEOARTHRITIS

Overview: Osteoarthritis, also referred to as **degenerative joint disease,** occurs as a result of degeneration of the articular cartilage, with a gradual onset of symptoms after 40 years of age.

Pathogenesis of primary osteoarthritis: Normal articular cartilage undergoes turnover; however, in osteoarthritis, this turnover does not occur. Osteoarthritis is due to wear and tear and other factors, including genetic factors. Osteoarthritis can also be secondary, as a result of trauma and other causes.

Joints involved: Weight bearing, including hips and knees; lower lumbar and cervical vertebrae; and proximal and distal interphalangeal joints.

Morphology of osteoarthritis (Figure 19-9 A and B)

- **Gross**
  - **Eburnation:** Term for thickened and polished subchondral bone.
  - **Subchondral cysts:** Synovial fluid leaks through defects in cartilage and into underlying bone.
  - **Osteophytes:** Include bony excrescences at the distal interphalangeal joint (**Heberden nodes**) and the proximal interphalangeal joint (**Bouchard nodes**).
  - **Joint mice:** Loose fragments of cartilage and/or bone in the joint cavity.
- **Radiographic findings:** Joint space narrowing, subchondral sclerosis and cysts, and osteophyte formation.
- **Microscopic:** Fibrillation of the cartilage (i.e., splitting of cartilage).

Clinical presentation of osteoarthritis: Aching pain, decreased mobility, mild and brief (< 30 minutes) morning stiffness; pain with movement and remission of pain with rest, joint crepitus, and "theater sign" (pain and knee joint locking when arising from a prolonged seated position). With progressive disease, pain occurs at night and with rest. Patients can have symptoms due to compression of nerves.

RHEUMATOID ARTHRITIS

Overview: Rheumatoid arthritis is an autoimmune disorder with an unknown antigen–antibody combination. Patients with HLA-DRB1*0401 and *0404 alleles have increased incidence of disease. Rheumatoid arthritis occurs in 1% of the population. Most patients are 40–70 years of age. It is more common in females than males, with a ratio of 3:1.

Joints affected: Metacarpophalangeal and proximal interphalangeal joints, and feet, wrist, ankle, elbows, and knees.

Morphology of rheumatoid arthritis

- **Gross:** Edematous and thick synovium (**pannus**); surface is rough, with projections.
- **Radiographic finding:** Osteopenia; bony erosion with narrowing of joint space.
- **Microscopic:** Increased number of B cells and T cells, vessels, fibrin, and neutrophils form the pannus. Rheumatoid nodule consists of central fibrinoid necrosis rimmed with histiocytes and lymphocytes; located in areas subject to pressure and can be in viscera.

Clinical presentation of rheumatoid arthritis

- **Symptoms:** Morning stiffness for > 1 hour, three or more affected joints, and arthritis of the hands with symmetric involvement of joints. Systemic signs such as weight loss, fatigue, and fever may be present.
- **Signs:** Warm tender joints; radial deviation of wrist and ulnar deviation of phalanges; **"swan neck" deformity, Dupuytren contracture, boutonnière deformity;** and stiffness after inactivity.

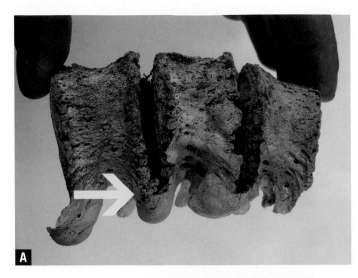

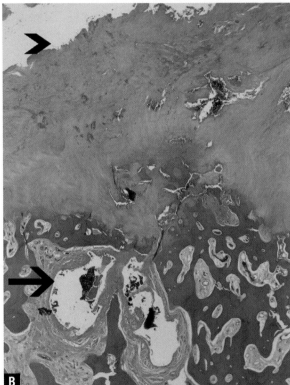

Figure 19-9. Osteoarthritis. **A,** Although osteoarthritis (i.e., degenerative joint disease) is not associated with ankylosis of the joint as is rheumatoid arthritis, it is possible for osteophytes to cross a joint and fuse (*arrow*), producing immobility of the joint. **B,** The histologic features of osteoarthritis include fibrillation and loss of basophilia of the cartilage (*arrowhead*) and subchondral cysts (*arrow*). Hematoxylin and eosin, 40×.

Laboratory findings: Rheumatoid factor (IgM versus Fc portion of IgG) is positive in 70–80% of patients.

Complications of rheumatoid arthritis: The pannus erodes cartilage and may bridge bones, causing ankylosis (Figure 19-10). Extra-articular manifestations are not unusual. The triad of rheumatoid arthritis, leukopenia, and splenomegaly is referred to as **Felty syndrome.** Pulmonary involvement may cause pleural effusions, interstitial fibrosis, or nodular disease (**Caplan syndrome**). Anemia of chronic disease is common.

Differentiation of osteoarthritis versus rheumatoid arthritis (Table 19-3): Osteoarthritis is degeneration of articular cartilage, and is often associated with wear and tear; therefore, symptoms will improve with rest. However, in rheumatoid arthritis, the disease is caused by the formation of a pannus, which causes fusion of the joint. Rest allows the fusion to progress and causes the joint to become stiffer; thus, conversely, use will keep the joint more mobile and decrease stiffness.

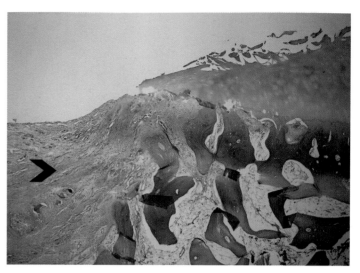

Figure 19-10. Rheumatoid arthritis. The inflammation associated with rheumatoid arthritis can lead to fibrosis (*arrowhead*) and fusion of the joint (ankylosis). Hematoxylin and eosin, 40×.

OTHER DISEASES OF THE JOINTS

ANKYLOSING SPONDYLITIS

Basic description: *HLA-B27*-associated seronegative spondyloarthropathy related to **Reiter syndrome** and psoriatic arthritis, and characterized by inflammation of axial joints (e.g., spine and sacroiliac joints).

Epidemiology: Second and third decades of life; prevalence in males more than females, with ratio of 3:1.

Important point: Approximately 90% of patients have *HLA-B27*.

Clinical presentation of ankylosing spondylitis: Gradual onset of back pain, loss of mobility, and tenderness on palpation of the sacroiliac joints. Sacroiliitis with "pseudo-widening" and eventual fusion of sacroiliac joints, and prominent involvement of spine with squaring and fusion of the vertebrae ("bamboo spine"). Erythrocyte sedimentation rate is elevated.

GOUT

Basic description: Arthritis due to deposition of uric acid crystals.

TABLE 19-3. Comparison and Contrast of Osteoarthritis and Rheumatoid Arthritis

Feature	Osteoarthritis	Rheumatoid arthritis
Joints affected	Weight-bearing (hips, knees); PIP, DIP	MCP, PIP, feet, wrists, ankles, elbow, knees
Morning stiffness	< 30 minutes	> 1 hour
Symptoms	Pain occurs with movement and is better after rest	Stiffness and pain are worst after inactivity
Physical examination	Heberden and Bouchard nodes	Rheumatoid nodules; radial deviation of wrist and ulnar deviation of phalanges

PIP, proximal interphalangeal; DIP, distal interphalangeal; MCP, metacarpophalangeal.

Types of gout

- **Primary gout:** About 85–90% of total number of cases of gout. Results from an unknown enzyme deficiency that causes either increased production of uric acid or normal production of uric acid with decreased excretion. Most patients with primary gout have normal production with decreased excretion of uric acid.

- **Secondary gout (causes)**
  - Increased nucleic acid turnover (e.g., in leukemia).
  - Chronic renal disease.

Risk factors for gout: Increasing age, alcohol use, obesity, thiazide diuretics (thiazide diuretics completely inhibit secretion of uric acid).

Pathogenesis of gout

- Urate crystals are precipitated in the synovium; trauma leads to their release into the synovial fluid. The uric acid crystals are chemotactic for neutrophils, and they activate complement.

- Uric acid levels must be elevated for 20–30 years to cause gout.

Forms of gout

- **Acute arthritis:** Occurs as a result of the neutrophilic infiltrate associated with uric acid crystals in the joint.

- **Chronic tophaceous arthritis:** Urates coat the surface of synovium and deposit within synovium, which causes hyperplasia of synovium.

- **Tophi:** Term for aggregates of urates rimmed with macrophages, lymphocytes, and giant cells (Figure 19-11). Tophi form in tendons and ligaments.

- **Gout nephropathy**
  - Formation of uric acid stones, which can precipitate pyelonephritis.
  - Deposition of uric acid crystals in interstitium.

Microscopic morphology: Uric acid crystals are needle shaped and have strong negative birefringence when polarized.

Clinical presentation of gout

- **Important point:** About 50% of the time, the first attack of gout occurs in the first metatarsophalangeal joint. The next joints involved are those in the instep, ankle, and heel.

- **Stages of gout in order of occurrence**
  - Asymptomatic hyperuricemia
  - Acute gouty arthritis
  - Asymptomatic period between acute attacks; then chronic tophaceous gout.

- **Diagnosis of gout:** Joint aspiration with identification of needle-shaped, **negatively birefringent** crystals in synovial fluid.

Conditions associated with gout

- **Lesch-Nyhan syndrome:** Characterized by hyperuricemia, gout, mental retardation, and self-mutilation; caused by hypoxanthine guanine ribosyl-transferase deficiency (HGPRT).

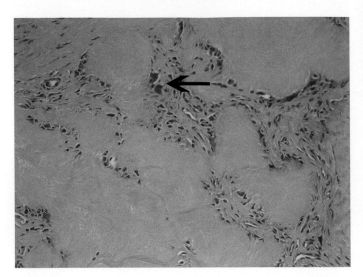

Figure 19-11. Gouty tophus. Deposition of the uric acid crystals within the synovium elicits a giant cell reaction (*arrow*). Hematoxylin and eosin, 400×.

- **Saturnine gout:** Caused by lead poisoning, and is characterized by gout, renal failure, and microcytic anemia. It is classically associated with homemade whisky ("moonshine") made from stills containing lead or old car radiators.

CALCIUM PYROPHOSPHATE CRYSTAL DEPOSITION (PSEUDOGOUT)

Epidemiology: Older than 50 years of age; occurs in patients with degenerative joint disease.

Microscopic morphology: Rhomboid **positively birefringent** crystals examined under polarized light.

Clinical presentation of pseudogout

- Mimics osteoarthritis.
- Affects large joints, such as the knee.

LENTIGO

Basic description: Hyperpigmented lesions occurring as a result of an increased number of melanocytes along the basement membrane.

Important point: A lentigo does not darken with sunlight.

MELANOCYTIC PROLIFERATIONS

Overview: Melanocytic proliferations vary from the benign melanocytic nevus to the highly aggressive malignant melanoma.

MELANOCYTIC NEVUS

Basic description: Benign proliferation of nevus cells, which are derived from melanocytes.

Types of melanocytic nevus

Junctional nevus: Proliferation of nevus cells confined to the basal portion of the epidermis.

Compound nevus: Proliferation of nevus cells at the basal portion of the epidermis and upper dermis.

Intradermal nevus: Proliferation of nevus cells confined to the dermis (Figure 20-1).

Microscopic morphology of melanocytic nevus: Nests of uniform round cells with inconspicuous nucleoli and few if any mitotic figures. As cells get deeper into the dermis, they acquire more of a neural appearance as a result of maturation of the cells.

DYSPLASTIC NEVUS

Basic description: Proliferation of dysplastic nevus cells; dysplastic nevi are precursors of malignant melanoma.

Morphology of dysplastic nevus

Gross: Variable pigmentation; > 5 mm in size; irregular borders.

Microscopic: Fusion and coalescence of nests of nevus cells in epidermis. Also, single nevus cells are present in basal portion of epidermis. The nevus cells have cytologic atypia.

MALIGNANT MELANOMA

Basic description: Malignant tumor of melanocytes.

Four types of malignant melanoma

Superficial spreading melanoma: Has a radial growth pattern for a significant period of time.

Lentigo maligna melanoma: Patients are older adults.

Nodular melanoma: Has a vertical growth pattern early in its development.

Acral lentiginous melanoma: Affects most commonly the nail bed, the sole of the foot, or the palms in African Americans.

Pathogenesis: Melanomas are caused by ultraviolet radiation that damages the DNA of melanocytes. Mutations in *CDKN2A*,

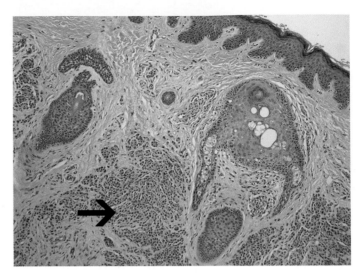

Figure 20-1. Intradermal nevus. Note the proliferation of nevus cells within the dermis only, surrounding the skin appendages. As the nevus cells penetrate deeper into the dermis, they acquire a more "neural" appearance (*arrow*). Hematoxylin and eosin, 100×.

which alter transcription and cell cycle control, are thought to play a prominent role in melanoma formation.

Growth patterns of melanoma

Radial: Grows horizontally; not associated with metastases.

Vertical: Grows downward into the dermis; is associated with metastases.

Risk factors for melanoma: Sun exposure, especially in fair skinned individuals. Although melanomas do not often arise from nevi, a history of atypical nevi, giant nevi (> 20 cm), or a large number of nevi are risk factors for melanoma.

Morphology of melanoma (Figure 20-2 A–C)

Gross: > 10 mm in size, variable pigmentation (can be hypopigmented), irregular borders.

Microscopic: Large cells with prominent nucleoli forming poorly defined nests; single cells are present. Neoplastic cells may or may not produce melanin.

Important point: For staging of a melanoma, depth of penetration into the dermis is crucial. The greater the depth of penetration, the more likelihood of metastases.

Clinical presentation of malignant melanoma

Warning signs of melanoma: Increasing size of nevus; itching and/or pain; change in size, shape, or color of nevus; growth of new nevus; irregular borders.

Favorable prognostic factors: Depth of invasion (**Breslow depth**) of < 1.7 mm; absence of mitotic figures.

Important point: S-100 and HMB-45 are commonly used tumor markers for melanoma.

OTHER PIGMENTED LESIONS
SEBORRHEIC KERATOSIS

Morphology (Figure 20-3 A and B)

Gross: Tan to dark brown papule or nodule with a "stuck-on" appearance.

Microscopic: Sheets of basal-like cells, hyperkeratosis, and keratin-filled cysts.

Epidemiology: Middle-aged and older adults.

Sign of Leser-Trélat: Sudden onset of multiple seborrheic keratoses, which is a cutaneous manifestation of internal malignancy (associated with adenocarcinoma of the gastrointestinal tract).

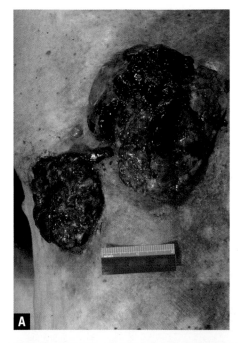

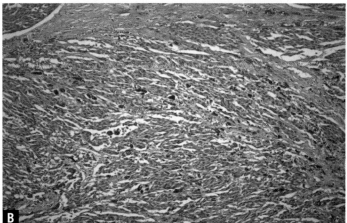

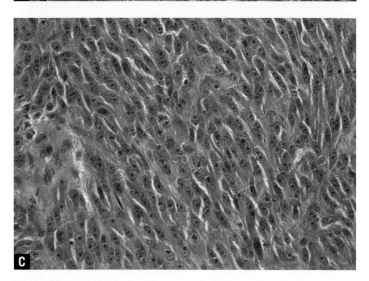

Figure 20-2. Malignant melanoma. **A,** This patient had two large, untreated and undiagnosed nodular malignant melanomas on her back. Malignant melanoma often produces pigment, which can be seen grossly as well as microscopically (**B**). However, not all malignant melanomas produce pigment, and this tumor must always be considered in the diagnosis of malignancies with large pleomorphic cells and prominent nucleoli (**C**). Hematoxylin and eosin, **B**, 200×; **C**, 400×.

ACANTHOSIS NIGRICANS

Morphology (Figure 20-4)

Gross and microscopic: Hyperplastic (i.e., acanthosis) and hyperpigmented papules.

Areas affected: Flexor regions, including the posterior neck, axilla, and groin.

Types of acanthosis nigricans

Benign: Commonly associated with insulin resistance and obesity.

Malignant: Can be a cutaneous manifestation of internal malignancy (associated with gastrointestinal adenocarcinoma).

NON–MELANOCYTIC PRENEOPLASTIC AND NEOPLASTIC LESIONS

ACTINIC KERATOSIS

Morphology

Gross: Rough, sandpaper-like lesion, which may have a keratin horn.

Microscopic: Dysplasia of keratinocytes in basal portion of epidermis; can have parakeratosis.

Risk factor: Actinic keratoses are caused by exposure to ultraviolet light and exposure to sun.

Important point: Actinic keratosis is a precancerous lesion that has the potential to develop into squamous cell carcinoma.

Mutations: Commonly of *p53* gene.

CUTANEOUS SQUAMOUS CELL CARCINOMA

Risk factors: Sun exposure; older patients. Other risk factors include chronic ulcers, osteomyelitis, and burns (**Marjolin ulcer**).

Incidence: Second most common type of skin cancer (80–100,000 cases per year).

Important point: Cutaneous squamous cell carcinoma rarely metastasizes (only 5% of cases metastasize). Multiple squamous cell carcinomas may arise at the sites of arsenic exposure.

Precursors of cutaneous squamous cell carcinoma

Actinic keratosis

Squamous cell carcinoma in situ: Full-thickness dysplasia of the epidermis. The only histologic difference between squamous cell carcinoma and squamous cell carcinoma in situ is that carcinoma in situ lacks features of invasion.

Mutations: Loss of heterozygosity of chromosomes 3, 9, 17; *p53* mutations.

Morphology of cutaneous squamous cell carcinoma

Location: Most commonly head, hands, and face.

Gross: Painless nodule with possible evidence of keratin formation; may ulcerate.

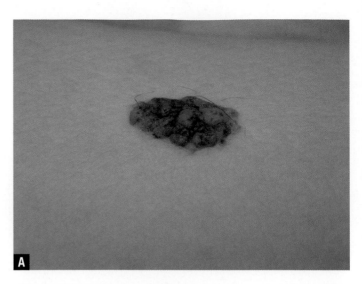

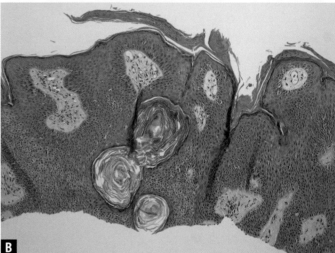

Figure 20-3. Seborrheic keratosis. **A**, Seborrheic keratosis has a nodular, "stuck-on" gross appearance. **B**, Microscopically, the tumor is composed of basaloid cells associated with hyperkeratosis and keratin-filled cysts. Hematoxylin and eosin, 40×.

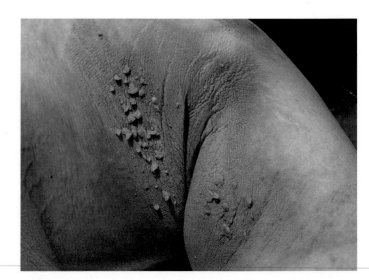

Figure 20-4. Acanthosis nigricans. The hyperplastic papules in the axilla of this patient are acanthosis nigricans. Acanthosis nigricans is found in obese persons, patients with diabetic mellitus, and in patients with a gastrointestinal neoplasm.

Microscopic: Invasive squamous-appearing cells in dermis. Keratin pearls and intercellular bridges are evidence of squamous differentiation.

BASAL CELL CARCINOMA

Risk factors: Sun exposure; older persons.

Important points: Locally invasive, but rarely metastasize. Most commonly develop on sun-exposed areas (e.g., nose, lip).

Mutations: *PTCH, p53.*

Morphology of basal cell carcinoma: Figure 20-5 *A–C*

Gross: Pearly papule with dilated subepidermal blood vessels; can ulcerate; formerly called **"rodent ulcers."**

Microscopic: Nests of neoplastic cells resembling basal cells of the epidermis. The nests have peripheral palisading and separation clefts and are embedded in mucoid matrix.

INHERITED SKIN NEOPLASIA SYNDROMES

BASAL CELL NEVUS SYNDROME

Inheritance pattern: Autosomal dominant.

Manifestations of basal cell nevus syndrome: Disfiguring disorder characterized by multiple basal cell carcinomas before 20 years of age; associated with dental and maxillofacial abnormalities (e.g., cleft palate, keratocysts of the jaw). Pitting of the palms and soles is a classic finding.

Mutation: *PTCH* ("patched") gene on chromosome 9q22.3. The protein product of the *PTCH* gene is the receptor for the protein produced by the sonic hedgehog gene. The mutation leads to uninhibited activation of *SMO* ("smoothened").

DYSPLASTIC NEVUS SYNDROME (FAMILIAL MELANOMA SYNDROME)

Mutation: *p16INK4a* on 9p21, which leads to unrestricted phosphorylation of RB and subsequent release of E2F.

Other mutations: *CDK4, BRAF* (part of RAS/RAF/MAP kinase pathway).

Inheritance: Autosomal dominant with high penetrance.

Clinical presentation: Fair-skinned, fair-complexioned patient with multiple irregular nevi with variegated color. High risk for malignant melanoma and increased risk for pancreatic cancer.

ACUTE INFLAMMATORY DERMATOSES

Overview: The acute inflammatory dermatoses are a group of inflammatory skin disorders with a general time course lasting days to weeks. Microscopically, the conditions have neutrophils, edema, and epidermal, vascular, or subcutaneous injury. The number of acute inflammatory dermatoses is large; however, only three common forms, urticaria, acute eczematous dermatitis, and erythema multiforme, are discussed here.

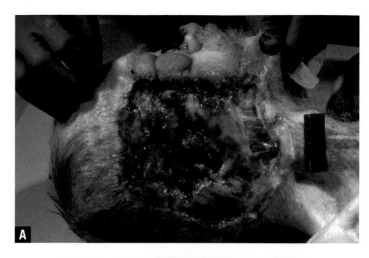

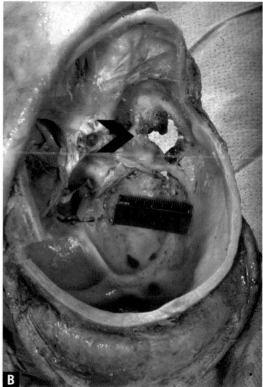

Figure 20-5. Basal cell carcinoma. Basal cell carcinoma is a slow-growing malignant neoplasm, which invades locally but almost never metastasizes. Often, patients will present for treatment many years after they first identified the neoplasm, some with incurable locally aggressive tumors. **A** and **B**, This patient has a large basal cell carcinoma on the right side of the head, which has invaded into and perforated the skull (*arrowhead*).

URTICARIA (HIVES)

Pathogenesis: Mast cell degranulation with resultant increased vascular permeability.

Epidemiology: Occurs most commonly in patients 20–40 years of age.

Types of urticaria

■ **IgE dependent:** A type I hypersensitivity reaction associated with pollens, drugs, and insect venom.

■ **IgE independent:** Some substances (e.g., opiates, some antibiotics) can directly cause degranulation of mast cells.

Morphology of urticaria

Gross: Pruritic, erythematous, edematous plaques ("wheals").

Microscopic: Perivascular edema.

ACUTE ECZEMATOUS DERMATITIS

Basic description: A group of skin disorders characterized in the acute period by red oozing and crusting papules and vesicles, and in the chronic stage by raised plaques.

Types: Allergic contact dermatitis, atopic dermatitis, drug-related eczematous dermatitis, photoeczematous dermatitis, and primary irritant dermatitis.

Pathogenesis of acute eczematous dermatitis: Antigen taken up by the dendritic Langerhans cell is presented to the T cell. Upon reexposure to the antigen, the memory T cells release cytokines.

Morphology of acute eczematous dermatitis

Gross: Red, papulovesicular rash with oozing and crusting lesions.

Microscopic

○ **Early stages:** Edema progressing to spongiosis.

○ **Later stages:** Parakeratosis and hyperkeratosis.

ERYTHEMA MULTIFORME (FIGURE 20-6)

Pathogenesis: Due to hypersensitivity to infections (e.g., herpes simplex virus [HSV], mycoplasma) and to drugs (e.g., sulfonamides, penicillin, salicylates); also seen in patients with carcinomas and collagen vascular diseases. Approximately 90% of cases of erythema multiforme are associated with HSV infection.

Gross morphology of erythema multiforme: Macules, papules, vesicles, and bullae; hence the term multiforme. The characteristic **target lesion** is a red macule or papule with a central pale center. The extremities are usually involved symmetrically.

Variants of erythema multiforme: Stevens-Johnson syndrome and toxic epidermal necrolysis

1. **Stevens-Johnson syndrome (i.e., erythema multiforme major):** An extensive form seen in children. Patients are febrile, and changes involve the lips and oral mucosa. Patients often develop a secondary infection leading to sepsis.

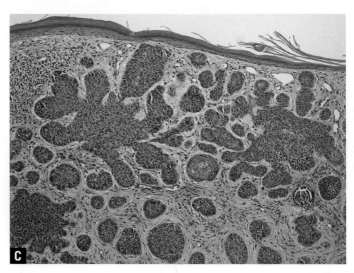

Figure 20-5. (*Continued*) **C**, Basal cell carcinoma is composed of nests of neoplastic cells, which resemble basal cells of the epidermis. The nests have peripheral palisading. Images **A** and **B** are provided courtesy of Dr. Sheila Spotswood, Dallas County Medical Examiner's Office, Dallas, TX. **C**, Hematoxylin and eosin, 100×.

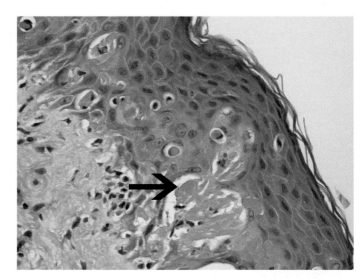

Figure 20-6. Erythema multiforme. There is a sparse infiltrate of lymphocytes at the dermal-epidermal junction. The arrow indicates a subepidermal vesicle. Hematoxylin and eosin, 400×.

2. **Toxic epidermal necrolysis**

  Basic description: Diffuse sloughing and necrosis of cutaneous and mucosal epithelium.

  Microscopic morphology: Diffuse epidermal necrosis, leading to blister formation; also perivascular lymphocytes and dermal edema (Figure 20-7 *A* and *B*).

CHRONIC INFLAMMATORY DERMATOSES

Overview: The chronic inflammatory dermatoses are a group of inflammatory skin disorders with a general time course lasting months to years. Microscopically, the conditions have epidermal changes (e.g., atrophy or hyperplasia) and dermal fibrosis. Although there are many conditions that fall under this category of skin disorders, only a few of the common forms (psoriasis and seborrheic dermatitis) will be discussed below.

PSORIASIS

Incidence: 1–2% of the population in the United States is affected.

Important points: Two thirds of patients with psoriasis have HLA-Cw*0602. Psoriasis rarely is pustular. The two forms of pustular psoriasis are benign and generalized.

  Benign pustular psoriasis: Involves the hands and feet.

  Generalized pustular psoriasis: Life threatening due to secondary infections and electrolyte abnormalities.

Morphology of psoriasis (Figure 20-8 *A* and *B*)

  Gross: Red plaque covered with silvery-white scales. Removal of the scale causes petechial bleeding (**Auspitz sign**). Brown discoloration ("oil spots") and pitting of nails is classic.

  Areas affected: Elbows, knees, scalp, and lumbosacral region; may involve the nails.

  Microscopic: Acanthosis; elongated dermal papillae with thinning of overlying epidermis and parakeratosis; neutrophils clustered in parakeratosis (i.e., **Munro microabscesses**).

Associated condition: Psoriatic arthritis is one of the seronegative spondyloarthropathies related to Reiter disease and ankylosing spondylitis. It occurs in 5% of patients with psoriasis. Patients are positive for *HLA-B27*. Psoriatic arthritis is characterized by psoriasis, arthritis, and spondylosis.

SEBORRHEIC DERMATITIS

Pathogenesis: Unknown; some cases may be due to *Malassezia furfur*.

Morphology of seborrheic dermatitis

  Gross: Moist or "greasy" macules and papules on an erythematous base; has scaling and crusting.

  Areas affected: Areas with sebaceous glands such as the scalp, face, anterior chest, and intertriginous areas.

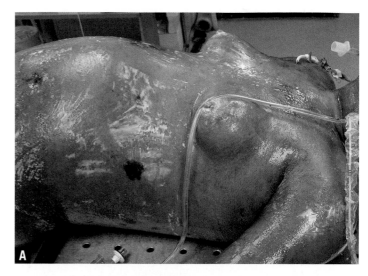

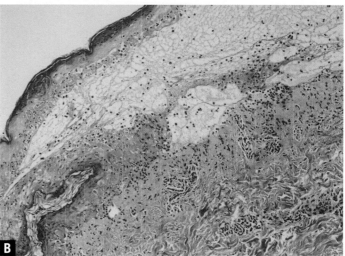

Figure 20-7. Toxic epidermal necrolysis. **A**, This patient had toxic epidermal necrolysis and underwent diffuse sloughing of the epidermis. The creamy white material represents therapeutic intervention. The loss of an extensive amount of epidermis predisposes the patient to electrolyte imbalances and infection. **B**, There is necrosis of the epidermis, with subepidermal blister formation. Hematoxylin and eosin, 100×.

- **Microscopic**
  - ○ **Early stages:** Spongiosis.
  - ○ **Later stages:** Acanthosis.
  - ○ Can have parakeratosis, neutrophils, and serum near the hair follicles; lymphocytes and neutrophils are in a perivascular distribution.

Important points: Dandruff in adults and cradle cap in infants are forms of seborrheic dermatitis.

BLISTERING (BULLOUS) DISEASES

Overview: The general microscopic morphology of the blistering skin diseases is acantholysis. This microscopic change results in bullae formation; the bullae involve the oral mucosa and skin. The three major blistering skin diseases are pemphigus, bullous pemphigoid, and dermatitis herpetiformis (Table 20-1).

PEMPHIGUS

Forms of pemphigus: There are four forms of pemphigus: vulgaris, vegetans, foliaceous, and erythematosus.

1. **Pemphigus vulgaris**

Incidence: About 80% of cases.

Areas affected: Lesions classically begin on the oral mucosa and later involve skin of the scalp, face, chest, axillae, and groin.

Pathogenesis: IgG to desmoglein 3 (an intercellular cement substance) produces a net-like pattern on immunofluorescence.

Morphology of pemphigus vulgaris

- **Gross:** Flaccid bullae, which readily rupture leaving superficial erosions. **Nikolsky sign** is positive.
- **Microscopic:** Suprabasal bullae with intercellular deposits of IgG and C3.

2. **Pemphigus vegetans**

Areas affected: Groin, axillae, and flexural areas.

Gross morphology: Wart-like plaques.

3. **Pemphigus foliaceous**

Areas affected: Scalp, face, and chest.

Epidemiology: Seen in South America.

Morphology

- **Gross:** Superficial bullae.
- **Microscopic:** Subcorneal bullae.

4. **Pemphigus erythematosus:** Affects the malar area of the face.

BULLOUS PEMPHIGOID

Epidemiology: Older patients.

Pathogenesis: Antibody against hemidesmosomes; produces linear pattern at the basement membrane on immunofluorescence.

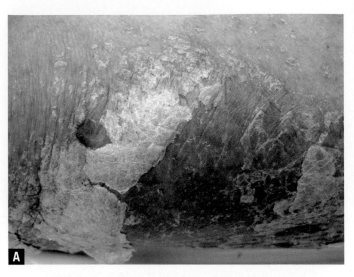

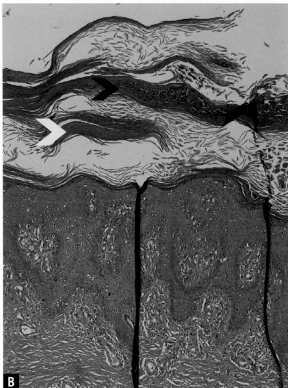

Figure 20-8. Psoriasis. **A,** Note the red plaque covered with white scales. Commonly, the flexural regions (e.g., elbows, knees, lumbosacral region) are involved. **B,** Microscopically, there is acanthosis (thickening of the epidermis), parakeratosis (*white arrowhead*), Munro microabscesses (*black arrowhead*), and elongation of the dermal papillae. Hematoxylin and eosin, 100×.

TABLE 20-1. Blistering Diseases of the Skin

Feature	Pemphigus Vulgaris	Bullous Pemphigoid	Dermatitis Herpetiformis
Areas involved	Oral mucosa (prominent), scalp, face and chest	Extremities, axillae and groin; oral mucosain 10–15%	Extensor surfaces; buttocks
Antibody target	Desmoglein 3	Hemidesmosomes	Gliadin and reticulin
Pattern on immunofluorescence	Net-like pattern	Linear pattern at basement membrane	IgA positive clusters at tips of dermal papillae
Nikolsky sign	Positive	Negative	

Morphology of bullous pemphigoid

Gross: Tense, up to 2.0-cm bullae. The bullae do not rupture as easily as those of pemphigus; thus the **Nikolsky sign** is negative.

Areas affected: Inner thighs, flexor surface of forearms, axillae, and groin; can involve oral mucosa (10–15% of patients), but not as often as in pemphigus.

Microscopic: Subepidermal nonacantholytic bullae; basal cell vacuolation; can have perivascular neutrophils, lymphocytes, and eosinophils.

DERMATITIS HERPETIFORMIS

Epidemiology: Affects males more frequently than females; third and fourth decades of life.

Pathogenesis: Antibodies versus gliadin (is associated with celiac disease) and reticulin.

Important point: Responds to gliadin-free diet.

Morphology of dermatitis herpetiformis

Gross: Extremely pruritic plaques and vesicles.

Areas affected: Bilateral and symmetrical; affects extensor surfaces and buttocks.

Microscopic: In the early stages, clusters of neutrophils and fibrin at the tips of dermal papillae; by immunofluorescence, these clusters at the tips of dermal papillae stain positive for IgA; subepidermal blisters are formed.

OTHER INFLAMMATORY SKIN DISEASES

Overview: As stated above, this chapter covers only a few of the inflammatory skin disorders. Two additional disorders that do not fall under the categories of acute or chronic inflammatory dermatoses or under blistering diseases are granuloma annulare and erythema nodosum, which are discussed briefly in this section.

GRANULOMA ANNULARE

Epidemiology: Most cases are diagnosed in patients younger than age 30 years; more common in females.

Morphology: May be localized or disseminated, and most often affects the dorsal surfaces of feet and hands and extensor surfaces of legs and arms. Lesion begins as an annular ring of small, firm, flesh-colored or red papules. The ring expands outward with time, with involution and resolution of central involvement.

Causes of granuloma annulare: Associated with a variety of conditions, including tuberculosis, trauma, human immunodeficiency virus (HIV) and HSV infections, and insect bites.

ERYTHEMA NODOSUM

Basic description: An acute form of panniculitis.

Morphology of erythema nodosum

   Gross: Poorly defined, tender, erythematous plaques. They are often felt but not seen. Over a few weeks, the plaques flatten and become bruise-like.

   Microscopic

   ○ **Early stages:** Edema, fibrin, and neutrophils in connective tissue septae.

   ○ **Later stages:** Lymphocytes, macrophages, and multinucleated giant cells in connective tissue septae.

Important point: Erythema nodosum arises in association with β-hemolytic streptococcal upper respiratory tract infections, tuberculosis, sulfonamide therapy, oral contraceptive use, and inflammatory bowel disease. Erythema nodosum is the most common cutaneous lesion associated with sarcoidosis.

INFECTIOUS DISORDERS OF THE SKIN

Overview: There are many infectious disorders of the skin; however, only verrucae vulgaris and impetigo will be discussed here.

VERRUCAE VULGARIS

Epidemiology: Occurs in children and adolescents.

Pathogenesis: Infection with the human papillomavirus.

Microscopic morphology: Epidermal hyperplasia with koilocytic changes.

IMPETIGO

Pathogenesis: Infection with group A *Streptococcus* or *Staphylococcus aureus;* due to toxin that cleaves desmoglein 1.

Morphology of impetigo

   Gross: Erythematous macules forming pustules; associated with honey-colored crust.

   Areas commonly affected: Face and hands.

   Microscopic: Neutrophils in stratum corneum; can form pustules.

CUTANEOUS MANIFESTATIONS OF SYSTEMIC DISEASE

Overview: Some systemic diseases produce lesions of the skin. Four disorders specifically associated with an underlying systemic disease are necrobiosis lipoidica, pyoderma gangrenosum, ecthyma gangrenosum, and porphyria cutanea tarda. All are discussed in this section.

NECROBIOSIS LIPOIDICA

Basic description: Uncommon disorder associated with diabetes mellitus.

Morphology

    Gross: Oval-shaped, yellow-brown plaques on the anterior surfaces of the lower legs.

    Microscopic: Histiocytomas, PAS-positive areas of necrobiosis.

PYODERMA GANGRENOSUM

Basic description: Seen in 5% of patients with ulcerative colitis.

Morphology: Progressive ulceration with well-defined margins. Classically, have purple base with surrounding red border.

Clinical presentation: Initially presents similar to cellulitis with erythema and pain. Patients do not respond to antibiotic therapy and are treated with steroid drugs.

ECTHYMA GANGRENOSUM

Basic description: Cutaneous manifestation of sepsis, classically due to *Pseudomonas*.

Morphology: Pustules with central hemorrhagic bullae that develop into necrotic ulcers.

PORPHYRIA CUTANEA TARDA

Basic description: Chronic blistering disease caused by deficiency of uroporphyrinogen decarboxylase. Most cases are acquired in association with liver disease due to alcohol use, viral hepatitis, or exposure to estrogen. Familial forms are less common.

Morphology: Blistering and erosions on sun-exposed areas, including the hands and face.

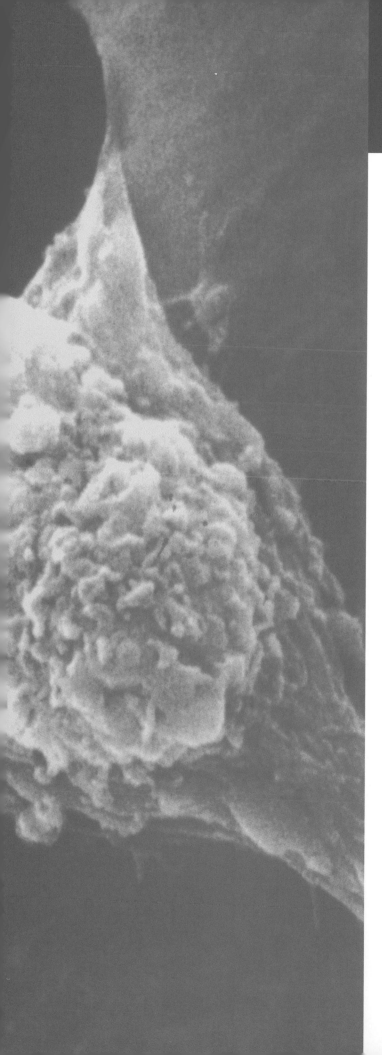

CHAPTER 21

PRACTICE EXAMINATION

DIRECTIONS

Each numbered item or incomplete statement is followed by options. Select the best answer to each question. Some options may be partially correct, but there is only **ONE BEST** answer.

PRACTICE EXAMINATION QUESTIONS

1. A 35-year-old marathon runner died in a motor vehicle accident while driving to work. At the time of the autopsy, which of the following features could be identified through gross and microscopic examination of the organs?

    A. Atrophy of the skeletal muscle
    B. Pathologic hyperplasia of the heart
    C. Physiologic hypertrophy of the heart
    D. Physiologic hyperplasia of the heart

2. A 72-year-old man suddenly developed weakness of his left leg, causing him to fall to the ground while shopping with his wife. An ambulance is called, and he is rushed to the hospital. He spends 4 days in the hospital, but the weakness in his left leg does not resolve. Which of the following is the most likely diagnosis?

    A. Global hypoxic ischemic encephalopathy
    B. Transient ischemic attack
    C. Acute infarct in the distribution of the right middle cerebral artery
    D. Acute infarct in the distribution of the right anterior cerebral artery

3. A 53-year-old man with a history of hypertension and diabetes mellitus routinely has chest pain after climbing five flights of stairs. When he rests, the chest pain subsides. He has had such chest pain for the past 5 months, and it has not changed in frequency. Which of the following is the most likely cause of his symptoms?

A. Atherosclerotic plaque in the left anterior descending coronary artery causing 75% stenosis of the vessel's lumen

B. Atherosclerotic plaque in the left anterior descending coronary artery causing 45% stenosis of the vessel's lumen

C. Atherosclerotic plaque in the left anterior descending coronary artery that causes 75% stenosis and has a large cluster of intact red blood cells within its core

D. Ruptured atherosclerotic plaque in the left anterior descending coronary artery associated with a nearly occlusive thrombus

4. A 30-year-old man with a history of a cerebellar tumor that was resected when he was 20 years of age presents to his physician because of blood in his urine. He is concerned because his father's brother died early in life from complications of a metastatic tumor. He is evaluated with an ultrasound and found to have a mass in the left kidney. The kidney is removed, and the mass is diagnosed as a renal cell carcinoma. This patient most likely has a mutation at which of the following sites?

A. 13q14

B. 5q21

C. 3p25

D. 17p13

5. A 29-year-old man falls 15′ while rock climbing and strikes his head. After a brief period of unconsciousness, he awakens and states that his head hurts. Within 30 minutes, he is flown by helicopter to the nearest hospital. En route, he becomes unconscious and his right pupil becomes fixed and dilated. Shortly thereafter, he sustains a cardiac arrest, and resuscitative efforts fail. Which of the following best describes the most likely findings at autopsy?

A. Fracture of the squamous portion of the right temporal bone

B. Fracture of the occipital bone

C. Torn bridging vein associated with a < 0.2-cm thick subdural hemorrhage

D. Diffuse subarachnoid hemorrhage

6. A 13-year-old white girl is brought to the emergency department by her parents, who relate her symptoms of fever, shortness of breath, and cough to the attending physician. A chest radiograph reveals complete consolidation of the lower lobe of the left lung. Cultures of the lower lobe of the left lung would most likely reveal which organism?

A. *Streptococcus pneumoniae*

B. *Staphylococcus aureus*

C. *Klebsiella pneumoniae*

D. *Pseudomonas aeruginosa*

7. A 45-year-old homeless man who is hospitalized on a mental illness warrant is having difficulty with speech and walking. On physical examination, he appears confused and has nystagmus, bilateral lateral rectus palsies, and a broad-based ataxic gait. Most of his symptoms resolve over the course of hospitalization, but he has a permanent footdrop. What is the most likely diagnosis?

A. Korsakoff psychosis

B. Wernicke encephalopathy

C. Herpes encephalitis

D. Bacterial meningitis

8. A 25-year-old man presents to his physician because of the recent unexpected death of his brother. His brother died suddenly while playing basketball. His autopsy report said the cause of death was an aortic dissection and also mentioned that he had a myxomatous mitral valve. The patient remembers that his brother was diagnosed with a heart murmur, and that he also has a murmur. He is concerned that he may die suddenly, similar to his brother's death. This patient is at most risk for which one of the following conditions?

A. Subarachnoid hemorrhage due to a ruptured berry aneurysm

B. Intracerebral hemorrhage centered on the basal ganglia or thalamus

C. Dislocation of the lens of his right or left eye

D. Aortic stenosis due to degenerative calcification of a bicuspid aortic valve

9. A 38-year-old white woman presents to her physician because of complaints of a persistent headache. She also has noted multiple episodes of double vision in the past several months. She has not seen a physician before this point because of her fears that she has a brain tumor. Physical examination reveals weakness of the lateral rectus muscle of the left eye. A CT scan reveals no intracerebral mass; however, the cortex of the skull is focally thickened. Histologic examination of the bone would likely reveal

A. neoplastic cells intermixed with lacy osteoid

B. granulomatous inflammation

C. hypercellular cartilage

D. mosaic pattern of the lamellar bone

10. A 31-year-old man presents to his family physician because of a palpable mass in his right testis identified upon self-examination. As a child, his right testis remained undescended until he was 3 years of age. Which of the following tests would be LEAST useful in presurgical assessment of the mass?

A. Serum human chorionic gonadotropin (hCG)

B. Alkaline phosphatase

C. Ultrasound

D. Serum α-fetoprotein (AFP)

11. A 51-year-old man who has diabetes mellitus and has a history of smoking two packs of cigarettes a day for 30 years presents to his family physician with complaints of pain in his legs when he walks. He describes the pain as an ache that it is relieved when he stops walking. Physical examination reveals the man to have a blood pressure of 151/93 mm Hg. Laboratory tests show a glucose level of 223 mg/dL and a normal CBC. What is the most likely diagnosis?

A. Diabetic peripheral neuropathy

B. Peripheral vascular disease

C. Raynaud phenomenon

D. Diabetes-induced dermatomyositis

12. A 1-year-old girl with a history of several infections since birth, including pneumonia and otitis media, is evaluated for a defect in her immune system. The extensive laboratory testing reveals that her white blood cells are incapable of crossing the endothelium into the surrounding tissue. Further testing reveals the abnormality. She is most likely deficient in which of the following cellular mediators?

A. LFA-1

B. ICAM-1

C. Sialyl-Lewis-X molecules

D. CD31

13. A 50-year-old man is in the hospital for treatment of an infected aortic graft, which was placed 4 years ago for treatment of an abdominal aortic aneurysm. During the night, he develops massive hematemesis. He has no history of gastric ulcers or cirrhosis. During resuscitation efforts, the physician attempts to place an endotracheal tube. At this time, the anesthesiologist sees a large amount of fluid blood exuding from the esophagus. Despite resuscitation and emergent exploratory surgery, the patient experiences heavy blood loss and dies. An autopsy is most likely to reveal which of the following conditions?

A. Multiple acute gastric ulcers

B. Duodenal peptic ulcer

C. Aortoduodenal fistula

D. Abscess of the stomach wall with erosion into a vessel

14. A 52-year-old man presents to his family physician with complaints of fatigue. His physical examination and laboratory work-up reveal pancytopenia and splenomegaly. Flow cytometric analysis of his blood reveals cells with CD11c and CD103 positivity. The cells are positive for tartrate-resistant acid phosphatase. What is the most likely diagnosis?

A. B-cell chronic lymphocytic leukemia

B. Hairy cell leukemia

C. Chronic myelogenous leukemia

D. T-cell chronic lymphocytic leukemia

15. A 15-year-old boy who is mentally retarded is noted by his family physician to have a long face and a large mandible. Physical examination reveals large testicles. Neither his father nor his grandfathers had mental retardation. Chromosomal analysis reveals more than 250 trinucleotide repeats on the X chromosome. What is the most likely composition of the trinucleotide repeats?

A. CGG

B. CTG

C. CAG

D. CCG

16. A 3-day-old infant develops bilious vomiting, abdominal distention, and intestinal obstruction. Plain films of the abdomen reveal dilated air filled loops of small intestine without air fluid levels and the appearance of "soap bubbles" in the bowel. The colon is small on contrast enema, and there is obstruction of the terminal ileum. Which of the following is the most likely underlying cause of this disorder?

A. Defect of cAMP-activated ion channel

B. Absence of ganglion cells in the large bowel

C. Benign hypertrophy of the pylorus

D. β-Glucosidase deficiency

17. A 9-year-old boy has puffy eyes and swollen extremities. He is brought by his parents to the hospital, where a urinalysis reveals proteinuria (4+) and no blood. Subsequent testing reveals a 24-hour urine with 10.5 grams of protein. What is the next best step in the treatment of this patient?

A. Admit the child for close monitoring

B. Perform a kidney biopsy to diagnose his condition

C. Perform a kidney biopsy to confirm the diagnosis is minimal change disease

D. Treat the child with steroid therapy

18. A 17-year-old girl who is pregnant says that she usually smokes about 15 cigarettes a day. Despite being advised to abstain from smoking during her pregnancy, she has not been able to stop. During her third trimester, she suddenly develops abdominal pain and vaginal bleeding. Her boyfriend brings her to the emergency department, where she rapidly deteriorates into shock. An emergent cesarean section is performed. What is the most likely diagnosis?

A. Placental abruption

B. Placenta previa

C. Premature rupture of the fetal membranes

D. An undiagnosed ectopic pregnancy

19. A 65-year-old woman who lives by herself on a very limited budget is brought to the emergency department by a neighbor. He states that he found her wandering outside unable to find her house, which was only two blocks away. He walked her there and upon entering the house he noticed a terrible smell, which turned out to be several large spots of liquid brown fecal material on the furniture in various states of drying. He also noticed there was very little food in the house. Upon examination, the emergency department physician notes several areas of inflammatory dermatitis. What is the most likely diagnosis?

A. Deficiency of vitamin B_1

B. Deficiency of vitamin B_2

C. Deficiency of vitamin B_3

D. Deficiency of vitamin B_6

20. A 50-year-old man presents to the hospital after a brief episode of chest wall pain. An ECG and cardiac enzyme tests reveal no abnormalities. A routine chest radiograph reveals only a single 2-cm coin lesion in the right lower lobe of the lung with a "popcorn" pattern of calcifications. The man is scheduled for surgery, and the lesion is removed. The pathology report describes the mass as a disorganized nodule of cartilage, with no cellular features of malignancy. What is the general term for this lesion?

A. Choristoma

B. Hamartoma

C. Adenoma

D. Sarcoma

21. A 55-year-old man presents to his family physician because of complaints of headaches and difficulty concentrating. He has also noticed an intermittent, slightly pink discoloration of his urine. A CBC reveals hemoglobin of 21.0 g/dL and normal white blood cell and platelet counts. Which of the following tests is most likely to detect the source of his symptoms?

A. Bone marrow biopsy

B. CT scan of the head

C. Chest radiograph

D. CT scan of the abdomen and pelvis

22. A 37-year-old woman presents to her family physician with complaints of increased shortness of breath. She is tachypneic but is not cyanotic. Additional physical examination reveals a yellow discoloration of the conjunctivae. A chest radiograph shows bilateral hyperlucency of the lower lung fields, an elevated right hemidiaphragm, and an infiltrate in the right lower lobe. Despite appropriate medical treatment, she dies and an autopsy is performed. Upon examination of the lungs, which pathologic condition will most likely be identified?

A. Centriacinar emphysema

B. Panacinar emphysema

C. Asthma

D. Bronchiectasis

23. A 24-year-old woman, who is in her 31st week of pregnancy, runs a red light and is struck on the side of her car. She sustains trauma to the abdomen, including premature separation of the placenta from the uterus. Because of her proximity to a hospital, she is able to undergo an emergent cesarean section. The infant has an initial Apgar score of 4, but with aggressive resuscitation, it survives. This infant will most likely develop which of the following complications?

A. Meconium ileus

B. Asymmetric growth retardation

C. Pink acellular membranes lining the alveolar septae

D. Intracerebral hemorrhage centered in the basal ganglia

24. A pathology resident is reviewing the slides from a pediatric neoplasm with his attending. The tumor is composed of small round blue cells. Molecular testing of the tumor revealed a t(11;22). Immunohistochemical staining of the tumor cells is positive for CD99. These findings are most consistent with a tumor that originated

A. in the vagina

B. in the diaphysis of the tibia

C. in the kidney

D. in a jaw mass

25. A 42-year-old man with a history of hypertension and 50 pack years of tobacco use presents to the emergency department because of chest pain, which he describes as "tightness." He also has nausea and some difficulty breathing. An ECG reveals ST depression. While being evaluated in the emergency department, the chest pain subsides approximately 18 minutes after it started. Cardiac enzyme tests completed at the time of admission to the emergency department and later at 3-hour and 6-hour intervals reveal normal levels of CK-MB and troponin I. What is the most likely diagnosis?

A. Non-ST elevation myocardial infarct

B. Prinzmetal angina

C. Unstable angina

D. Stable angina

26. A 60-year-old woman is brought to the emergency department by her family after they witnessed seizure activity at home. Laboratory testing in the emergency department reveals normal electrolyte and glucose levels and no evidence of toxic levels of a medication or drug. A CT scan reveals a mass in the left cerebral hemisphere. Prior to surgical biopsy of the mass, the patient's left pupil becomes dilated. Which of the following has most likely occurred in this patient?

A. Cerebellar tonsillar herniation

B. Overmedication with an opiate

C. Herniation of the left uncus

D. Herniation of the left cingulate gyrus

27. A 26-year-old white man with no significant past medical history presents to the emergency department because of sudden onset of shortness of breath and chest pain. An arterial blood gas reveals that he is hypoxic. A ventilation-perfusion scan of the chest is consistent with a pulmonary thromboembolus. He has no identifiable risk factors for deep venous thrombi. This patient is most likely to have

A. an antiphospholipid antibody

B. a mutation in the cleavage site for protein C

C. a mutation in the prothrombin gene

D. an undiagnosed pancreatic adenocarcinoma

28. A 72 year-old man who works for a mine in Libby, Montana, has a clinical history of pulmonary function tests that show a decreased FEV_1 and FVC, with a normal FEV_1/FVC ratio. He dies and an autopsy is performed. The autopsy reveals a tumor in the right pleural cavity, which completely encases the lung. He also has tan-white pleural plaques in the right pleural cavity. Upon histologic examination of the lung, prominent alveolar septal fibrosis with honeycomb change is identified. This patient was most likely exposed to which of the following agents?

A. Cigarette smoke

B. Beryllium

C. Coal

D. Asbestos

29. A 38-year-old woman presents to her physician with complaints of having no menstrual period for 7 months. A β-hCG is negative. Her prolactin level is markedly elevated, at 430 ng/mL (normal range 2–17 ng/L). Which of the following is most likely to be identified on a CT scan of the head?

A. A 0.7-cm nodule in the adenohypophysis of the pituitary gland

B. An 8.0-cm nodule in the sella turcica, which compresses the infundibulum

C. A 5.0 cm nodule in the pituitary gland, which compresses the optic chiasm

D. A mass in the sella turcica, with a mammogram revealing a mass in the left breast

30. A 48-year-old man is brought to the emergency department by his family because he has been acting disoriented and confused. A complete blood cell count reveals hemoglobin of 20 g/dL. A urinalysis indicates hematuria (2+). A CT scan of the abdomen reveals a mass in the right kidney. What is the most likely cause of his disorientation and confusion?

A. Relative erythrocytosis

B. Polycythemia rubra vera

C. Secondary polycythemia

D. Pure red cell aplasia

31. A 32-year-old woman who weighs 125 kg (275 lb) is in the hospital for open reduction and internal fixation of a fractured ankle. She states that the only medication she is taking is an oral contraceptive. Four days after the surgery, she suddenly complains of chest pain and is noted to have difficulty breathing. Pulse oximetry reveals an arterial pO$_2$ of 75%. She becomes unresponsive. During resuscitation, she is noted to have pulseless electrical activity. Despite aggressive efforts, she dies. An autopsy is most likely to reveal which of the following conditions?

    A. Saddle pulmonary thromboembolus occluding the bifurcation of the pulmonary trunk

    B. Thromboembolus occluding the branch of the left pulmonary artery to the left upper lobe

    C. Acute myocardial infarct of the anterior wall of the left ventricle

    D. Fat vacuoles within the alveolar capillaries

32. A 24-year old man is involved in a motor vehicle collision and sustains a fracture of his left femur. While in the hospital, 2 days after the accident he is noted to be dyspneic and disoriented, and he develops petechiae on his trunk and axilla. What is the most likely diagnosis?

    A. Fat embolism

    B. Pulmonary thromboembolus

    C. Septic emboli

    D. Air embolus

33. A 65-year-old man with diabetes mellitus is brought to the emergency department by Emergency Medical Services because of increased confusion and gangrene of the left leg. Upon evaluation in the emergency department, he is noted to have an increased heart rate, increased respiratory rate, and decreased blood pressure. A Foley catheter is placed; however, no urine can be obtained for culture. His skin is noted to be warm to the touch. Further evaluation is most likely to reveal which of the following?

    A. Elevated CK-MB and troponin I levels

    B. Bilateral pulmonary infiltrates on radiograph of the chest

    C. Elevated central venous pressures

    D. Hypoglycemia

34. A 1-year-old boy with a history of several infections since birth, including pneumonia, is evaluated for a defect in his immune system. The extensive laboratory testing reveals that his white blood cells are unable to engulf material because of an inability to recognize opsonins coating the surface of the foreign substance. Further testing reveals the abnormality. This infant is most likely to be deficient in which of the following cellular constituents?

    A. CD31 on white blood cells

    B. CR1 on white blood cells

    C. Sialyl-Lewis-X molecules on white blood cells

    D. ICAM-1 on white blood cells

35. A 25-year-old woman presents to her family physician for an annual check-up. She is noted to have a normal heart rate and respiratory rate and blood pressure of 164/91 mm Hg. Laboratory studies show hemoglobin of 12.3 g/dL and normal electrolytes. Physical examination reveals a bruit upon auscultation of the abdomen. Which of the following treatments is most appropriate for this patient?

    A. Prescription of a β blocker

    B. Dietary supplementation with iron

    C. Radiologic imaging of the renal arteries

    D. Nothing at this time

36. A 39-year-old woman who smokes presents to her family physician because of weight gain. She has gained about 9 kg (20 lb) since her last visit 8 months ago. On physical examination, she has marked truncal obesity with abdominal stretch marks. Laboratory testing reveals elevated levels of cortisol and adrenocorticotropic hormone (ACTH), and suppression of ACTH secretion with high-dose, but not low-dose, dexamethasone. What is the most likely cause of these laboratory results?

    A. Pituitary adenoma

    B. Bilateral nodular adrenocortical hyperplasia

    C. Functioning adrenal adenoma

    D. Small cell lung cancer

37. A 23-year-old pregnant women is seeing her obstetrician for a routine visit during her third trimester. Her only complaint is some swelling of her arms and legs. She reports no other difficulties with the pregnancy. She has not experienced any headaches, sweating, or vaginal bleeding. Her physical examination reveals a blood pressure of 157/93 mm Hg. Laboratory studies show hemoglobin of 12.6 g/dL. Urinalysis is negative for glucose, but does show an elevated level of protein. This patient is at most risk for

    A. a third trimester stillbirth

    B. seizures

    C. an intracerebral hemorrhage

    D. placental abruption

38. A 54-year-old woman presents to her family physician because of a left temporal headache and diminished vision in the left eye. Upon physical examination, the patient is febrile with tenderness over the left temple. A CT scan of the head does not reveal any abnormalities. Which of the following is the best next step in management of this patient?

A. Obtain an erythrocyte sedimentation rate (ESR)

B. Make the diagnosis of a migraine headache and treat appropriately

C. Perform a biopsy of the temporal artery

D. Start the patient on a course of steroids

39. A 52-year-old man has been seen several times in the past several months by his family physician for recurrent episodes of sinusitis. However, over the past few weeks, he has developed increasing shortness of breath with exertion, and in the past 24 hours, has had blood in his urine as well as experiencing nausea and vomiting. Physical examination reveals a blood pressure of 165/95 mm Hg (he was previously always normotensive), and a urine dipstick of proteinuria (2+). Which of the following is the most likely diagnosis?

A. Goodpasture syndrome

B. Wegener granulomatosis

C. Membranous glomerulonephropathy

D. Undiagnosed diabetes mellitus

40. A neonate is noted to have a holosystolic murmur on examination. An echocardiogram is performed, and the pulmonary valve is noted to have a normal structure, and the great vessels arise from the heart as they normally should. The boy is followed by his pediatrician until the age of 10 years, at which point the murmur has disappeared. What was the most likely diagnosis for the abnormalities noted upon examination of the heart?

A. Ventricular septal defect

B. Atrial septal defect

C. Tetralogy of Fallot

D. Congenital bicuspid aortic valve

41. A 62-year-old woman with diabetes mellitus and hypertension presents to her family physician because of complaints of difficulty breathing while walking 30 yards to her mailbox. She also reports that she requires four pillows to sleep at night. She states that if she doesn't stay propped up that she has difficulty breathing. Physical examination reveals bibasilar crackles, pitting edema of the lower extremities, and pressure in the right upper quadrant of the abdomen causing distension of the right internal jugular vein to 6 cm above the sternal angle. Which of the following is the most likely underlying cause of her symptoms?

A. Severe pulmonary emphysema due to cigarette use

B. Chronic restrictive lung disease due to sarcoidosis

C. Chronic ischemic heart disease due to coronary artery atherosclerosis

D. Mitral regurgitation due to myxomatous mitral valve

42. A 37-year-old woman with rheumatoid arthritis had what was clinically diagnosed as an adrenal crisis. She does not have increased perioral pigmentation. She dies, and an autopsy reveals atrophic adrenal glands. How might her death have possibly been prevented?

A. Less rapid withdrawal of her steroid therapy

B. More rapid withdrawal of her steroid therapy

C. Replacement of her glucocorticoids with dexamethasone

D. Treatment of her Addison disease

43. A 35-year-old homeless man presents to the public hospital with complaints of a non-healing wound of his right leg, which has gotten progressively more swollen and painful over the past several days. Physical examination reveals the patient to be febrile, and he has a non-healing laceration of the right leg, overlying the tibia, with bone visible in the depths. Laboratory testing reveals a white blood cell count of 21,000 cells/mm³. A radiograph reveals destruction of the underlying bony cortex. This patient is NOT at risk for which of the following?

A. Development of a sarcoma

B. Pathologic fracture

C. Amyloidosis

D. Fatty emboli

44. A 15-year-old boy notices a swelling around his left knee, which has been progressive over the past few months. The swelling is associated with pain, which becomes unbearable. He is brought by his parents to the emergency department. Radiographic analysis of his left knee reveals an elevation of the periosteum and an infiltrative mass in the distal femur. What is the most likely diagnosis?

A. Osteosarcoma

B. Ewing sarcoma

C. Chondrosarcoma

D. Metastatic colonic adenocarcinoma

45. A 64-year-old woman presents to her family physician because of pain in her hips. She has also noted a gradual decrease in her ability to walk and climb stairs over the past several months to a year or more. She relates that the pain is worse at the end of the day and sometimes keeps her up late into the evening. Which of the following best explains this patient's disease process?

A. Physical examination may reveal Heberden or Bouchard nodes

B. The articular cartilage within her hip joints is rough, with evidence of pannus formation

C. She most likely had some form of accident as a young child that involved trauma to her hips

D. Laboratory testing will reveal IgM versus the Fc portion of IgG

46. A 42-year-old man presents to his family physician because of complaints of severe pain in the great toe of his left foot. Which of the following statements best explains this patient's condition?

A. The condition is not related to his obesity or alcohol use

B. Most likely he has some underlying condition that is causing him to produce an excessive amount of uric acid

C. This disease process will never cause him to lose renal function

D. Histologic analysis of the synovium would reveal needle-shaped, strongly negatively birefringent crystals

47. A 46-year-old man is found by his wife unresponsive on the floor. She immediately calls 911. An interview with the wife by Emergency Medical Services reveals that her husband has complained of a headache for several months now, and that she has noticed some changes in his memory. However, despite her requests, he refused to see a physician. Physical examination reveals left-sided pupillary dilation. Which of the following might a CT scan of the head reveal?

A. An infarct of the patient's right cerebral hemisphere in the distribution of the right middle cerebral artery

B. An infarct of the patient's left cerebral hemisphere in the distribution of the left anterior cerebral artery

C. An infarct of the patient's left cerebral hemisphere in the distribution of the left posterior cerebral artery

D. An infarct of the left olivary nucleus in the medulla

48. A 42-year-old woman presents to the hospital with complaints of nasal drainage and a stuffy nose. In the past day, she has also had a red discoloration of her urine. Upon physical examination, her blood pressure is noted to be 180/95 mm Hg, when normally it is 110/70 mm Hg. She is positive for c-ANCA. A biopsy of the kidney would most likely show which of the following?

A. Crescentic glomerulonephritis

B. Membranous glomerulonephropathy

C. Hyperplastic arteriolosclerosis

D. An extensive infiltrate of neutrophils

49. A 35-year-old white woman presents to her physician with complaints of fatigue. She recently has noticed weight loss, which she attributes to feeling full sooner than usual when consuming a meal. She says that when she eats fatty foods, she often has pain on the right side of her abdomen, which gradually subsides. Her family history includes her mother and her mother's father who were diagnosed with some form of anemia. Which laboratory test, in addition to a peripheral blood smear, would help confirm the diagnosis?

A. A karyotype, looking for a t(9;22)

B. An osmotic fragility test

C. A hemoglobin electrophoresis

D. A direct Coombs test

50. A 73-year-old woman sustains an infarct of her right parietal lobe due to an embolic occlusion of the right middle cerebral artery due to atherosclerosis of the internal carotid artery. She dies 1 year later, and an autopsy is performed. Examination of the brain will most likely reveal

A. a 4.5 cm cavity in the right parietal lobe

B. an ill-defined softening of the right parietal lobe

C. a well-defined friable area in the right parietal lobe

D. a tiny (< 1.0 cm) cavity in the pons

51. A 3-year-old child is being evaluated by his physician during an office visit. Over the past 2 years, the child has had several bouts of ostitis media and one severe case of pneumonia, which required hospitalization. At the time of the examination, the physician also notes that the child's skin is generally very white. The child's mother mentions that one of the child's grandmother's sisters died at a young age from recurrent infections. After further laboratory testing, the physician makes a diagnosis of

   A. chronic granulomatous disease

   B. Chédiak-Higashi syndrome

   C. severe combined immunodeficiency syndrome

   D. hyper-IgM syndrome

52. A pathologist is viewing a slide of the cerebral cortex, which shows a large collection of foamy macrophages near the surface. Overlying this collection of macrophages, between the macrophages and the meninges, is a thin rim of cerebral parenchyma. No neurons are scattered among the macrophages. What is the pathologist looking at?

   A. A recent resolving contusion

   B. An organizing infarct

   C. An active plaque in a patient with multiple sclerosis

   D. A resolving small intracerebral hemorrhage

53. A 38-year-old man presents with depression and has uncontrollable writhing movements of the extremities. His uncle died of a similar disease. What would confirm the diagnosis?

   A. Chromosomal analysis looking for CGG repeats in chromosome 4

   B. Chromosomal analysis looking for CAG repeats in chromosome 4

   C. Chromosomal analysis looking for CAG repeats in chromosome 8

   D. Autopsy of the brain looking for spongiform changes

54. A 7-year-old child is brought to his pediatrician because his parents have noticed a mass in his abdomen. The child has a history of mental retardation, and required surgery on his bladder at a young age to correct a malformation. An ultrasound is performed, and reveals a 10.0 cm mass in the left kidney. Histologic examination of the renal mass following excision reveals three histologic patterns—epithelial cells, immature-appearing cells, and stroma. What is the most likely diagnosis?

   A. Denys-Drash syndrome

   B. WAGR syndrome

   C. Beckwith-Wiedemann syndrome

   D. A sporadic Wilms tumor

55. An 8-year-old girl is brought by her parents to her pediatrician because of complaints of a headache and rash all over her body. Upon physical examination, her physician notes she has a diffuse petechial rash and also determines that the child has neck stiffness. The physician admits the young girl to the hospital and begins antibiotic treatment. Despite treatment, she dies and an autopsy is performed. The adrenal glands are noted to be markedly hemorrhagic and are described as bags of blood. What organism is causing her symptoms?

   A. *Streptococcal pneumonia*

   B. Group B streptococcus

   C. *Escherichia coli*

   D. *Neisseria meningitidis*

56. A 56-year-old obese man with a history of a recent ankle fracture, which has impaired his mobility, develops chest pain and difficulty breathing while walking to the bathroom. He is taken to the emergency department by Emergency Medical Services, where an ECG and cardiac enzyme testing are performed, both of which reveal no evidence of an acute myocardial infarct. He is admitted to the hospital for further testing. The next day, 24 hours after his initial pain, the patient has chest pain and dyspnea and then collapses. Despite resuscitation, he dies. An autopsy reveals a large saddle pulmonary thromboembolus and a pleural-based wedge of firm, red-tan parenchyma. Microscopic examination of this wedge-shaped area will reveal

   A. sheets of lipid-laden macrophages

   B. intact alveolar septae with increased eosinophilia of the cytoplasm and loss of nuclear basophilia

   C. giant cells surrounding granulomas with a central area of necrosis

   D. neoplastic cells lining the alveolar septae, with focal areas of invasion into the pulmonary parenchyma

57. A 42-year-old patient presents to his family physician because of complaints of weight loss despite a good appetite. His other complaints are rapid heart rate and diarrhea. He is subsequently identified to have a thyroid-stimulating hormone-secreting pituitary adenoma. A transsphenoidal resection of the mass is performed. The pathologist evaluating the tumor must identify which of the following conditions to reliably diagnose the mass as malignant?

   A. A loss of the reticulin framework of the gland

   B. Multiple mitotic figures

   C. Nuclear and cytoplasmic pleomorphism

   D. Evidence of invasion of surrounding tissue

58. A 26-year-old woman presents to the hospital with complaints of a rapid heart rate and palpitations. She has lost about 14 kg (30 lb) in the past 5 months despite having a good appetite. She complains of left lower abdominal pain. Laboratory evaluation reveals that her thyroid-stimulating hormone (TSH) level is barely detectable and her T_4 level is elevated. No autoantibodies are detected in her serum. A brain MRI reveals no masses in the pituitary gland. An ultrasound of her thyroid gland is interpreted as normal. A CT scan of the abdomen and pelvis shows a 7-cm complex cystic mass of the left ovary, but is otherwise unremarkable. What is the most likely diagnosis?

A. Graves disease

B. Toxic goiter

C. Struma ovarii

D. Ectopic production of TSH

59. A 10-year-old boy develops knee pain while playing soccer. A radiograph reveals a mass in the proximal portion of the tibia. A biopsy is performed, and the diagnosis of osteosarcoma is made. The patient had a brother who was diagnosed with an osteosarcoma and also a tumor of his eye. What is the normal role of the protein product of the gene involved with his tumor?

A. Down-regulation of β-catenin

B. Binding of E2F

C. Arresting of cell cycle by transcription of p21

D. Arresting of cell cycle by transcription of p27

60. A 46-year-old man has a nodule in the left lobe of his thyroid gland. The nodule is surgically excised, and the diagnosis of a follicular carcinoma is made by the pathologist based upon histologic identification of invasion of the capsule. If a fine needle aspirate (FNA) had been performed prior to the surgery, the diagnosis would have been

A. follicular carcinoma

B. follicular adenoma

C. follicular neoplasm

D. no thyroid nodules can be effectively diagnosed by FNA

61. A 54-year-old white woman falls at home and sustains an ankle fracture. During her subsequent hospitalization, she is found to have a white blood cell count of 50,000 cells/μL composed predominantly of lymphocytes. Flow cytometry reveals the cells to be positive for CD5. Which of the following is his most likely diagnosis?

A. Chronic lymphocytic leukemia

B. Mantle cell lymphoma

C. T-cell acute lymphoblastic leukemia

D. Follicular lymphoma with leukemic phase

62. During an assault, a 15-year-old boy is struck on the head with a baseball bat, producing a large 6-inch laceration that requires 25 sutures. He returns to his physician in 3 weeks for removal of the sutures and in 6 months for a follow-up appointment to assess for any neurologic changes and other sequelae of the blow to his head. Evaluation of the scar at 6 months will reveal

A. a barely visible line in the skin

B. a scar that is the same size as the original wound

C. a scar that has the strength of the original intact skin

D. an easily visible scar that is smaller than the original laceration

63. A 25-year-old woman with a history of phenylketonuria (PKU) has been on a less restrictive diet for a few years. However, she recently has been advised by her family physician to return to a phenylalanine-free diet for a period of 1 year or more. Which of the following best explains her advised change in diet?

A. She is planning on becoming pregnant

B. She has developed cirrhosis of the liver

C. She has developed acute renal failure

D. She is planning on having elective weight-reduction surgery

64. A 42-year-old African-American man has been diagnosed with hypertension for the past 10 years and treated with medication. One morning, he is found unresponsive by his wife. He is taken to the emergency department and pronounced dead by the physician. An autopsy revealed cardiac hypertrophy and a narrowing of the aorta just distal to the ligamentum arteriosum, with dilation of the intercostal artery's ostia. How could the death have possibly been prevented?

A. Better management of his hypertension with prescription medication

B. Early diagnosis of the cause of his hypertension by physical examination

C. Evaluation of the aortic valve with an echocardiogram

D. The death could not have been prevented

65. A 17-year-old girl develops an infection that is documented to be caused by *Neisseria gonorrhoeae*. Which of the following is she NOT at risk for in the future?

A. An ectopic pregnancy

B. Tubo-ovarian adhesions and possible torsion and infarction of an ovary

C. Infertility

D. A surface epithelial serous cystadenocarcinoma

66. A 42-year-old woman with 12 lifetime sexual partners presents to her family physician because of vaginal bleeding. During her visit, a colposcopic examination is performed and a biopsy of an acetowhite lesion on her cervix is taken, which reveals invasive squamous cell carcinoma. Which of the following statements is FALSE?

    A. The lesion most likely resulted from infection with human papillomavirus (HPV) type 11

    B. Her condition could have been prevented by having regular PAP smears

    C. The virus responsible for her condition produces a protein (E7), which hinders the ability of the RB protein to bind elongation factor

    D. A biopsy of the cervix prior to the development of invasive tumor would have shown cervical intraepithelial neoplasia (CIN) grade III

67. On his day for covering frozen sections, a pathology resident received a large uterus that has multiple well-circumscribed nodules within the myometrium, some of which bulge into the endometrium and some of which project from the serosal surface. Which of the following is NOT a common complication of this condition?

    A. Metastases to the lungs

    B. Pelvic pain

    C. Vaginal bleeding

    D. Infertility

68. A 39-year-old woman has a biopsy performed of a mass in the left breast. The biopsy reveals sclerosing adenosis, fibrocystic changes, and lobular carcinoma in situ. No evidence of an invasive carcinoma or ductal carcinoma in situ component is identified. What is the next best step in the treatment of this patient?

    A. Counsel the patient regarding the possibility of a bilateral mastectomy

    B. Schedule her for surgery again and remove more tissue from the site to prevent a recurrence and possible progression to invasive lobular carcinoma

    C. Perform a radial mastectomy, followed with chemotherapy and radiation therapy

    D. Nothing, because the lesion is not invasive and was completely removed by the biopsy

69. A 50-year-old man is witnessed to veer off the road and collide with a telephone pole. He is conscious when the ambulance arrives and is taken to the hospital. He tells the physician in the emergency department that he just passed out at the wheel. Auscultation of the chest reveals a crescendo-decrescendo, ejection-type systolic murmur. If he had died in the motor vehicle accident, which of these would have most likely been identified in his heart at the time of autopsy?

    A. Iron accumulations within the myocardium

    B. Vacuolated myocardial cells containing glycogen

    C. Firm yellow nodules on the aortic valve cusps

    D. A dilated aortic valve ring due to prominent cholesterol accumulation

70. A 40-year-old man presents to the emergency department because of sudden onset of severe sharp substernal pain in his chest, which radiates to his back. On physical examination, his blood pressure is 200/120 mm Hg, and he has a harsh decrescendo diastolic murmur at the left sternal border. Which of the following is the most likely diagnosis?

    A. An aortic dissection

    B. An acute myocardial infarct

    C. A pulmonary thromboembolus

    D. Acute pancreatitis

71. A 53-year-old white man who uses alcohol frequently and takes nonsteroidal anti-inflammatory drugs (NSAIDs) for his knee pain presents to the emergency department with acute abdominal pain. On physical examination, he is pale. His blood pressure is 88/43 mm Hg, and his pulse is 130 beats/min. Laboratory testing shows a hemoglobin of 12.5 g/dL. He is taken to the operating room, where he dies just prior to the start of surgery. An autopsy is performed and will most likely reveal

    A. a perforated gastric peptic ulcer

    B. diverticulitis

    C. an ulcerated and bleeding intestinal type gastric adenocarcinoma

    D. an infarcted segment of small intestine due to a volvulus

72. A 49-year-old white man who smokes, drinks six cans of beer per day, and eats plenty of fatty foods presents to his family physician with complaints of long-standing indigestion. After an ECG and cardiac enzyme testing rule out a myocardial infarct, an esophagogastroduodenoscopy (EGD) is performed. The EGD reveals a reddened esophageal mucosa just proximal to the gastroesophageal junction. A biopsy of this area is most likely to reveal

    A. fungal hyphae

    B. adenocarcinoma

    C. glandular metaplasia

    D. nuclei with viral inclusions

73. A 60-year-old non-alcoholic woman presents to her family physician because of pallor and consistent fatigue after walking six blocks to work. A CBC reveals a hemoglobin of 7.0 g/dL with an MCV of 122. A peripheral blood smear has oval macrocytes and segmented neutrophils. She reports eating a normal healthy diet. A rectal examination reveals stool guaiac test is negative. Evaluation of her gastrointestinal tract will most likely reveal

A. a perforated duodenal ulcer

B. an ulcerated and bleeding intestinal adenocarcinoma

C. atrophic gastric mucosa with focal intestinal metaplasia

D. atrophic duodenal villi

74. A 43-year-old woman presents to the emergency department because of two episodes of vomiting blood. An emergent EGD reveals two ulcers, one recent and one healed on the greater curvature of the stomach, and a third ulcer in the duodenum. Hypertrophic gastric folds are present throughout the stomach. Which of the following will additional history, physical examination, laboratory testing, and diagnostic studies most likely reveal?

A. A history of heavy nonsteroidal anti-inflammatory drug (NSAID) use

B. An elevated level of gastrin and a mass in the head of the pancreas

C. Heavy infection of gastric mucosa with *Helicobacter pylori*

D. Antimitochondrial and antiparietal cell antibodies

75. A widowed 78-year-old woman with a history of diabetes mellitus is admitted for elective hip replacement. She tolerates her procedure well, but during her second postoperative night she becomes confused and experiences visual hallucinations. Her pulse is 130 beats/min, and her blood pressure increases from 125/80 mm Hg to 190/120 mmHg. Her oxygen saturation remains stable at 97% on room air. Which of the following is most likely responsible for the patient's alteration in mental status?

A. Acute alcohol withdrawal

B. Fat embolism

C. An acute myocardial infarct

D. Dementia

76. A 30-year-old woman presents to her family physician because of complaints of stiffness in her fingers. She works as a transcriptionist, and lately her work has caused her a great deal of discomfort. She is afraid of losing her job because of reduced turn-around time on reports. She relates that the stiffness is worse in the morning, but gets better as the day progresses. Which of the following is her most likely diagnosis?

A. Osteoporosis

B. Osteoarthritis

C. Rheumatoid arthritis

D. Gout

77. A 9-year-old boy is brought by his parents to their pediatrician because of the boy's history of diarrhea and foul-smelling stool. Comparison of the boy's height and weight to a normal growth curve indicates that he is in the less than 5% percentile categories (small for age). A biopsy of his duodenum shows a mucosa with flattened villi. How should this patient be managed?

A. Contact Child Protective Services because of suspected neglect

B. Perform segmental resection of the duodenum

C. Increase his caloric intake and reduce the amount of fat in his diet

D. Remove food that is wheat-based from his diet

78. A 27-year-old man who is an IV drug user presents to the emergency department because of abdominal pain. He reports red discoloration of his urine. On examination, he is hypertensive and has no dyspnea, chest pain, or hemoptysis. After initial evaluation in the clinic, the patient is admitted to the hospital. A chest radiograph and radiographic imaging of the kidneys, bladder, and pelvis reveal no abnormalities. Laboratory studies reveal elevated levels of amylase and lipase and an elevated level of creatinine. The patient is positive for hepatitis B surface antigen. Which of the following is the most likely diagnosis?

A. Polyarteritis nodosa

B. Kawasaki disease

C. Goodpasture syndrome

D. Acute pancreatitis

79. A 37-year-old woman presents to the emergency department with complaints of right lower quadrant pain. A review of symptoms reveals that she also has pain in her joints and a skin lesion on the foot. She undergoes surgery, and her appendix is removed. Pathologic evaluation of the appendix reveals granulomas in the submucosa and clusters of lymphocytes throughout the wall. What is her diagnosis?

A. Ulcerative colitis

B. Crohn disease

C. Acute tuberculous appendicitis

D. *Entamoeba histolytica*

80. A 28-year-old woman presents to her physician because of complaints of a mass on her left shoulder that has grown rapidly in size over the past several months. The nodule is nontender, and the patient is afebrile. She has multiple large (> 2 cm) hyperpigmented macules on her skin, and small brown dome-shaped elevations on her irises. Which of the following conditions is the most likely diagnosis for her rapidly growing mass?

A. A malignant peripheral nerve sheath tumor

B. A hamartoma composed of smooth muscle

C. A benign tumor of Schwann cells

D. An angiomyolipoma

81. A 63-year-old man presents to his family physician with complaints of abdominal pain and constipation. A subsequent barium enema reveals an "apple-core" lesion in the sigmoid colon. The barium enema also reveals multiple diverticula. The patient is scheduled for surgery. At the time of the surgery, the segment of bowel with the "apple-core" lesion noted on the barium enema is resected. When the pathologist opens the bowel, no mucosal lesions are identified. Which of the following statements is correct?

A. The surgeon must operate again because the tumor was not resected

B. Despite the segmental colonic resection, this condition can recur in this patient

C. The patient most likely has segmental loss of Meissner plexus

D. The patient most likely has Crohn disease

82. A 53-year-old alcoholic with a history of multiple falls is brought to the hospital by his family, who reports the patient has developed psychiatric symptoms. While in the hospital, he sustains an episode of ventricular fibrillation and is unable to be revived. At autopsy, he is found to have a dilated cardiomyopathy and an extracerebral hemorrhage. Which type is this hemorrhage most likely to be?

A. An acute subdural hemorrhage

B. A chronic subdural hemorrhage

C. An acute epidural hemorrhage

D. Subarachnoid hemorrhage

83. A neuropathologist is summoned to the pathology gross room by the neurosurgical team to perform a frozen section on a cerebral neoplasm that they are currently resecting. All of the features required for a diagnosis are present on the slide the pathologist will review. Based on the grading criteria, which of the following tumors will be the most difficult for the pathologist to diagnose?

A. A low-grade astrocytoma

B. A glioblastoma multiforme

C. A gliosarcoma (glioblastoma multiforme with sarcomatous pattern)

D. An anaplastic astrocytoma

84. A 48-year-old white woman with a history of Hashimoto thyroiditis presents to the emergency department because of right upper quadrant abdominal pain. During her subsequent evaluation, a biopsy of the liver is performed. The liver biopsy reveals a prominent number of lymphocytes within the portal tract, some extending beyond the limiting plate. Serologies for viral hepatitis reveal no evidence of an acute or chronic infection. Additional serologies would most likely reveal which antibody that is responsible for the liver disease?

A. Anti-mitochondrial

B. Anti-smooth muscle or anti–liver-kidney

C. Anti-TSH receptor

D. Anti-scl70

85. A 13-year-old boy is brought to his pediatrician by his parents because of his complaints of fatigue. A CBC reveals a white blood cell count of 200,000 cells/μL. Analysis of the cells reveals hypodiploidy and a t(9;22) translocation. What should the physician tell the family about this boy's condition?

A. He has acute leukemia with multiple good prognostic indicators

B. If he has a recurrence, it is unlikely to involve the central nervous system

C. He has acute lymphoblastic leukemia (ALL) with multiple bad prognostic indicators

D. He has chronic myelogenous leukemia (CML) with a good prognosis

86. A 3-month-old male infant is placed by his mother face down in his crib. Upon waking the next morning and checking on her child, the mother notices that he is unresponsive. She immediately calls for an ambulance. Upon arrival, the emergency medical technicians determine that the infant is not revivable and do not transport him to the hospital. The death is reported to the medical examiner, who subsequently performs an autopsy. The only gross or microscopic finding is petechial hemorrhages of the thymus and pleurae. Police investigation of the scene and questioning of the parents does not reveal any suspicious circumstances. What is the most likely cause of death?

A. Sudden infant death syndrome

B. Intentional suffocation by the mother

C. Accidental suffocation due to the infant being placed into the crib face down

D. Accidental ingestion of the mother's prescription medication by the infant

87. A 47-year-old man presents to his family physician because of recent onset of yellow eyes and a generalized feeling of malaise, with some right upper quadrant abdominal pain. As part of his evaluation, his physician orders a biopsy of the liver. The liver biopsy reveals a neutrophilic infiltrate of the parenchyma, ropy and eosinophilic condensations within the hepatocytes, and sclerosis of the central veins. What is the most likely etiology of his condition?

   A. Alcohol abuse
   B. Hepatitis B infection
   C. Hepatitis E infection
   D. Bacterial colitis with hematogenous dissemination to the liver

88. A 58-year-old white man presents to his family physician because of complaints of early satiety. A physical examination reveals splenomegaly. A complete blood cell count indicates a white blood cell count of 73,000 cells/μL. Laboratory testing of his blood reveals a t(9,22) translocation. Which of the following statements regarding his condition is NOT true?

   A. A smear of the peripheral blood will show an increased number of basophils
   B. The level of leukocyte alkaline phosphatase may be decreased
   C. A peripheral blood smear will show a large number of myeloblasts
   D. A smear of his peripheral blood will show a large number of myelocytes, metamyelocytes, and bands

89. A 41-year-old woman presents to her family physician because of intolerable pain upon swallowing. During the physical examination, the physician notices the patient winces upon palpation of her thyroid gland. If a fine needle aspirate (FNA) were performed, what would most likely be identified?

   A. Lymphocytes and follicular epithelial cells with oncocytic change
   B. Multinucleated giant cells
   C. Cells with pseudoinclusions and optically clear nuclei
   D. Papillary collections of follicular epithelial cells without fibrovascular cores

90. A 28-year-old pregnant woman in her third trimester collides with another vehicle while driving to the store. She sustains a compound fracture of the left femur and loses approximately 2.5 L of blood. Because of rapid response by the local ambulance service, she receives blood in a short amount of time and survives the incident. During her subsequent hospitalization, she develops cold intolerance and hypoglycemia. Previously, she had no evidence of gestational diabetes mellitus. What is her most likely diagnosis?

   A. Sudden onset of type 2 diabetes mellitus
   B. Sheehan syndrome
   C. Metastatic breast cancer
   D. An undiagnosed craniopharyngioma

91. A 28-year-old woman has been taking clindamycin for 1 week for cellulitis. She develops a fever and nonbloody diarrhea. Fecal leukocytes are present. A colonoscopy is most likely to reveal

   A. a patchy layer of thin tan material on the mucosa
   B. flask-shaped ulcers
   C. mucosal erythema and oval ulcers in the rectum
   D. patchy mucosal erythema associated with deep linear ulcers

92. A 51-year-old man has a history of hypertension, a 12-year history of diabetes mellitus type 2, and he also has hyperlipidemia. He has smoked one pack of cigarettes a day for 35 years. He takes a β blocker for his hypertension and insulin therapy for his diabetes. He complains of abdominal pain to his wife. She wants to take him to the hospital, but he refuses. Several hours after the pain begins, he becomes unresponsive. Emergency Medical Services are called, and on arrival at the emergency department, the patient's blood pressure is 75 mm over palpable with a pulse of 90 beats per minute. What is the most likely cause of this patient's death?

   A. A ruptured acute myocardial infarct
   B. Acute pancreatitis
   C. A ruptured abdominal aortic aneurysm
   D. An intestinal volvulus, with resultant infarction of the small bowel

93. A 16-year-old girl presents to her family physician with concerns because she has never had a menstrual period. On physical examination, she has Tanner stage 1 breast development with normal axillary and pubic hair development. Her blood pressure is significantly higher in her arms than in her legs. A pelvic examination is unremarkable. Her parents are both phenotypically normal, and she has no brothers or sisters with any type of hereditary condition. What is the most likely diagnosis?

   A. Turner syndrome
   B. Androgen insensitivity syndrome
   C. Polycystic ovarian disease
   D. Hypogonadotrophic hypogonadism

94. An 11-year-old child is brought to the hospital by his parents because of a red discoloration of his urine. He is also having blood in his stool and complaints of joint and abdominal pain. A biopsy of the kidney is performed. Which of the following is most likely to be found on the biopsy?

    A. Spikes on the silver stain

    B. Tram-tracks on the silver stain

    C. IgA positivity on immunofluorescence

    D. Fusion of the foot processes

95. A 16-year-old boy is brought to the emergency department by his parents because of his complaints of pain on urination. His work-up includes a urine culture that subsequently grows *Escherichia coli* 2 days after his visit to the emergency department. On the day he was seen in the emergency department, he was placed on antibiotics, which would adequately treat the *E coli* that subsequently grew. How should this boy be followed up?

    A. He needs no follow-up because he received appropriate antimicrobial therapy for his urinary tract infection

    B. A second antibiotic should be added to ensure coverage of *E coli* and prevent pyelonephritis

    C. Subsequent renal ultrasound to ensure that the infection did not spread to kidney

    D. His genitourinary tract should be evaluated for any congenital abnormalities

96. A 15-year-old boy develops acute lymphoblastic leukemia. Shortly after birth, he was diagnosed with duodenal atresia, which was treated with surgical intervention. Which of the following factors most likely contributed to the development of his condition?

    A. Maternal tobacco use

    B. Maternal alcohol use

    C. Maternal age of 48 years

    D. Maternal exposure to ionizing radiation

97. A 13-year-old girl experiences severe leg pain while playing soccer. She reports no falls or recent trauma. A radiograph taken when she is in the emergency department reveals a soft tissue density and fracture of the diaphysis of her right femur. What is the most likely cause of the fracture?

    A. Trauma

    B. Osteosarcoma

    C. Ewing sarcoma

    D. Chondrosarcoma

98. A 23-year-old man with a recent history of a viral-type illness presents to the emergency department because of complaints of weakness in his legs. He is admitted to the hospital and the weakness progresses into his thighs and hips. What is his prognosis?

    A. Fair, with treatment the progression of the muscle weakness will stop, but the weakness will remain for the remainder of his life

    B. Good, with treatment the muscle weakness will definitely stop and not progress further

    C. Good, with treatment the condition will run its course, and his life can be saved and he should have no residual sequelae

    D. Dismal, the condition will continue to progress, involving his respiratory muscles, causing his death even if treated

99. A 67-year-old man with a long history of smoking presents to the hospital with complaints of increasing shortness of breath. During his evaluation, a small mass is identified in the lower lobe of the left lung. Laboratory testing reveals an elevated level of cortisol, a decreased level of ferritin, and increased total iron-binding capacity. A colonoscopy reveals a mass in the descending colon. The patient is taken to the operating room, where a wedge resection of the pulmonary nodule is performed. A frozen section reveals cells with a high nuclear to cytoplasmic ratio and evidence of nuclear molding. What should the surgeon do next?

    A. End the operation; he has removed the pulmonary metastatic nodule derived from the colon carcinoma

    B. End the operation and inform the clinical team to proceed with radiation and chemotherapy in the treatment of the pulmonary nodule

    C. Perform a left-sided pneumonectomy to ensure a cure for the pulmonary nodule

    D. Ask the pathologist if the margins are clear; if not, remove more lung

100. A 5-year-old child is brought to his pediatrician because his parents have noticed that his hands and feet are swelling, and they can feel lumps in his neck. In addition, his mouth appears redder than normal. A physical examination reveals a blood pressure of 110/71 mm Hg, a temperature of 41°C (105°F), and cervical lymphadenopathy. Which of the following complications is this child at most risk for in the future?

    A. A restrictive cardiomyopathy

    B. Thoracic aortic aneurysm

    C. Coronary artery aneurysm

    D. Mitral stenosis

101. A 79-year-old man with Alzheimer disease aspirates a large bolus of food during a meal. The food does not occlude his airway. However, shortly afterward he develops severe dyspnea. He is taken to the hospital and despite therapy, he dies. An autopsy is performed. What will be identified in the lungs of this patient?

A. Prominent alveolar septal lymphocytic infiltrate

B. Thick bands of eosinophilic, proteinaceous material layered on the alveolar septae

C. Pulmonary edema

D. Most likely nothing of significance

102. A 25-year-old woman presents to the hospital because of blindness in her right eye. She has a twin sister with a similar condition. Many years ago, her sister went blind in one eye, but the blindness resolved and she has never had any other neurologic symptoms. The physician obtains cerebrospinal fluid and submits it for laboratory testing. The laboratory testing reveals oligoclonal bands. What should the physician tell the patient regarding her condition?

A. The blindness is most likely not caused by the same condition that your sister had, so we need to test you for antinuclear antibodies

B. This may be your only episode of neurologic dysfunction, but most likely you will have other episodes in the future, not necessarily involving the eyes

C. Like your sister, this will be the only episode you have like this

D. Unlike your sister, you will probably have multiple neurologic episodes and end up wheelchair bound

103. A 20-year-old man is being evaluated by his family physician because of an inability to conceive a child with his wife, despite numerous attempts. His physician notices the patient has atrophic testicles and a reduced amount of body hair. Of the following, what further testing should be done to evaluate this patient?

A. Evaluation of cognitive abilities, looking for mental retardation

B. Breast examination

C. Echocardiogram, looking for coarctation of the aorta

D. Body mass index determination and evaluation of eating habits

104. A 56-year old man with a long-standing history of hypertension presents to his family physician because of complaints of dyspnea on exertion. A physical examination reveals bibasilar crackles. An ECG reveals left ventricular hypertrophy by voltage criteria, but no evidence of ST elevation or depression. Cardiac enzymes levels are within normal limits. An echocardiogram of the heart reveals dilation of the left ventricle. Which of the following is the most likely diagnosis?

A. Low-output, left-sided congestive heart failure due to systolic dysfunction

B. High-output, left-sided congestive heart failure due to diastolic dysfunction

C. Low-output, right-sided congestive heart failure due to systolic dysfunction

D. High-output, left-sided congestive heart failure due to systolic dysfunction

105. A 38-year-old African-American woman marketing executive has bilateral hilar lymphadenopathy on a plain chest radiograph performed during a health insurance examination. The lung fields are otherwise unremarkable, and her PPD skin test is negative. Which of the following statements concerning her diagnosis is correct?

A. She may have a decreased level of angiotensin-converting enzyme (ACE)

B. Involvement of the lymph nodes is more serious than involvement of the lungs

C. The disease process is confined to the lungs and lymph nodes

D. The condition may be associated with hypercalcemia

106. A 43-year-old woman underwent an exploratory laparotomy following a motor vehicle accident. At the time of the surgery, she was found to have a right ovarian mass, which was subsequently diagnosed as a granulosa cell tumor. She is nulligravida with a history of diabetes mellitus and obesity. Which of the following is NOT a possible complication of her above-mentioned conditions?

A. Vaginal bleeding

B. Complex hyperplasia of the endometrium

C. Invasive ductal carcinoma of the breast

D. Invasive endometrial adenocarcinoma

E. All of the following are possible complications

107. A 28-year-old woman of Mediterranean descent presents to her family physician with complaints of heavy menstrual periods. She reports increased fatigue on review of systems, and she says "anemia" runs in her family. Laboratory testing reveals a hemoglobin of 8.0 g/dL, MCV of 82, and a low MCHC. What additional information would be most helpful in determining if this woman has a genetic cause of anemia?

A. Sickle index

B. Meltzer index

C. HbA_2

D. Osmotic fragility test

108. An 80-year-old man has experienced a progressive decline of cognitive function over the past 5 years. Currently, he does not remember any family members, with the exception of his wife. He sometimes gets lost within his own house. Evaluation of his brain will reveal cellular accumulations of

A. iron

B. fat

C. protein

D. lipofuscin

109. A 43-year-old man who is a chronic alcoholic presents to the hospital with fatigue and a burning sensation in his feet. Laboratory testing is performed, and a peripheral blood smear reveals anemia with hypersegmented neutrophils and oval macrocytes. The patient is given folate, and the anemia resolves. However, the burning sensation in his feet worsens. Which of the following statements best explains this patient's symptomatology?

A. The patient had megaloblastic anemia due to folate deficiency, and the worsening of the sensation in his feet is unrelated

B. The patient lacks the ability to absorb the folate due to pancreatic insufficiency from chronic pancreatitis

C. The patient had a vitamin B_{12} deficiency, and the treatment with folate partially masked its effects, treating the anemia but not the neurologic changes

D. The patient's peripheral neuropathy is secondary to thiamine deficiency, and addition of folate to the diet without thiamine supplementation caused increased demand for thiamine and acute worsening of his neuropathy

110. A 48-year-old man presents to the hospital with back pain. A full-body CT scan reveals a single osteolytic lesion in the vertebral column at the level of the seventh thoracic vertebra. Serum protein electrophoresis does not reveal an M spike. A biopsy of the mass reveals basophilic cells with eccentric nuclei and a clear, perinuclear area. What is the most likely diagnosis?

A. Solitary plasmacytoma

B. Monoclonal gammopathy of undetermined significance (MGUS)

C. Multiple myeloma

D. Diffuse large B-cell lymphoma

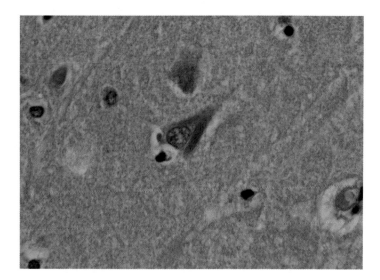

111. How would the patient shown in the above image present?

A. Memory loss

B. Seizure activity

C. Choreiform movements

D. Flat affect and shuffling gait

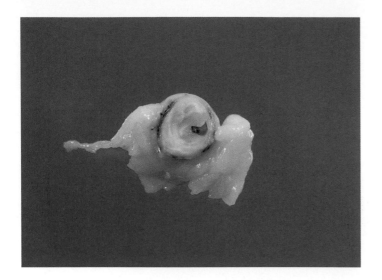

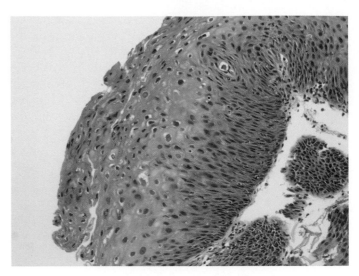

112. At autopsy, the above specimen was taken from a 57-year-old man who died suddenly at home. The lesion above was the direct cause of his death. What symptoms would this man have complained of prior to his death?

A. Sudden onset of chest pain with radiation to the left arm, associated with nausea and vomiting

B. Shortness of breath after climbing two flights of stairs, when he normally only becomes short of breath after climbing five flights of stairs

C. Shortness of breath after climbing four flights of stairs, which is unchanged from his normal pattern

D. Difficulty breathing at night and swelling of the ankles

114. The patient in this image was most likely exposed to which of the following infectious agents?

A. Human papillomavirus type 6 (HPV-6)

B. HPV-33

C. Herpes simplex virus

D. *Neisseria gonorrhoeae*

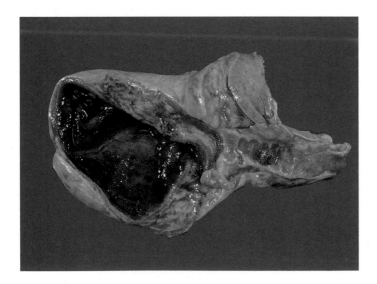

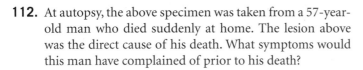

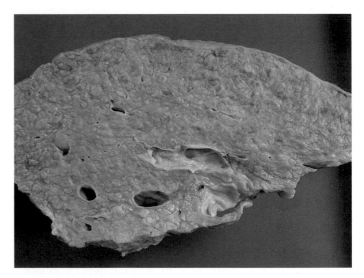

115. Of the following, which is a likely cause of death of a patient with the condition shown in the image?

A. Tumor metastases to the brain and lungs

B. Congestive heart failure

C. Gastrointestinal hemorrhage

D. Bowel obstruction

113. Which of the following is a likely complication of the condition shown in this image?

A. Metastases to the liver

B. Peritonitis

C. Acute pancreatitis

D. Gastric peptic ulcer

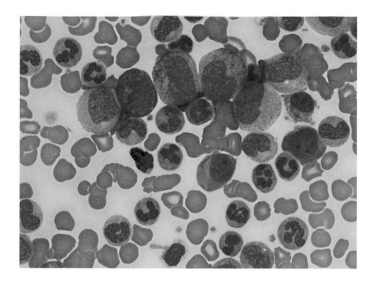

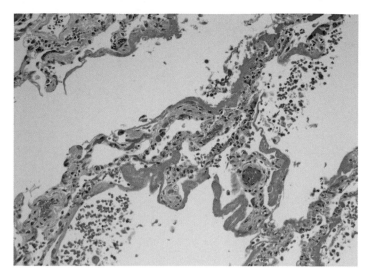

116. A patient with the condition shown in the image would most likely have which of the following?

   A. A t(15;17) translocation

   B. CD5 positive neoplastic cells

   C. A decreased or normal leukocyte alkaline phosphatase level

   D. An eosinophilia

118. Which of the following conditions is NOT a common cause of the changes featured in the image?

   A. Sepsis

   B. Metastatic neoplasm

   C. Head injuries

   D. Aspiration of gastric contents by a patient with dementia

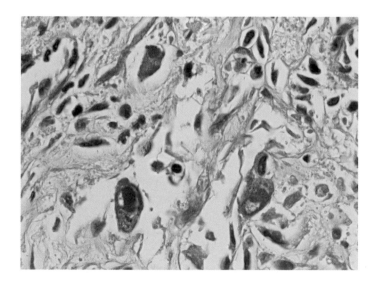

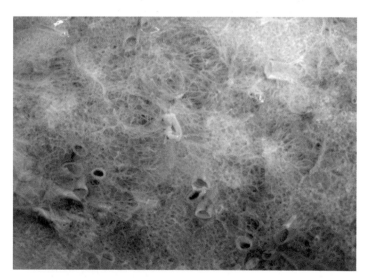

117. Which of the following conditions does the patient in this image have?

   A. An infection with cytomegalovirus

   B. An infection with herpes simplex virus

   C. A nodular sclerosis type Hodgkin lymphoma

   D. Infection with *Entamoeba histolytica*

119. Which of the following is the etiology for the disease process shown in the above image?

   A. Hypersensitivity to inhaled allergens

   B. Cigarette smoking

   C Beryllium exposure

   D. An obstructing tumor in the main stem bronchus

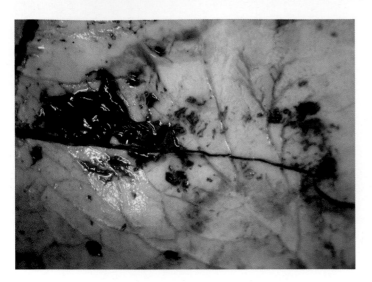

120. Which of the following statements best explains the condition shown in this image?

A. It commonly occurs in alcoholics and the elderly who fall and strike their head

B. Patients become unconscious immediately and remain unconscious indefinitely

C. The hemorrhage is most commonly from tears of the sagittal sinus

D. The condition results most commonly from a fracture of the temporal bone

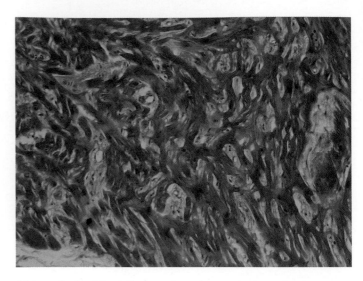

122. Which of the following clinical scenarios bests fits the image?

A. A 32-year-old woman with no recent complaints or significant past medical history found dead in bed by her husband

B. A 45-year-old chronic alcoholic with congestive heart failure

C. A 77-year-old man with amyloidosis

D. A 56-year-old man with hypertension and diabetes mellitus who complains of chest pain while bike riding with friends

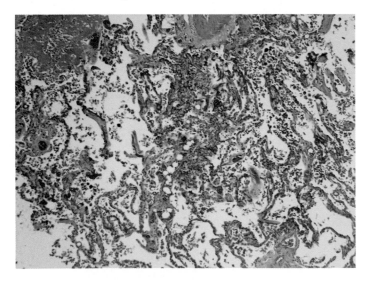

121. Which of the following is the most likely clinical scenario for the condition in the image?

A. A hospitalized patient who suddenly becomes unresponsive 12 days after a motor vehicle accident that resulted in a femur fracture

B. Dyspnea and mental status changes in a patient 1 day after a motor vehicle accident, which resulted in a fractured femur

C. Aspiration of gastric contents by a neuromuscularly impaired individual

D. A pregnant woman who suddenly becomes short of breath after the delivery of her infant

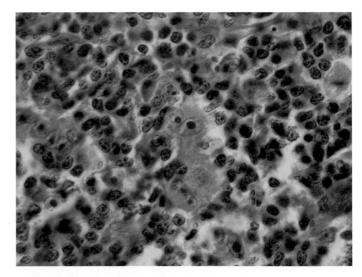

123. The patient in this image has which of the following conditions?

A. An infection with cytomegalovirus

B. An infection with herpes simplex virus

C. The nodular sclerosis variant of Hodgkin lymphoma

D. Burkitt lymphoma

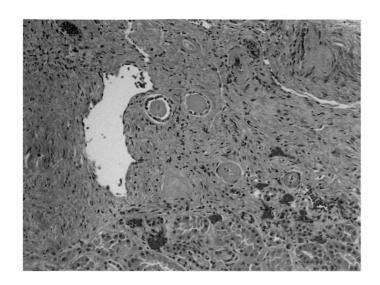

124. This image depicts which of the following conditions?

  A. Hyperplastic arteriolosclerosis

  B. Kimmelstiel-Wilson lesion

  C. Hyaline arteriolosclerosis

  D. A neurofibroma

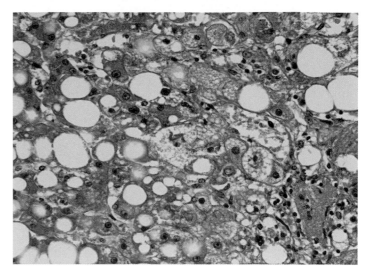

126. What most likely accounted for the microscopic changes in this patient's liver?

  A. Chronic hepatitis C infection

  B. Acute hepatitis B infection

  C. Alcohol use

  D. α_1-Antitrypsin deficiency

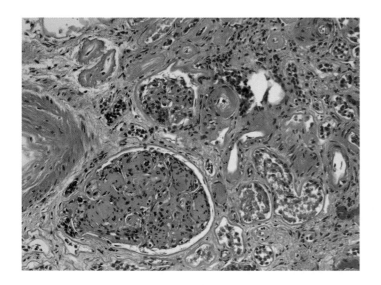

125. Physical examination and laboratory evaluation of a patient with the disease process represented by this image would most likely reveal

  A. a blood glucose level of 250 mg/dL

  B. a 24-hour urine protein level of 5.5 grams, hematuria (2+), and a blood pressure of 195/100 mm Hg

  C. schistocytes in the peripheral blood smear

  D. anemia, thrombocytopenia, and elevated BUN and creatinine

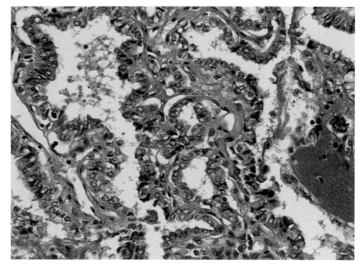

127. This tissue shown in the image was taken from a resected thyroid mass. Examination of other areas of this tumor would most likely reveal

  A. amyloid deposition

  B. psammoma bodies

  C. extensive hemosiderin deposition

  D. numerous mitotic figures

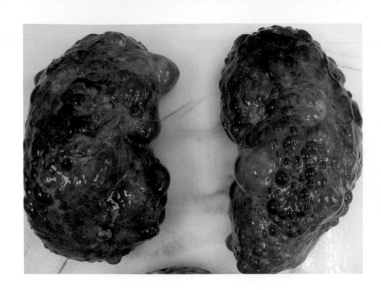

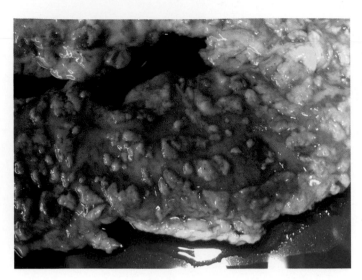

128. The kidneys shown in this image are from a 24-year-old man. What would have been the most likely cause of his death?

A. A subarachnoid hemorrhage due to a ruptured berry aneurysm

B. A hypertensive crisis

C. Chronic renal failure

D. Metastatic renal cell carcinoma

130. Which of the following statements best explains the condition shown in this image?

A. The patient has a 100% chance of developing an invasive colonic adenocarcinoma during his lifetime

B. The condition can affect any segment of the gastrointestinal tract

C. The patient recently finished a course of antibiotic therapy

D. The patient is most likely septic and hypotensive

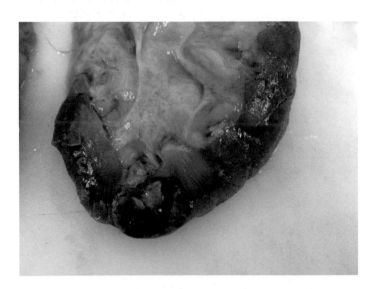

129. The kidney shown in the image was resected from a 63-year-old man with a history of smoking two packages of cigarettes a day for 40 years, who presented with hematuria. What is the most likely diagnosis?

A. Papillary necrosis

B. Renal cell carcinoma

C. Angiomyolipoma

D. Hemangioma

PRACTICE EXAMINATION ANSWERS

Question 1

Answer: C. Due to conditioning, the marathon runner will have physiologic hypertrophy of the heart. Because physical exercise is a normal process, the changes in the heart are physiologic. The myocardial cells cannot divide, so the heart cannot undergo hyperplasia. A marathon runner would have hypertrophy of skeletal muscle, not atrophy.

Question 2

Answer: D. The sudden focal change in neurologic function is consistent with a stroke. It has lasted longer than 24 hours, so it is not a transient ischemic attack, and it is not global in nature. Weakness of the left leg can be caused by an infarct in the distribution of the right anterior cerebral artery.

Question 3

Answer: A. The patient has stable angina. Stable angina is caused by a fixed (i.e., no recent change) obstruction of the coronary artery, which causes ≥ 75% stenosis. Choice C (atherosclerotic plaque in the left anterior descending coronary artery that causes 75% stenosis and has a large cluster of intact red blood cells within its core) and choice D (ruptured atherosclerotic plaque in the left anterior descending coronary artery associated with a nearly occlusive thrombus) describe atherosclerotic plaques with recent changes (e.g., hemorrhage and thrombus formation).

Question 4

Answer: C. The location of the retinoblastoma gene is 13q14, and in familial cases, it is associated with retinoblastoma and osteosarcoma. 5q21 is the location of the *APC* gene, and in familial cases, it is associated with colonic adenocarcinoma. 17p13 is the location of the *p53* gene, and in familial cases, it is associated with various sarcomas and with breast carcinoma. 3p25 is the location of the von Hippel-Lindau gene and in familial cases, it is associated with renal cell carcinomas and cerebellar hemangioblastomas.

Question 5

Answer: A. A young healthy patient who sustains head trauma with a lucid interval (a period of consciousness between the injury and subsequent unconsciousness) and subsequently becomes unresponsive with evidence of a space-occupying lesion in the right side of the cranial cavity most likely has an epidural hemorrhage. The epidural hemorrhage can produce a midline shift and uncal and cerebellar tonsillar herniation. An epidural hemorrhage is most commonly due to a fracture of the temporal bone, with subsequent tearing of the middle meningeal artery.

Question 6

Answer: A. The history and findings are consistent with a lobar pneumonia. The most common etiologic agent of lobar pneumonia is *Streptococcus pneumoniae*.

Question 7

Answer: B. Patients with Wernicke encephalopathy have ataxia, disturbed cognition, and ophthalmoplegia. The disorder is caused by a deficiency of thiamine and is classically seen in chronic alcoholics. The three clinical manifestations of thiamine deficiency are peripheral neuropathy, wet beriberi (high output cardiac failure), and Wernicke-Korsakoff syndromes. Overlap exists between Wernicke encephalopathy and Korsakoff syndrome, but Korsakoff syndrome is usually associated with amnesia and is not reversible.

Question 8

Answer: C. The patient's brother most likely had Marfan syndrome. Of the possible choices, patients with Marfan syndrome are most likely to have dislocation of the lens.

Question 9

Answer: D. The patient most likely has Paget disease. Her symptoms are being caused by the compressive effects of bony overgrowth on the cranial nerves, including the left abducens nerve (CN VI). The mosaic pattern of the lamellar bone is characteristic of Paget disease.

Question 10

Answer: B. Choriocarcinomas and seminomas with giant cells produce hCG. Yolk sac tumors produce AFP. An ultrasound would help to determine whether the mass was solid or was a fluid-filled cyst.

Question 11

Answer: B. The patient is describing claudication, which is the characteristic symptom of peripheral vascular disease, a form of atherosclerotic cardiovascular disease. The patient has numerous risk factors for atherosclerosis.

Question 12

Answer: D. The patient's white blood cells are incapable of transmigration, which requires the presence of PECAM (CD31) on both the white blood cells and endothelial cells.

Question 13

Answer: C. A fistula is a possible complication of an acute inflammatory process. In this case, a fistula developed between the infected aortic graft and the duodenum, allowing blood to enter the gastrointestinal tract and move retrograde through the esophagus.

Question 14

Answer: B. The clinical symptomatology, clinical findings, and the flow cytometry results are consistent with hairy cell leukemia.

Question 15

Answer: A. The question describes a patient with fragile X syndrome. Patients with fragile X syndrome have CGG repeats on the X chromosome.

Question 16

Answer: A. The patient has a meconium ileus. The "soap bubble" pattern is caused by air trapped within the thickened meconium and is highly suggestive, but not pathognomonic, of meconium ileus. Pyloric stenosis (C) is associated with bilious vomiting, but gaseous dilation of the small bowel would not be expected, and most cases of pyloric stenosis occur after 3 weeks of life. Hirschsprung disease (B) can cause delayed passage of meconium and may be associated with a small colon initially, but most cases of meconium ileus are associated with cystic fibrosis.

Question 17

Answer: D. The patient has the signs and symptoms of nephrotic syndrome. The most common cause of nephrotic syndrome in children is minimal change disease. Minimal change disease is treated with steroids, rarely requiring a biopsy for diagnosis. If a child with suspected minimal change disease responds to steroids, the diagnosis of minimal change disease can be made. If the child does not respond to steroid therapy, a kidney biopsy is warranted to diagnose the cause of the nephrotic syndrome.

Question 18

Answer: A. Of the listed conditions, the most likely to be occurring in this patient is a placental abruption. Cigarette smoking during pregnancy, trauma, and possibly cocaine use increase the risk for placental abruption. Placenta previa causes painless vaginal bleeding during the third trimester. An ectopic pregnancy is unlikely to be carried to term.

Question 19

Answer: C. The question describes a patient with pellagra, which is a complication of niacin (vitamin B_3) deficiency. The manifestations are diarrhea, dermatitis, and dementia.

Question 20

Answer: B. Hamartomas are the third most common cause of a solitary pulmonary nodule "coin lesion." A hamartoma is a benign disorganized collection of a tissue type normally found in the organ in which the mass occurred. Most pulmonary hamartomas are solitary, peripherally located, and often have a "popcorn" or stippled pattern of calcification.

Question 21

Answer: D. The patient is experiencing symptoms from sluggish blood flow due to the high red blood cell count. The pink discoloration of the urine is due to blood. The elevated red blood cell count is due to abnormal erythropoietin production. Both of these features indicate a renal cell carcinoma, which, of the above choices, would be diagnosed with a CT scan of the abdomen and pelvis.

Question 22

Answer: B. The patient had emphysema, and the icteric conjunctivae indicate possible liver damage. In a young person with this combination, α_1-antitrypsin deficiency is a possible diagnosis.

Question 23

Answer: C. Hyaline membrane disease, necrotizing enterocolitis, and germinal matrix hemorrhage are well-known potential complications of prematurity. Pink acellular membranes lining the alveolar septae describe the histologic features of hyaline membrane disease.

Question 24

Answer: B. The histologic and molecular features of the tumor are most commonly associated with Ewing sarcoma. A common location for Ewing sarcoma is the diaphysis of the tibia.

Question 25

Answer: C. The lack of elevation in cardiac enzymes indicates that no damage was done to the heart. However, the symptoms are suggestive of a myocardial infarct; therefore, the patient had unstable angina. Unstable angina is also referred to as preinfarct angina. The patient may have had a change in an atherosclerotic plaque (e.g., hemorrhage or thrombus), which resolved prior to causing irreversible damage to the heart.

Question 26

Answer: C. A mass in the left cerebral hemisphere will cause swelling, which can lead to herniation. Herniation of the left uncus can impinge on the oculomotor nerve, damaging parasympathetic fibers and leading to pupil dilation. Herniation of the uncus can also impinge on the posterior cerebral artery, causing ipsilateral occipital lobe infarcts.

Question 27

Answer: B. Any of the above conditions are possible causes of a hypercoagulable state. The most common inherited hypercoagulable condition is factor V Leiden, which is an inherited mutation in factor V that removes the cleavage site for protein C; thus, protein C cannot inactivate activated factor V.

Question 28

Answer: D. The gross appearance of the tumor is consistent with a malignant mesothelioma. A pleural malignant mesothelioma is consistent with a history of asbestos exposure until proven otherwise. The pleural plaques are also an indication of asbestos exposure, and the histology of the lung and clinical testing is consistent with asbestosis.

Question 29

Answer: A. The patient's symptoms are consistent with a prolactinoma. The prolactin level could be increased by a nodule in the sella turcica that compresses the infundibulum (stalk effect) and blocks the inhibitory effects of dopamine. However, stalk effect causes a lower level of hyperprolactinemia (100–200 ng/L) compared to a prolactinoma. In most cases, hormone-producing adenomas present with symptoms at a much smaller size than adenomas that do not secrete a hormone (i.e., null cell adenomas), because of the clinical effects of the hormones produced. Null cell adenomas usually present at a much larger size because they require mass effects to present.

Question 30

Answer: C. Given the history, this patient most likely has a secondary erythrocytosis due to erythropoietin production by a renal cell carcinoma.

Question 31

Answer: A. The signs and symptoms combined with the clinical scenario (obese woman taking oral contraceptives who dies suddenly) are characteristic of a pulmonary thromboembolus. To cause sudden death, a pulmonary thromboembolus must obstruct > 60% of the pulmonary artery vasculature.

Question 32

Answer: A. The clinical scenario is characteristic for fatty emboli. The classic clinical triad is dyspnea, mental status changes, and petechial hemorrhages (often axillary) following a traumatic fracture of a long bone.

Question 33

Answer: B. The patient's clinical features are consistent with septic shock. In hypovolemic or cardiogenic shock, patients will have increased heart rate and decreased blood pressure, but will have cold skin. Septic shock causes a generalized vasodilation, producing the symptoms. However, in response to hypovolemic or cardiogenic shock, the peripheral arteries will constrict to facilitate shunting of blood to the vital organs and cause cold extremities. Acute respiratory distress syndrome (ARDS) is a common complication of septic shock, and is characterized by development of bilateral infiltrates and consolidation on chest radiograph. There is no evidence that this patient has suffered a myocardial infarction (A). Central venous pressures would be expected to be low, secondary to vasodilation in the setting of septic shock. The stress response, the infection, and this patient's diabetes mellitus all make hyperglycemia more likely than hypoglycemia.

Question 34

Answer: B. CR1 molecules on the surface of leukocytes are used to recognize C3b (an opsonin) coating the surface of the material to be engulfed. CD31 is used for transmigration of white blood cells. Sialyl-Lewis-X molecules and ICAM-1 are used, respectively, for rolling and pavementing of white blood cells.

Question 35

Answer: C. The physical findings are suggestive of renal artery stenosis, possibly due to renal artery dysplasia. The patient has hypertension, which is secondary to another underlying disorder and potentially can be treated and cured.

Question 36

Answer: A. Of the choices, only the pituitary adenoma and small cell lung cancer would produce elevated cortisol levels and elevated ACTH level. Ectopic ACTH production as a paraneoplastic process, however, would not result in suppression of ACTH production with dexamethasone challenge. The two processes within the adrenal gland (hyperplasia and adenoma) may produce an elevated cortisol level, but negative feedback would result in a decreased ACTH level.

Question 37

Answer: B. The patient has features of preeclampsia. Preeclampsia can progress to eclampsia with the development of seizures.

Question 38

Answer: D. These symptoms suggest the possibility of a temporal arteritis. The definitive diagnosis of temporal arteritis requires a biopsy, although the ESR is usually elevated. However, diagnostic tests should not delay treatment with corticosteroids since the risk for blindness is significant.

Question 39

Answer: B. The patient's signs and symptoms are most consistent with Wegener granulomatosis. Although the patient has both upper respiratory and renal abnormalities, patients with Goodpasture syndrome often have hemoptysis, and it is the lower respiratory tract that is involved (i.e., the alveolar basement membranes).

Question 40

Answer: A. The most common congenital cardiac malformation is a ventricular septal defect. The signs and symptoms are consistent with the diagnosis of a ventricular septal defect, and, as happened with this child, many ventricular septal defects close spontaneously.

Question 41

Answer: C. The patient has features of congestive heart failure. Given her age and history of diabetes mellitus and hypertension, her congestive heart failure likely resulted from multiple ischemic events over the past several years.

Question 42

Answer: A. Patients with Addison disease usually have increased pigmentation (especially oral) and atrophic adrenal glands. Secondary hypoadrenalism will produce atrophic adrenal glands, but not the increased pigmentation. Secondary hypoadrenalism is commonly due to steroid therapy. Steroids must be withdrawn slowly to allow the atrophic adrenal gland to increase in size and restore normal function.

Question 43

Answer: D. Patients with osteomyelitis are at risk for future development of a sarcoma, a pathologic fracture, and systemic amyloidosis. Fatty emboli syndrome arises a few days after fracture of a long bone, and has also been associated with diffuse fatty liver and pancreatitis.

Question 44

Answer: A. Based upon the patient's demographics and location of the mass, of the given choices, the most likely diagnosis is an osteosarcoma.

Question 45

Answer: A. The patient has symptoms of osteoarthritis. Pannus formation and rheumatoid factor (IgM versus the Fc portion of IgG) are characteristic of rheumatoid arthritis. Although osteoarthritis can be secondary to a traumatic incident, most cases are primary, with wear and tear as one contributory factor.

Question 46

Answer: D. The patient's clinical presentation is characteristic for gout. Alcohol use and obesity are risk factors for gout. Most patients are underexcretors of uric acid, and not overproducers. Gout can contribute to the development of uric acid stones in the kidney, and also to the precipitation of uric acid into the renal interstitium.

Question 47

Answer: C. The patient has a rapidly growing, left-sided intracerebral neoplasm, which has resulted in left uncal herniation. Compression of the left oculomotor nerve, with subsequent involvement of the parasympathetic nerve fibers caused the pupillary dilation. Uncal herniation can also compress the posterior cerebral artery.

Question 48

Answer: A. The patient has features consistent with Wegener granulomatosis (sinusitis, features of nephritic syndrome, positive for c-ANCA). Wegener granulomatosis is associated with type III crescentic glomerulonephritis (pauci-immune type).

Question 49

Answer: B. The question describes a patient with hereditary spherocytosis. Patients with hereditary spherocytosis have increased osmotic fragility, and can develop splenomegaly (causing early satiety) and gallstones.

Question 50

Answer: A. Answer A, a 4.5-cm cavity in the right parietal lobe, refers to the appearance of a remote infarct. Answer B, an ill-defined softening of the right parietal lobe, refers to the appearance of an acute infarct. Answer C, a well-defined friable area in the right parietal lobe, refers to the appearance of an organizing infarct. Answer D, a tiny (< 1.0-cm) cavity in the pons, refers to the appearance of a lacunar infarct.

Question 51

Answer: B. Chédiak-Higashi syndrome is an autosomal recessive disorder (hence skipping generations) that causes increased susceptibility to infections because of impaired transport of bacteria from phagocytic vesicles to lysosomes. Patients can also have albinism.

Question 52

Answer: B. The thin rim of parenchyma represents subpial sparing, which rules out a contusion. The subpial parenchyma receives its nutrients from the cerebrospinal fluid and meningeal vessels and, in an infarct, will be spared; however, in a contusion, where the force is delivered to the cortical surface, the subpial parenchyma would not be spared. An active plaque in multiple sclerosis is a demyelinating process, but neurons are spared and would be present on the slide.

Question 53

Answer: B. The history is consistent with Huntington chorea. Spongiform changes would be associated with Creutzfeldt-Jakob disease (CJD).

Question 54

Answer: B. The histologic features of the tumor are consistent with a Wilms tumor. In combination with the other features the child has (i.e., mental retardation and bladder malformation), the most likely diagnosis is WAGR syndrome.

Question 55

Answer: D. The age range and clinical and autopsy findings are consistent with *Neisseria meningitidis*. The patient has Waterhouse-Friderichsen syndrome.

Question 56

Answer: B. The wedge-shaped pleural-based firm red-tan tissue is most likely a pulmonary infarct caused by a smaller pulmonary thromboembolus that occurred 24 hours prior to his saddle thromboembolus. The dead tissue at the site of the infarct would be characterized by coagulative necrosis, which is described in answer B.

Question 57

Answer: D. In general, the diagnosis of malignant neoplasms of the endocrine system requires documentation of invasion or metastases. Cellular features such as pleomorphism and mitotic figures do not consistently predict malignancy in endocrine neoplasms.

Question 58

Answer: C. Struma ovarii is a monodermal teratoma of the ovary that produces ectopic thyroid hormone. The complex cystic mass composed of both cystic and solid components that is present in this young female patient is most likely a teratoma (dermoid cyst). A patient with Graves disease would have a detectable autoantibody. A toxic goiter would be identified on ultrasound. The TSH level is not consistent with answer D, ectopic production of TSH, for example, by a small cell lung carcinoma.

Question 59

Answer: B. The question is describing a family with familial retinoblastoma. Familial retinoblastoma is caused by a mutation of the retinoblastoma (*RB*) gene, whose function is to bind E2F, thereby preventing (and subsequently controlling) progression of the cell cycle.

Question 60

Answer: C. The differentiation of follicular carcinoma from follicular adenoma (unless metastases are present) requires evaluation of the tumor for capsular or blood vessel invasion—two features that usually are not identifiable with an FNA. The nuclear features of papillary thyroid carcinoma can be easily evaluated with an FNA of a thyroid gland nodule.

Question 61

Answer: A. The initial diagnosis of chronic lymphocytic leukemia (CLL) is commonly made in patients who are being evaluated or treated for another disease process. Although most cases of CLL are B cell in origin, the neoplastic cells are positive for CD 5.

Question 62

Answer: D. The nature of the wound (i.e., large laceration), although sutured to prevent blood loss and infection, implies that it will heal, at least partially, through the process of second intention. The scar will be smaller than the original wound due to wound contraction, but will most likely be easily visible and reduced in strength.

Question 63

Answer: A. After childhood, patients with PKU can use a less restricted diet. However, in pregnant females, an uncontrolled level of phenylalanine can adversely affect fetal neurologic development; therefore, prior to and during pregnancy, women with PKU should return to a phenylalanine-free diet.

Question 64

Answer: B. The patient has a secondary cause of hypertension, an aortic coarctation. An aortic coarctation can often be identified with an appropriate physical examination, including recording of the blood pressure of both the upper and lower extremities. Once a coarctation is identified, it can potentially be treated with surgery.

Question 65

Answer: D. Infections caused by *Neisseria gonorrhoeae* or *Chlamydia trachomatis* place a patient at risk for pelvic inflammatory disease (PID). Complications of PID include ectopic pregnancy, tubo-ovarian adhesions, and infertility.

Question 66

Answer: A. HPV types 6 and 11 are associated with condyloma acuminatum. Types 16, 18, 31, 33, and 35 are associated with high-grade lesions, such as CIN II and III, which more frequently progress to invasive squamous cell carcinoma.

Question 67

Answer: A. The patient has multiple uterine leiomyomas. Uterine leiomyomas can produce pelvic pain, ulceration of overlying endometrium leading to vaginal bleeding, and infertility due to inability of uterus to expand in size, as is normally required during pregnancy. Although rare case reports of metastasizing benign leiomyomas have been reported, it is definitely *not* a common complication.

Question 68

Answer: A. Lobular carcinoma in situ is a marker that indicates the patient is at increased risk for the future development of an invasive carcinoma (either lobular or ductal carcinoma) in either breast (i.e., not necessarily in the same breast as the site of the biopsy). Therefore, some women diagnosed with lobular carcinoma in situ will voluntarily elect to undergo a prophylactic bilateral mastectomy to prevent future development of an invasive breast carcinoma.

Question 69

Answer: C. The patient has aortic stenosis. Given his relatively young age, the stenosis is most likely due to dystrophic calcification of a bicuspid aortic valve.

Question 70

Answer: A. The symptoms are suggestive of an aortic dissection. The diastolic murmur and widened pulse pressure indicates aortic regurgitation from a dilated aortic root.

Question 71

Answer: A. Patients who use NSAIDs are at risk for development of a gastric peptic ulcer. The hypotension, tachycardia, and pallor are due to an acute hemorrhagic shock. The cause of this patient's death is an acute bleeding peptic ulcer. In the setting of acute hemorrhage, hemoglobin and hematocrit are normal prior to fluid resuscitation.

Question 72

Answer: C. The EGD would most likely reveal glandular metaplasia. Smoking, excessive alcohol intake, and fatty foods are among the list of things that increase the risk for gastric reflux. Gastric reflux can lead to glandular metaplasia of the distal esophagus (i.e., Barrett esophagus).

Question 73

Answer: C. The patient most likely has megaloblastic anemia. Of the choices, atrophic gastric mucosa with focal intestinal metaplasia is the histologic description of autoimmune gastritis, which is one cause of megaloblastic anemia.

Question 74

Answer: B. Zollinger-Ellison syndrome is due to a gastrin-secreting endocrine tumor in the head of the pancreas or duodenum. These patients have a history of multiple ulcers, and ulcers in unusual locations such as the jejunum. Hypertrophic gastric folds are a classic finding in Zollinger-Ellison syndrome.

Question 75

Answer: A. Patients with delirium tremens will have confusion, disorientation, hallucinations, tremor, and signs of autonomic instability. This patient most likely has a history of surreptitious drinking. Dementia can predispose a patient to sundowning, but it is not an acute alteration in mental status.

Question 76

Answer: C. The symptoms are consistent with rheumatoid arthritis.

Question 77

Answer: D. This patient has celiac sprue. Celiac sprue is caused by sensitivity to gluten in wheat, and is treated by alteration of the diet to remove gluten-containing substances.

Question 78

Answer: A. Polyarteritis nodosa (PAN) is characterized by segmental necrotizing vasculitis of small and medium sized arteries. PAN can present with a broad constellation of findings, including renal disease but not pulmonary disease. Up to 30% of cases of PAN are associated with hepatitis B. The clinical scenario is not suggestive of Kawasaki disease. The lack of upper respiratory symptoms, including the lack of hemoptysis, and the patient's young age is less suggestive of Goodpasture syndrome. Acute pancreatitis would not easily explain his hematuria.

Question 79

Answer: B. The histologic description and location (appendix) are consistent with Crohn disease. Both Crohn disease and ulcerative colitis can have many extra-intestinal manifestations, which account for the patient's joint pain and skin lesion.

Question 80

Answer: A. The patient has neurofibromatosis type 1. The macules are café au lait spots, and the lesions on her iris are Lisch nodules. Patients with neurofibromatosis are prone to malignant degeneration of neurofibromas (especially plexiform neurofibromas) with subsequent development of a malignant peripheral nerve sheath tumor. Angiomyolipomas are associated with tuberous sclerosis.

Question 81

Answer: B. The lesion in the colon is the result of acute diverticulitis. The "apple-core" lesion seen on barium enema is the result of segmental constriction of the lumen of the colon. An "apple-core" lesion is suggestive of colonic adenocarcinoma, but can also be seen with acute diverticulitis. The segmental resection removed the area of acute inflammation, but because the patient has other diverticuli in the colon, he is at risk for another episode of diverticulitis in the future.

Question 82

Answer: B. Chronic subdural hemorrhages are known for causing psychiatric symptoms and should always be considered in elderly patients who present with such symptoms. Elderly patients and alcoholic patients are especially at risk for subdural hemorrhages, because atrophy of the brain facilitates easier tearing of the bridging veins due to less extensive head trauma.

Question 83

Answer: A. The four criteria for grading astrocytomas are mitotic figures, necrosis, angiogenesis, and pleomorphism. A low-grade astrocytoma has only pleomorphism, making the differential diagnosis between a reactive process and a low-grade astrocytoma difficult on frozen section. Mitotic figures, angiogenesis, and necrosis are more easily identified on the slide.

Question 84

Answer: B. The patient has histologic features of autoimmune hepatitis (i.e., similar histology to chronic viral hepatitis but with negative viral serologies). Autoimmune hepatitis is associated with anti-smooth muscle and anti–liver-kidney antibodies.

Question 85

Answer: C. Recurrences of ALL often involve the central nervous system. The age of the boy (> 12 years), hypodiploidy, and t(9;22) translocation are all unfavorable prognostic indicators.

Question 86

Answer: A. The diagnosis of sudden infant death syndrome (SIDS) is made after complete investigation of the death, including examination of the scene of death and a full autopsy. Thymic petechial hemorrhages are nonspecific findings seen with a SIDS death. A prone sleeping position is felt to be a risk factor for SIDS.

Question 87

Answer: A. The histology describes alcoholic hepatitis (neutrophilic infiltrate, Mallory hyaline, and central vein fibrosis).

Question 88

Answer: C. The patient has chronic myelogenous leukemia (CML). Although patients with CML may have a few myeloblasts, the peripheral smear will consist mainly of more mature myelocytes, with an associated basophilia. One differential diagnosis is a leukemoid reaction (a profound reactive increase in white blood cells), but a leukemoid reaction will have an elevated leukocyte alkaline phosphatase (LAP).

Question 89

Answer: B. A painful thyroid gland is consistent with subacute (de Quervain) thyroiditis. Histologic examination of the thyroid gland in these patients will reveal multinucleated giant cells. Lymphocytes and oncocytic change are consistent with Hashimoto thyroiditis, a usually painless condition. Pseudoinclusions and optically clear nuclei are consistent with papillary thyroid carcinoma, which is usually painless.

Question 90

Answer: B. During pregnancy, the anterior pituitary gland increases in size due to hyperplasia of prolactin-producing cells. Because of the increased size of the gland, the blood supply becomes tenuous and an event that reduces the blood supply, such as an acute hemorrhage, can lead to ischemia and resultant necrosis of the gland. This damage to the gland results in decreased levels of the anterior pituitary hormones, a condition referred to as Sheehan syndrome.

Question 91

Answer: A. The patient has pseudomembranous colitis due to *Clostridium difficile* following antibiotic treatment. Flask-shaped ulcers are seen in *Entamoeba histolytica* infections.

Question 92

Answer: C. The patient has all four modifiable risk factors for atherosclerosis. The abdominal pain and subsequent shock suggest a ruptured abdominal aortic aneurysm. Despite hemorrhagic shock, the patient's heart rate remains relatively stable because of the β blocker.

Question 93

Answer: A. Turner syndrome is a common cause of primary amenorrhea. It is associated with coarctation of the aorta, a webbed neck, short stature, and wide-spaced nipples.

Question 94

Answer: C. The patient has Henoch-Schönlein purpura (HSP). One component of HSP is an IgA nephropathy. Other systemic manifestations, including arthritis and gastrointestinal involvement, are found in patients with Henoch-Schönlein purpura.

Question 95

Answer: D. Urinary tract infections in males, especially young males, are uncommon and are often due to an anomaly in the genitourinary tract.

Question 96

Answer: C. The question is describing two well-known complications for patients with Down syndrome, acute lymphoblastic leukemia, and duodenal atresia. Of the choices, Down syndrome is associated with increased maternal age.

Question 97

Answer: C. A pathologic fracture implies that the fracture is secondary to another lesion in the bone and not just the result of trauma. Of the tumors listed, Ewing sarcoma is the most likely to occur in the diaphysis of a long bone in a 13-year-old child.

Question 98

Answer: C. The patient has the symptoms of Guillain-Barré syndrome (ascending paralysis). If the patient's airway is managed, the symptoms will pass and there will be no residual sequelae.

Question 99

Answer: B. The histology is consistent with small cell carcinoma. Small cell carcinoma of the lung can produce ACTH, resulting in increased cortisol level, and is considered to have metastasized at the time of diagnosis. Therefore, once the diagnosis was made by frozen section, no further resection of the lung would have been performed.

Question 100

Answer: C. The patient has Kawasaki syndrome (edema of the hands and feet, cervical lymphadenopathy, oral erythema, and fever). A possible late-term complication of this disease is a coronary artery aneurysm.

Question 101

Answer: B. The patient has diffuse alveolar damage (clinically termed acute respiratory distress syndrome, or ARDS). The four main causes of diffuse alveolar damage are diffuse pulmonary infection, head trauma, sepsis, and aspiration.

Question 102

Answer: B. The patient most likely has multiple sclerosis (MS). In most cases, MS has a waxing and waning course, but the clinical history can vary from patients having one episode with no subsequent episodes to patients having multiple episodes one after the other, leaving them wheelchair bound or worse. Patients often present with visual symptoms.

Question 103

Answer: B. The question is describing a patient with Klinefelter syndrome. These patients usually have normal intelligence. They are at increased risk for breast cancer. A gynecoid habitus, breast enlargement, and long legs are common physical manifestations of Klinefelter syndrome. Coarctation of the aorta is associated with Turner syndrome.

Question 104

Answer: A. The patient has features of congestive heart failure. Given his long-standing history of hypertension, he most likely has a low-output, left sided form of congestive heart failure with predominant systolic dysfunction.

Question 105

Answer: D. The patient most likely has sarcoidosis. In the United States, sarcoidosis is 10 times more common in African Americans than in whites. Fewer than 5% of patients with sarcoidosis have normal chest radiographs. Patients with sarcoidosis often have an elevated level of ACE. Lung involvement is more serious than lymph node involvement, and the disease can affect many other organs, including the skin and heart. Sarcoidosis may be associated with hypercalcemia due to secretion of 1,25-OH-vitamin D, and the histology is noncaseating granulomas.

Question 106

Answer: E. Granulosa cell tumors produce large amounts of estrogen. Elevated levels of estrogen are risk factors for breast carcinoma and endometrial adenocarcinoma. Complex hyperplasia of the endometrium is a risk factor for endometrial adenocarcinoma and can result from prolonged elevated levels of estrogen. Either hyperplasia of the uterus or endometrial adenocarcinoma can present with vaginal bleeding.

Question 107

Answer: C. β-Thalassemia is found in people of Mediterranean and African descent. Patients with β-thalassemia major have severe disease and, from childhood, are dependent upon transfusions. This patient has a hypochromic microcytic anemia, and may have either iron deficiency, thalassemia minor, or both, based on her history. The Meltzer index may be useful in distinguishing iron deficiency from thalassemia minor, but in this patient with menorrhagia and a family history of anemia, it would be of questionable use. In β-thalassemia, the excess α chains pair with δ chains, resulting in elevated hemoglobin A_2.

Question 108

Answer: C. The patient has Alzheimer disease, which is characterized by the intracellular accumulations of tau protein.

Question 109

Answer: C. Both vitamin B_{12} and folate deficiency will cause a megaloblastic anemia. A vitamin B_{12} deficiency (not a folate deficiency) is associated with neurologic symptoms. If a patient with a vitamin B_{12} deficiency is treated with folate supplementation, the treatment will resolve the anemia, but it will not prevent the effects of vitamin B_{12} deficiency on the nervous system. In alcoholics or otherwise malnourished patients with altered mental status, supplementation with both vitamin B_{12} and thiamine is advisable. Always give thiamine before dextrose in the DONT algorithm (dextrose, oxygen, naloxone, thiamine), because a large glucose load in a thiamine-deficient patient will acutely increase the metabolic need for thiamine and may precipitate Korsakoff syndrome.

Question 110

Answer: A. In multiple myeloma, the patient would almost always have an M spike (unless the clone was a nonsecretor) and osteolytic bone lesions. In MGUS, the patient has an M spike, but not osteolytic bone lesions. Patients with MGUS and those with a solitary plasmacytoma can later develop multiple myeloma.

Question 111

Answer: A. The image depicts a neurofibrillary tangle, characteristic of Alzheimer disease.

Question 112

Answer: C. The image depicts a stable atherosclerotic plaque in a coronary artery, causing > 75% stenosis. The patient most likely died of an arrhythmia related to his cardiac disease. An acute myocardial infarction would be associated with acute plaque change such as rupture or hemorrhage, resulting in occlusion of the vessel.

Question 113

Answer: C. The image depicts a gallstone in the cystic duct. One of the two main causes of acute pancreatitis is a gallstone. If this gallstone had become lodged in the common bile duct (choledocholithiasis), obstruction would have resulted in gallstone pancreatitis.

Question 114

Answer: A. The image depicts cervical intraepithelial neoplasia (CIN) grade I. The dysplastic changes only involve the lower third of the mucosa. Within the upper layers of mucosa can be seen several koilocytes. CIN I is associated with low-grade types of HPV, such as type 6.

Question 115

Answer: C. The image depicts cirrhosis. Patients with cirrhosis are prone to develop esophageal varices, which can lead to fatal gastrointestinal hemorrhages.

Question 116

Answer: C. The image depicts chronic myelogenous leukemia (CML). Patients with CML will have a decreased or normal leukocyte alkaline phosphatase (LAP) level, which helps distinguish the condition from a leukemoid reaction, in which patients will have an elevated LAP.

Question 117

Answer: A. The enlarged cells with the large intranuclear inclusion with a clear peripheral halo are characteristic of infection with cytomegalovirus.

Question 118

Answer: B. The image depicts hyaline membranes in the lung, characteristic of diffuse alveolar damage (histologic correlate of acute respiratory distress syndrome). Metastatic neoplasms are *not* a common cause of diffuse alveolar damage.

Question 119

Answer: B. The image depicts pulmonary emphysema. The most common cause of pulmonary emphysema is tobacco use.

Question 120

Answer: D. The image depicts a small epidural hemorrhage. The fracture line in the temporal bone involves the distribution of the middle meningeal artery.

Question 121

Answer: B. The image depicts fatty emboli (vessel in center of image). Patients with fatty emboli usually develop dyspnea, mental status changes, and petechial hemorrhages shortly (within a few days) after a motor vehicle accident in which long bones are fractured.

Question 122

Answer: A. The image depicts myocardial disarray, which is the characteristic histologic feature of hypertrophic cardiomyopathy.

Question 123

Answer: C. In the center of the image is a Reed-Sternberg cell, which is characteristic of Hodgkin lymphoma.

Question 124

Answer: C. The vessel with the thick acellular eosinophilic wall is characteristic of hyaline arteriolosclerosis.

Question 125

Answer: A. The glomerulus has nodular glomerulosclerosis (Kimmelstiel-Wilson lesion), which is characteristic of diabetes mellitus.

Question 126

Answer: C. The hepatocyte in the center of the image has Mallory hyaline (the ropy, eosinophilic condensation in the cell). In combination with the macrovesicular and microvesicular steatosis, of the choices given, the Mallory hyaline is most likely due to alcohol use.

Question 127

Answer: B. The tumor is a papillary thyroid carcinoma (note the optically clear, overlapping nuclei). Another common histologic feature of papillary thyroid carcinoma is psammoma bodies.

Question 128

Answer: C. Although patients with autosomal dominant polycystic kidney disease can have an associated berry aneurysm, the most common cause of death for these patients is chronic renal failure.

Question 129

Answer: B. The yellow (glycogen) and red (hemorrhage) coloration of this tumor are characteristic gross features of renal cell carcinoma.

Question 130

Answer: C. The patient has pseudomembranous colitis, which is most frequently the result of a course of antibiotic therapy that unintentionally causes the death of gut flora and allows overgrowth of *Clostridium difficile*.

INDEX

Page numbers followed by "*f*" indicate figures; page numbers follow by "*t*" indicate tables.

Abnormal uterine bleeding, 320
Abortion, 326–327
Abrasions, 50, 50*f*
Absence seizures, 137
Acalculous cholecystitis, acute, 278
Acanthosis nigricans, 323, 382, 382*f*
Achalasia, 236
Achondroplasia, 361–362
Acid-base disorders
    metabolic acidosis, 305*t*, 306
    metabolic alkalosis, 305*t*, 306
    respiratory acidosis, 305, 305*t*
    respiratory alkalosis, 305, 305*t*
Acidophil bodies, 270
Acoustic schwannoma, 57
Acquired Immunodeficiency Syndrome (AIDS), 33–34
Acromegaly, 339
ACTH. See Adrenocorticotropic hormone
ACTH-secreting adenoma, 339
Acute disseminated encephalomyelitis, 168
Acute fatty liver of pregnancy, 265
Acute interstitial pneumonia, 220
Acute lymphoid leukemia (ALL), 191–192, 191*t*, 192*f*,
    403, 418
Acute multiple sclerosis (Marburg), 167
Acute myeloid leukemia (AML), 193–194, 193*t*, 194*f*
    megakaryoblastic, 66, 194
    myelomonocytic, 194
    promyelocytic, 194, 194*f*, 207
Acute necrotizing hemorrhagic encephalomyelitis, 168
Acute respiratory distress syndrome (ARDS), 210, 215
Acute tubular necrosis, 90–91, 298, 298*f*
Addison disease, 286, 356, 357*f*
Adenocarcinoma
    colonic, 257–258, 257*f*–258*f*
    endometrial, 321–322, 321*f*
    esophageal, 240
    gallbladder, 279
    gastric, 244–245, 244*f*–245*f*
    pancreatic, 281
    prostatic, 315–316, 315*f*
    pulmonary, 227, 227*f*–228*f*
Adenomas
    adrenal, 358
    fibroadenoma, 332, 332*f*
    hepatic, 277
    intestinal, 256–257, 256*f*
    liver, 277
    parathyroid, 8, 349*t*, 350, 350*f*
    pituitary, 338*f*, 339
    pleomorphic, 234–235, 235*f*
    thyroid follicular, 347–348, 348*f*

Adenoma sebaceum, 58
Adenomyosis, 319, 319*f*
ADPCKD (autosomal dominant polycystic kidney disease),
    302, 302*f*
Adrenal disorders
    Addison disease, 356, 357*f*
    adenoma, 358
    congenital adrenal hyperplasia, 357
    Cushing syndrome, 354–355, 355*f*, 355*t*
    hyperaldosteronism, 358
    hypoadrenalism, 356, 356*f*–357*f*
    neoplasms, 358–360, 359*f*
        adrenal adenoma, 358
        adrenocortical carcinoma, 358
        multiple endocrine neoplasia, 359–360
        pheochromocytoma, 358–359, 359*f*
Adrenocortical carcinoma, 358
Adrenocorticotropic hormone (ACTH), 40, 338–339,
    354–358, 355*t*
Adult T-cell leukemia/lymphoma, 202
Agyria, 141
AIDS (acquired immunodeficiency syndrome), 33–34
Alanine aminotransferase, 261, 262*t*
Alcoholic liver disease. *See also* Hepatitis
    hepatic stenosis, 271, 271*f*
    Mallory hyaline, 9, 9*f*, 271*f*, 272
Alcohol withdrawal, 48, 402, 417
Alkaline phosphatase, 261, 262*t*
Alkaptonuria, 61
ALL. *See* Acute lymphoid leukemia
Allergic asthma, 212
ALP (alkaline phosphatase), 261, 262*t*
Alobar holoprosencephaly, 140
α-Fetoprotein, 44*t*, 45*t*, 311, 311*f*
α-Thalassemia, 177–178
α-Thalassemia trait, 177
α₁-Antitrypsin deficiency, 58, 211, 267, 273
Alport syndrome, 290, 296
ALS (amyotrophic lateral sclerosis), 166
ALT (alanine aminotransferase), 261, 262*t*
Alzheimer disease, 9, 162–163, 163*f*-164*f*
Amenorrhea, 318–319
AML. *See* Acute myeloid leukemia
Amnesia, 135–136
Amniotic band syndrome, 71
Amniotic fluid embolus, 87
Amyloid, 31, 31t, 32*f*, 130, 242, 353, 353*f*
Amyloidosis, 31, 31*t*, 32*f*
Amyotrophic lateral sclerosis (ALS) (Lou Gehrig disease), 166
Anaphylactic shock, 24, 90
Anaplastic carcinoma of the thyroid, 349, 349*f*
Anasarca, 83, 288

ANCA (antineutrophilic cytoplasmic antibody)
  c-ANCA, 102, 105, 294
  p-ANCA, 102, 105, 274
ANCA-mediated vasculitis, 102
Anemia, 173–187, 174*t*
  aplastic, 180–181, 180*f*
  clinical presentation of, 176
  hemolytic, 181–187, 184*t*
  macrocytic (megaloblastic), 179–180, 180*f*, 180*t*
  microcytic, 176–178, 176*f*, 176*t*, 178*f*
  morphology of, 175
  myelophthisic, 181, 181*f*
  paroxysmal nocturnal hemoglobinuria (PNH), 175
  pure red cell aplasia, 181, 181*f*
  sickle cell, 186–187, 186*f*
Anemia of chronic disease, 176*t*, 178
Anencephaly, 139, 140*f*
Aneurysm, 95, 100–101, 100*f*, 101*f*, 119, 121*f*
  berry, 148, 150*f*, 302
Angelman syndrome, 68
Angina
  stable, 113–114, 114*f*
  unstable, 113–117, 115*f*
  variant, 115
Angiodysplasia, 254
Angiomyolipoma, 58
Angiosarcoma
  liver, 277
  vascular, 107
Anhidrosis, 228
Ankylosing spondylitis, 27, 375
Anorexia, 51
Antibody
  anti-centromere, 27*t*, 30
  anti-desmoglein-3, 386, 387*t*
  anti-dsDNA, 27*t*, 28
  anti-endomysial, 249
  anti-gliadin, 249, 387, 387*t*
  anti-hemidesmosome, 386, 387*t*
  anti-histone, 27*t*, 28
  anti-liver/kidney, 270
  anti-mitochondrial, 273
  anti-scl70, 27*t*, 30
  anti-smooth muscle, 270
  anti-SSA/SSB, 27*t*, 30
Antibody-mediated red blood cell destruction
  ABO incompatibility, 182–183
  blood transfusion reactions, 183
  cold autoimmune hemolytic anemia, 184–185, 184*t*
  erythroblastosis fetalis, 183
  isohemagglutinin reaction, 182
  warm autoimmune hemolytic anemia, 184, 184*t*
Anticipation, 164
Antineutrophilic cytoplasmic antibody. *See* ANCA
Antiphospholipid antibody syndrome, 29
Aortic disorders
  coarctation, 112–113, 112*f*, 125
  dissection, 98–99, 99*f*, 100*f*, 125

Aortic valvular disorders
  regurgitation
    acute, 122*f*, 126–127
    chronic, 126–127
  stenosis, 112, 125–126
    congenital bicuspid aortic valve degenerative calcification, 125, 126*f*
    pulsus parvus et tardus, 126
    rheumatic valvulitis, chronic, 125
    tricuspid aortic valve degenerative calcification, 125, 125*f*
APC/β-catenin, 41*t*, 43–44
Aphasia, 135
Aplastic anemia, 180–181, 180*f*
Apoptosis, 5–6, 5*f*
Apoptosis genes, 44
Appendicitis, acute, 256, 256*f*
ARDS (acute respiratory distress syndrome), 210, 215
Argyll-Robertson pupils, 76
ARPCKD (autosomal recessive polycystic kidney disease), 302–303
Arteriolosclerosis, 93, 98, 98*f*
Arteriosclerosis, 93
Arteriovenous fistula, 101
Arteriovenous malformation, 141
Arthritis, 373*t*
  osteoarthritis, 373–374, 374*f*, 375*t*
  rheumatoid, 29–30, 374–375, 375*f*, 375*t*
Asbestosis, 217–218, 218*f*
Ascending acute cholangitis, 279
Aschoff nodules, 124
ASD (atrial septal defect), 111–112, 112*f*
Asherman syndrome, 318
Ash-leaf patches, 58
Aspartate aminotransferase (AST), 261, 262*t*
Aspergillus flavus, 276
Aspiration pneumonia, 224, 224*f*–225*f*
AST (aspartate aminotransferase), 261, 262*t*
Asterixis, 266
Asteroid bodies, 219, 220*f*
Asthma, 106, 212–213, 213*f*–214*f*
  allergic, 212
  mast cell tryptase, 213
  morphology, 213, 213*f*
  nonallergic, 212
Astrocytic reactions, 137
Astrocytomas, 158–159, 158*f*–159*f*
  grading criteria, 158
  pilocytic, 159, 159*f*
Asymptomatic hematuria, 295–296
  Alport syndrome, 296
  Henoch-Schönlein purpura, 296
  IgA nephropathy, 295–296
Ataxia-telangiectasia, 41*t*
Atelectasis
  compressive, 210, 210*f*
  contraction, 210
  microatelectasis, 210
  obstructive, 210

Atherosclerosis, 48, 93–95, 97
  complications of, 95
    aneurysm, 95
    emboli, 95
    peripheral vascular disease, 95
  vessels affected by, 94, 94f
Atrial myxoma, 132
Atrial septal defect (ASD), 111–112, 112f
Atrophy, 2
Atypical adenomatous hyperplasia, 227
Auer rods, 194, 194f
Auspitz sign, 385
Autoimmune disease(s)
  CREST syndrome, 27t, 30
  hemolytic anemias, 184–185, 184t
  hepatitis, 270–271
  mixed connective tissue disorder, 30
  Sjögren syndrome, 30, 30f
  systemic lupus erythematosus (SLE), 28–29, 29f, 131t, 132
  systemic sclerosis, 30
Autosomal disorders
  dominant, 55–58, 56f–58f, 56t
  recessive, 58–62, 59t
Autosomal dominant polycystic kidney disease (ADPCKD), 302, 302f
Autosomal recessive polycystic kidney disease (ARPCKD), 302–303
Avascular necrosis. See Osteonecrosis
Axonal neuropathy, 169
Azotemia, 283–285
  intrinsic, 284
  postrenal, 284
  prerenal, 284

B_{12} deficiency, 52, 179–180, 180t
Bacillary angiomatosis, 34
Bacterial meningitis, 151–153, 152f
Baló disease, 167
Barrett esophagus, 3, 3f, 238, 238f
Basal cell carcinoma, 383, 383f–384f
Basal cell nevus syndrome, 383
bcl-2, 44, 197t, 200
Becker muscular dystrophy, 65
Beckwith-Wiedemann syndrome, 80
Bence-Jones proteins, 203, 203f
Benign prostatic hyperplasia, 314, 314f
Berger disease. See IgA nephropathy
Berry aneurysm, 148, 150f, 302
β-Thalassemia, 177–178, 178f
Bicuspid aortic valve, 125, 126f
Biliary pain, 278
Biliary tract disorders, obstructive, 273–274, 274f, 274t
Bisferious pulse, 127
Bite cells, 187
Bitemporal hemianopsia, 339
Bladder, ureter disorders
  ureter obstruction, 305
  urothelial neoplasm, 304–305, 304f–305f

Blistering diseases of the skin, 387t
  bullous pemphigoid, 386–387
  dermatitis herpetiformis, 249, 387
  pemphigus, 386
Blueberry muffin baby, 76
Boerhaave syndrome, 236
Bone, joint disorders
  ankylosing spondylitis, 27, 375
  arthritis, 373, 373t
  fractures, 367, 367f
  gout, 375–377, 376f
  inherited diseases, 361–363
  osteoarthritis, 373–374, 374f
  osteodystrophy, renal, 366–367
  osteomyelitis, 364–365, 365f
  osteonecrosis, 364
  osteoporosis, 363–364
  Paget disease, 365–366, 366f
  pseudogout, 377
  rheumatoid arthritis, 29–30, 374–375, 375f, 375t
  tumors, 367–372, 368t
    chondroma, 368t, 370
    chondrosarcoma, 368t, 370–371, 371f
    giant cell tumor, 368t, 372, 372f
    metastases, 37, 39f–40f, 372–373
    osteochondroma, 368t, 370, 370f
    osteoid osteoma/osteoblastoma, 368–369
    osteoma, 368, 368t
    osteosarcoma, 41t, 368t, 369, 369f
    primitive neuroectodermal (PNET), 78, 368t, 372, 372f
Bouchard nodes, 374
Bowen disease, 313
Brain. See Central Nervous System; Neuropathology
  abscess, 153–154, 154f
Brainstem glioma, 159
BRCA1/BRCA2, 38, 334
Breast carcinoma, 334–336, 335f
  colloid, 335, 336
  inflammatory, 335
  invasive ductal, 335
  invasive lobular, 335, 336
  medullary, 335, 336
  tubular, 335, 336
Breast diseases, nonneoplastic, 331t
  fibroadenoma, 331t, 332, 332f
  fibrocystic change, 331–332, 331t, 332f
  intraductal papilloma, 333, 333f
  mastitis, acute, 331
  phyllodes tumor, 332–333
  sclerosing adenosis, 331t, 332
Brenner tumor, 325, 326f
Breslow depth, 381
Bridging necrosis, 262
Broca aphasia, 135
Brodie abscess, 365
Bronchiectasis, 214–215, 215f
Bronchioalveolar carcinoma, 227

Bronchitis, chronic, 214
Bronchopneumonia, 222, 222*f*
Bronchopulmonary dysplasia, 75
Brown tumors, 350
Brudzinski sign, 153
Budd-Chiari syndrome, 196, 275
Buerger disease. *See* Thromboangiitis obliterans
Bulimia, 52
Bullous pemphigoid, 386–387
Burkitt lymphoma, 38, 43, 78, 78*t*, 201, 201*f*

Cachexia, 39
Café-au-lait spots, 57
Calcium oxalate/phosphate kidney stones, 301
Calcium pyrophosphate crystal deposition.
          See Pseudogout
Calculous cholecystitis, acute, 278, 279*f*
Call-Exner bodies, 326
c-ANCA, 102, 105, 294
Cancer. *See also* Neoplasm/neoplasia; *specific types of*
          Tumors
Cancer stem cells, 37
CA-125, 44*t*
Capillary angioma, 142
Caplan syndrome, 375
Caput medusae, 267
Carcinogenesis. *See also* Neoplasm/neoplasia
     apoptosis genes, 40, 44
     DNA repair defects, 45
     DNA repair genes, 40
     initiators, 40
     nuclear transcription factors, 42–43
     oncogenes role, 42
     promoters, 40
     proto-oncogene conversion, 42
     proto-oncogenes, 40, 42–43
     tumor suppressor genes, 40, 43–44
     two-hit hypothesis, 43
Carcinoid syndrome, 259
Carcinoid tumor, 258–259, 259*f*
Carcinoma ex pleomorphic adenoma, 135
Carcinoma in situ, breast
     ductal (DCIS), 333–334, 333*f*–334*f*
     lobular (LCIS), 334
Cardiac death, sudden, 120
Cardiac disorders
     aortic valvular disease, 125–127, 125*f*–126*f*
     cardiomyopathies, 128–130, 129*f*–130*f*
     congenital heart disease, 110–113, 111–112*f*
     congestive heart failure, 9, 109, 121–122
     coronary syndromes, acute, 116
     endocarditis, 122–124, 122*f*–123*f*
     hypertensive cardiovascular disease, 120
     ischemic heart disease, 113–115, 114*f*–115*f*, 120, 121*f*
     mitral valvular disease, 127–128, 128*f*
     myocardial infarcts, 116–120, 116*f*, 117*t*, 119*t*,
          118*f*–120*f*
     pericardial disease, 119, 119*t*, 131–132, 131*f*–132*f*, 131*t*

     rheumatic fever, 124–125, 124*t*, 124*f*–125*f*
     sudden death, 120
     tumors, 132
Cardiac tamponade, 132
Cardiogenic shock, 89, 118, 118*f*
Cardiomyopathies, 128
     dilated, 48, 60, 129, 129*f*,130
     hypertrophic, 129, 129*f*
     restrictive, 130, 130*f*
Caspases, 5
Casts
     red blood cell, 292
     white blood cell, 299
Catalase, 4
Cavernous angioma, 142
CD markers of leukemia, lymphoma, 190, 191*t*,
          192–193, 197*t*, 200–202
CD10, 191, 191*t*
CD99, 372, 372*f*
CD117, 245
Celiac sprue, 249
Cellular disorders
     accumulations, 7–10
          calcium, 8, 8*f*
          cholesterol, 10
          fat, 9, 9*f*
          glycogen, 10
          iron, 9, 9*f*
          lipofuscin, 7–8, 8*f*
          pigments 10, 10*f*–11*f*
          protein, 9, 9*f*
     aging, 11
     apoptosis, 5–6, 5*f*
     atrophy, 2, 2*f*
     death, 5–7
          apoptosis, 5–6, 6*f*
          necrosis, 6–7, 6*f*–7*f*
     hyperplasia, 1
     hypertrophy, 2, 2*f*
     hypoplasia, 2
     injury, 3–5
          cellular system vulnerability, 3
          chemical injury, 4
          electron microscope morphologic changes, 5
          free radicals, 4
          hypoxia, 3–4
          irreversible, 5
          ischemia, 3
          light microscope morphologic changes, 5
          mitochondrial cytosolic calcium, 4
          reactive oxygen species, 4
          reversible, 4
     metaplasia, 3, 3*f*
     necrosis, 6–7, 6*f*–7*f*
Cellular rejection, 26, 26*f*
Central nervous system (CNS). *See also* Neuropathology
     infections, 150
          abscess, 153–154, 154*f*

encephalitis, 154–155, 155f
    meningitis, 151–153, 152f–153f, 151t, 154t
malformations
    associated with hydrocephalus, 140
    forebrain developmental disorders, 140–141
    neural tube defects, 139–140, 140f
    neuronal migration disorders, 141
morphologic changes
    astrocytic reactions, 137
    microglial reactions, 137
    neuronal, 137, 137f
tumors, 156–157, 156t
    astrocytoma, 158, 158f, 403, 418
    brainstem glioma, 159
    clinical presentation, 157
    ependymoma, 159
    lymphoma, 34, 160–161, 161f
    medulloblastoma, 160, 161f
    meningioma, 161, 162f
    oligodendroglioma, 159, 160f
    pilocytic astrocytoma, 159, 159f
Central pontine myelinolysis, 168
Centriacinar emphysema, 211
Centrilobular necrosis, 90, 90f
Cerebellar tonsillar herniation, 82, 138, 138f
Cerebral amyloid angiopathy, 145
Cerebral cortex, subpial sparing, 399, 416
Cerebral edema, herniation, 82, 138–139, 138f
    cerebellar tonsillar, 82, 138, 138f
    cingulate (subfalcine), 82, 139
    cytotoxic edema, 138
    Duret hemorrhage, 139, 139f
    transcalvarial, 139
    uncal (transtentorial) 82, 139, 139f
    vasogenic edema, 138
Cerebral infarcts, 143t
    borderzone, 144
    hemorrhagic, 143
    lacunar, 145, 146f
    morphology of, 143–144
    nonhemorrhagic, 143
Cervical intraepithelial neoplasia, 38, 41t, 42f, 316–317, 317f
C5a, 14t, 16
C5b, 14t, 16
Chalkstick-type fracture, 366
Chancre, 76
Charcot-Bouchard aneurysm, 145
Charcot-Leyden crystals, 213
Charcot triad, 279
Chédiak-Higashi syndrome, 17
Chemical injury, 4
Chemical meningitis, 151
Chemotaxis, 16
Cheyne-Stokes respirations, 139
Chiari syndrome, types I and II, 140
Chocolate cyst, 320
Cholangiocarcinoma, 276, 277f
Cholecystitis, chronic, 278–279

Cholelithiasis, 277–278, 279f
Cholestasis/jaundice, 11, 262–265, 262f, 263t, 264f
    neonatal, 264
Chondroma, 368t, 370
Chondrosarcoma, 368t, 370–371, 371f
Choreiform movement, 164
Chorioamnionitis, 327
Choriocarcinoma, 44t, 312, 312f, 327–329, 328t
Choristoma, 36
Chromophobe renal cell carcinoma, 303
Chronic granulomatous disease, 16–17
Chronic lymphoid leukemia (CLL), 192–193, 191t, 193f, 200
Chronic myeloid leukemia (CML), 194–195, 195f
Chronic obstructive pulmonary disease (COPD), 210, 215
Chronic passive congestion
    of liver, 84, 84f
    of lung, 83, 83f
Churg-Strauss syndrome, 106
Chvostek sign, 350
Cingulate (subfalcine) herniation, 82, 139
Circulatory disorders, liver, 274–275
Cirrhosis, 9, 48, 58, 60, 82, 262, 262t, 266–268, 266t, 266f–268f
    ascites in, 267, 268f
    cryptogenic cirrhosis, 267
    esophageal varices in, 267, 267f
    hepatocellular dysfunction in, 267
    portal hypertension in, 267, 267f
    primary biliary, 273–274, 274f, 274t
    spontaneous bacterial peritonitis, 267, 268f
CK-MB (creatine kinase-MB), 117
Claudication, 95
Clear cell adenocarcinoma of vagina, 316
Clear cell renal cell carcinoma, 303, 303f
CLL. See Chronic lymphoid leukemia
Clostridium difficile, 247
CML (chronic myeloid leukemia),194–195, 195f
CMV. See Cytomegalovirus
CNS. See Central nervous system
Coarctation of the aorta, 112–113, 112f, 125
Codman triangle, 369
Cold hemolysin hemolytic anemia, 185
Collapsing variant of focal segmental glomerulosclerosis (FSGS), 290
Colonic adenocarcinoma, 39f–40f, 41t, 44, 44t, 257–258, 257f–258f
Coma, 134–135
Common variable immunodeficiency, 32
Community-acquired atypical pneumonia, 223–224, 224f
Community-acquired typical pneumonia, 222–223, 222f–223f
Compressive atelectasis, 210, 210f
Concussion, 150
Condyloma lata, 76
Congenital bicuspid aortic valve degenerative calcification, 125, 126f
Congenital disorders
    adrenal hyperplasia, 357
    anomalies, 71–73

Congenital disorders (*continued*)
　heart disease
　　aortic coarctation, 112–113, 112*f*, 125
　　aortic stenosis, 112
　　atrial septal defect (ASD), 111–112, 112*f*
　　atrioventricular defect, 112
　　patent ductus arteriosus (PDA), 112
　　tetralogy of Fallot, 110
　　totally anomalous pulmonary venous return, 111
　　transposition of the great vessels, 111
　　tricuspid atresia, 110–111
　　truncus arteriosus, 111
　　ventricular septal defect (VSD), 111, 111*f*
　pyloric stenosis, 232
　rubella, 76
　syphilis, 76
Congestive heart failure, 9, 82, 109, 121–122
　left-sided , 121–122
　right-sided , 121–122
Consciousness disorders, 133–135
　coma, 134–135
　confusion, 133
　drowsiness, 133
　stupor, 134
Constipation/ diarrhea
　Entamoeba histolytica infection, 247, 247*f*
　mechanism, 245–246, 245*t*, 246*f*
　pseudomembranous colitis, 247, 247*f*
Contraction atelectasis, 210
Contrecoup contusion, 149, 151*f*
Contusions, 50, 50*f*, 149, 151*f*
Coombs test, 182
COPD (chronic obstructive pulmonary disease), 210, 215
Cor pulmonale, 211
Corrigan pulse, 127
Coup contusion, 149
Courvoisier sign, 281
Cowden syndrome, 44
Coxsackie B virus, 130, 130*f*, 131
Craniopharyngioma, 341
Creatine kinase-MB (CK-MB), 117
Creeping fat, 251, 252
Crescentic glomerulonephritis. *See* Rapidly progressive
　　glomerulonephritis
CREST syndrome, 27*t*, 30
Cretinism, 345
Creutzfeldt-Jakob disease, 155
Cri-du-chat syndrome, 67
Crigler-Najjar syndrome, 263*t*, 264
Crohn disease, 250–252, 250*t*, 251*f*
Crooke hyaline change, 355
Crypt abscesses, 252
Cryptococcal meningitis, 152, 153*f*
Cryptogenic cirrhosis, 267, 272
Cryptorchidism, 310
Curling ulcer, 243
Curschmann spirals, 213
Cushing disease, 354

Cushing syndrome, 40, 354–355, 355*f*, 355*t*
Cushing ulcer, 243
Cutaneous squamous cell carcinoma, 382–383
Cyclin-D1, 197*t*, 202
Cystic fibrosis, 59, 59*t*
Cystic medial degeneration, 57, 99, 100*f*
Cystic renal diseases
　autosomal dominant polycystic kidney(ADPCKD), 302, 302*f*
　autosomal recessive polycystic kidney (ARPCKD), 302–303
　cystic renal dysplasia, 302
　simple cysts, 302
Cystic teratoma, mature, 325–326, 327*f*
Cystitis, 298–299
Cytomegalovirus (CMV), 33*f*, 34, 76, 226
Cytotoxic edema, 138

DCIS. *See* Ductal carcinoma in situ
Degenerative joint disease. *See* Osteoarthritis
Dehiscence, 21
Delirium tremens, 48
Dementia, 162
Demyelinating disorders, 166
　central pontine myelinolysis, 168
　disseminated encephalomyelitis, acute, 168
　multiple sclerosis, 167–168, 167*f*
　necrotizing hemorrhagic encephalomyelitis, acute, 168
　progressive multifocal leukoencephalopathy, 168
De novo 5q- syndrome, 189
Denys-Drash syndrome, 80
Dependent edema, 83
De Quervain thyroiditis, 346–347
Dermatitis herpetiformis, 387, 387*t*
Dermatomyositis/polymyositis, 170
Dermatopathology
　blistering diseases. *See* Blistering diseases of the skin
　inflammatory dermatoses
　　acute, 383–385, 384*f*–385*f*
　　chronic, 385–386, 386*f*
　inherited skin neoplasia syndromes, 383
　melanocytic nevus, 380, 380*f*
　melanocytic proliferations, 380–382, 380*f*–382*f*
　nonmelanocytic lesions, 382–383, 383*f*–384*f*
　other skin diseases
　　infectious, 388
　　inflammatory, 387–388
　pigment disorders, 379–380
　systemic disease, cutaneous manifestations, 389
DES (diethylstilbestrol), 316
Devic disease, 167
Diabetes insipidus, 286, 307, 342
Diabetes mellitus, 9, 60, 72, 291–292, 292*f*, 295, 295*f*, 351, 363
　DKA, 351–352, 351*t*
　type 1, 351, 351*t*
　type 2, 352–354, 353*f*–354*f*
Diabetic ketoacidosis (DKA), 351–352, 351*t*
Diabetic nephropathy, 291–292, 292*f*
Diamond-Blackfan syndrome, 181
DIC. *See* Disseminated intravascular coagulation

Diethylstilbestrol, 316
Diffuse alveolar damage, 90, 215–216, 216*f*
Diffuse axonal injury, 149–150, 151*f*
Diffuse large B-cell lymphoma (DLBCL), 197*t*, 200–201, 201*f*
Diffuse Lewy body disease, 163
Diffuse pulmonary hemorrhage, 220–221
DiGeorge syndrome, 66–67
Dilated cardiomyopathy, 48, 60, 129, 129*f*, 130
Dimorphic fungi, 225
Direct antibody interaction-mediated vasculitis, 102
Disaccharidase deficiency, 248–250
Disseminated intravascular coagulation(DIC), 185, 206–207, 207*f*, 280, 280*f*
Diverticular disease, 254–255, 254*f*–255*f*
Diverticulitis, 255
Dizziness, 136
DKA (diabetic ketoacidosis), 351–352, 351*t*
DLBCL. *See* Diffuse large B-cell lymphoma
DNA repair defects, 45
Donath-Landsteiner antibody, 185
Down syndrome, 65–66, 66*f*, 112, 194, 232, 346
DPC4, 44
Dressler syndrome, 119
Drop metastases, 160
Drug-induced lupus, 29
Drug interactions, liver, 271
Dry beriberi, 52
Dubin-Johnson syndrome, 263*t*, 264
Duchenne muscular dystrophy, 64–65, 129
Ductal carcinoma in situ (DCIS), 331*t*, 333–334, 333*f*–335*f*
Duodenal atresia, 232
Dupuytren contracture, 374
Duret hemorrhage, 139, 139*f*
Dwarfism, 362
Dysgerminoma, 326
Dysplastic nevus, 380–381, 381*f*, 383
Dysplastic nevus syndrome, 383
Dyspnea, 109, 121
Dystrophic calcification, 8, 8*f*, 125*f*

EBV. *See* Epstein-Barr virus
Ecchymoses, 84
Eclampsia. *See* Toxemia of pregnancy
Ecthyma gangrenosum, 389
Ectopia lentis, 57
Ectopic kidney, 73
Ectopic pregnancy, 317, 318*f*, 329–330
Eczematous dermatitis, acute, 384
Edema, 81–83, 82*f*–83*f*
  decreased plasma osmotic pressure, 82
  increased vascular hydrostatic pressure, 82
Edward syndrome, 66
Eisenmenger syndrome, 110
Ehlers-Danlos syndrome, 65
Embolus
  amniotic fluid, 87
  fatty emboli, 87, 87*f*

  paradoxical, 110–112, 153
  pulmonary thromboembolus, 86–87, 86*f*–87*f*
Embryonal carcinoma, 311
Emphysema, 58, 211–212, 211*f*
  centriacinar, 211
  cor pulmonale, 211
  morphology of, 211, 211*f*
  panacinar, 211
  pulmonary, 211
Empty sella syndrome, 340
Empyema, 223, 223*f*, 226
Encephalitis
  cytomegalovirus (CMV), 154–155
  features of, 154, 154*f*
  HIV, 154–155
  HSV-1, 154–155
  HSV-2, 154–155
  rabies, 154–155
Endocarditis. *See also* Infective endocarditis
  Libman-Sacks, 28
Endocrine disorders
  adrenal neoplasms, 358–360, 359*f*
  diabetes mellitus, 351–354, 351*t*, 353*f*–354*f*
  goiter, 342–343, 343*f*
  hyperadrenalism, 354–355, 355*f*, 355*t*
  hyperaldosteronism, 358
  hyperparathyroidism, 349–350, 350*f*
  hyperpituitarism, 337–339, 338*f*
  hyperthyroidism, 343–344, 343*t*, 344*f*
  hypoadrenalism, 356–357, 356*f*-357*f*
  hypoparathyroidism, 350
  hypopituitarism, 340, 340*f*
  hypothyroidism, 343*t*, 345–346, 346*f*
  mass effect, 340–341
  posterior pituitary pathology, 341–342
  thyroiditis, 346–347
  thyroid neoplasms, 347–349, 347*f*–349*f*
Endogenous pigments, 10, 10*f*
Endometrial disorders
  adenocarcinoma, 321–322, 322*f*
  adenomyosis, 319, 319*f*
  endometriosis, 319–320, 320*f*
  endometritis, acute/chronic, 319
  hyperplasia, 320–321, 321*f*
  neoplasms, 321–323, 322*f*–323*f*
Endometrioid tumor, 325
Endometriosis, 319–320, 320*f*
Endometritis, acute/chronic, 319
Endothelial cell retraction, contraction, 15
Entamoeba histolytica infection, 247, 247*f*
Enterocolitis, necrotizing, 75, 75*f*
Environmental disorders
  physical trauma, 50–51, 50*f*–51*f*
  toxic substances, 47–50, 48*f*–49*f*
Ependymoma, 159
Epidural hemorrhage, 146, 148*f*
Epilepsy, 136–137
Epispadias, 73

Epstein-Barr virus (EBV), 38, 198, 201, 234
Erlenmeyer flask deformity, 363
Erosion, 18, 242
Erythema chronicum migrans, 124, 124t
Erythema multiforme
    Stevens-Johnson syndrome, 384, 384f
    toxic epidermal necrolysis, 385, 385f
Erythema nodosum, 219, 251–252, 388
Erythroblastosis fetalis, 24, 183
Erythropoiesis, ineffective, 180
Erythropoietin, 40
Esophageal disorders
    esophagitis, 237–238, 237f–238f
    motor function
        achalasia, 236
        hiatal hernia, 235–236
    neoplasms
        adenocarcinoma, 240
        morphology of, 240
        squamous cell carcinoma, 239–240
    varices, 237, 237f
Esophagitis
    Barrett esophagus, 238, 239f
    gastroesophageal reflux discasc (GERD), 237–238, 237f
Essential hypertension. See Primary essential hypertension
Essential thrombocytosis, 195–196
Ewing sarcoma, 78, 78t, 368t, 372, 372f
Exogenous pigments, 10, 10f
Exostosis. See Osteochondroma
Extracerebral hemorrhage
    epidural, 146, 148f
    subarachnoid, 148, 150f
    subdural, 146–147, 149f
Exudate, 83, 229

Factor V Leiden mutation, 85
False aneurysm, 100, 119
Familial adenomatous polyposis. See Familial polyposis coli
Familial hypercholesterolemia, 56, 56t
Familial melanoma syndrome. See Dysplastic nevus
        syndrome
Familial polyposis coli, 41t, 56, 56f, 257
Fatty streak, 95, 95f
Felty syndrome, 375
Female pseudohermaphrodite, 68
Female reproductive tract disorders, 309
    amenorrhea, 318–319
    breast carcinoma, 334–336, 335f
    breast diseases, nonneoplastic, 331–333, 331t, 332f–333f
    carcinoma in situ, breast, 333–334, 333f–334f
    cervical intraepithelial neoplasia, 38, 41t, 42f, 316–317, 317f
    fibroids, 322–323, 323f
    nonneoplastic uterine diseases, 319–321, 319f–321f
    ovarian disease, nonneoplastic, 323
    ovarian tumors, 324f–327f, 324–326, 324t
    pelvic inflammatory disease (PID), 317–318, 318f
    placental, pregnancy-related, 326–331, 328f, 328t, 330f
    squamous intraepithelial lesion, 316–317

uterine tumors, 321–323, 322f-323f
    vaginal tumors, 316
Ferruginous body, 218, 218f
Fetal alcohol syndrome, 48, 69
Fetal hydrops, 76–77, 76f
        immune/nonimmune causes, 77
Fetor hepaticus, 266
Fibrinous inflammation, 17
Fibroadenoma, 332, 332f
Fibrocystic change, 331t, 331–332, 332f
Fibroids. See Leiomyoma
Fibrothecoma, 326
Fibrous cortical defect, 371
Fibrous dysplasia, 371
Field effect, 230
Fistula, 18, 19f
    arteriovenous, 101
    tracheoesophageal, 72
Fitz-Hugh-Curtis syndrome, 318
Focal nodular hyperplasia, 276, 277f
Focal segmental glomerulosclerosis (FSGS), 290, 290f, 296
Folate deficiency, 52, 52t, 180, 180f, 180t
Follicular adenoma, carcinoma of the thyroid, 347–348, 348f
Follicular lymphoma, 197t, 200, 200f
Forebrain developmental disorders
    alobar holoprosencephaly, 140
    lobar holoprosencephaly, 141
    semilobar holoprosencephaly, 141
Foregut cysts, 72
Fractures, 367
Fragile X syndrome, 68
Freckles, 379
Free radicals, 4
Frontotemporal dementia, 163
FSGS. See Focal segmental glomerulosclerosis
Fungal meningitis, 153
Fusiform aneurysm, 100

Galactosemia, 60
Gamma-glutamyltransferase, 261, 262t
Gardner syndrome, 368
Gastric neoplasms
    adenocarcinoma, 244–245, 244f–245f
    gastrointestinal stromal tumor, 245
    polyps, 244
Gastric ulcers, acute, 91, 91f, 243
Gastrinoma triangle, 243
Gastritis
    acute, 240–241, 241f
    chronic, 241–242, 242f
Gastroesophageal reflux disease (GERD), 237–238, 237f, 239f
Gastrointestinal disorders
    abdominal pain, 231, 232t
    acute
        inflammation, 231, 232t
        obstruction, 231, 232t
        perforation, 231, 232t
        vascular disease, 231, 232t

chronic
   abdominal wall pain, 231, 232*t*
   functional, 231, 232*t*
   inflammation, 231, 232*t*
   metabolic disease, 231, 232*t*
   vascular disease, 231, 232*t*
appendicitis, acute, 256, 256*f*
bleeding, 231, 232*t*
constipation/diarrhea, 245–247, 245*t*, 246*f*–247*f*
diverticular disease, 254–255, 254*f*–255*f*
esophageal motor function, 235–236
esophageal neoplasms, 239–240
esophagitis, 237–238, 237*f*–239*f*
gastric neoplasms, 244–245, 244*f*–245*f*
gastric ulcers, acute, 243
gastritis, 240–242, 241*f*–242*f*
intestinal obstruction, 253*f*, 255, 255*f*
intestinal tumors, 256–259, 256*f*–259*f*
malabsorption, 248–253, 248*t*, 250*t*, 251*f*–252*f*
nonneoplastic disorders of esophagus alcohol-related,
      236–237, 236*f*–237*f*, 239
oral cavity, salivary glands, 234–235, 235*f*
pediatric, 232–233
peptic ulcer disease, 242–243, 243*f*
vascular disorders, 253–254, 253*f*
Gastroschisis, 73, 73*f*
Gaucher disease
   Type I, 62
   Type II, 62
   Type III, 63
GBM (glioblastoma multiforme), 158, 158*f*
Genetic disorders
   autosomal dominant, 55, 56*t*
      familial hypercholesterolemia, 56, 56*t*
      familial polyposis coli, 41*t*, 56, 56*f*, 257
      hereditary spherocytosis, 56, 56*t*, 186
      Marfan syndrome, 56–57, 56*t*, 98–99, 100*f*
      myotonic dystrophy type 1, 58
      NF-1, 44, 56*t*, 57, 57*f*
      NF-2, 56*t*, 57
      tuberous sclerosis, 56*t*, 58, 58*f*
      VHL disease, 41*t*, 44, 57
   autosomal recessive, 58, 59*t*
      alkaptonuria, 61
      α_1-Antitrypsin, 58, 211, 267, 273
      cystic fibrosis, 59, 59*t*
      galactosemia, 59*t*, 60
      hereditary hemochromatosis, 9, 9*f*, 59*t*, 60, 129–130, 266*t*,
         267, 272–273, 273*f*
      maple syrup urine disease, 59*t*, 61
      mucopolysaccharidosis (MPS), 62
      phenylketonuria(PKU), 59*t*, 60–61
      Wilson disease, 59*t*, 61, 266*t*, 267, 273, 276
   Cri-du-chat syndrome, 67
   Down syndrome, 65–66, 66*f*, 112, 194, 232
   Edward syndrome, 66
   genomic imprinting, Prader-Willi and Angelman
      syndromes, 68
glycogen storage
   hepatic forms, 63
   miscellaneous forms, 64, 64*f*
   myopathic forms, 64
lysosomal storage, 62
   Gaucher disease, 62–63
   Niemann-Pick disease, 63
   Tay-Sachs disease, 63
mixed inheritance patterns, Ehlers-Danlos
      syndrome, 65
Patau syndrome, 66
sex chromosome abnormalities
   fragile X syndrome, 68
   Klinefelter syndrome, 67
   Turner syndrome, 67, 67*f*
sexual differentiation
   female pseudohermaphrodite, 68
   male pseudohermaphrodite, 69
   true hermaphrodite, 68
22q11.2 deletion, 66–67
X-linked inheritance patterns
   Becker muscular dystrophy, 65
   Duchenne muscular dystrophy, 64–65
Genomic imprinting, 68
GERD. *See* Gastroesophageal reflux disease
Germ cell neoplasms, 35, 310, 310*t*
Germinal matrix hemorrhage, 75, 75*f*
Gestational hypertension, 97
Gestational trophoblastic disease. *See* Hydatidiform mole
GGT (gamma-glutamyltransferase), 261, 262*f*
Ghon complex/focus, 225, 226*f*
Giant cell arteritis, 103, 103*f*, 103*t*
Giant cell tumor of bone, 368*t*, 372, 372*f*
Giardia lamblia, 246, 246*f*
Gigantism, 339
Gilbert syndrome, 263–264
Glioblastoma multiforme (GBM), 158, 158*f*
Global hypoxic-ischemic encephalopathy, 90, 90*f*, 142–143
Glomerular disorders, 287–288
Glomerulonephritis
   chronic, 295, 295*f*
   membranoproliferative, 289*t*, 294–295, 294*f*
   postinfectious, 289*t*, 293, 293*f*
   rapidly progressive (RPGN), 289*t*, 293–294, 293*f*
Glucose-6-phosphate dehydrogenase deficiency
      (G6PD), 187
Glycogen storage disorders, 63–64, 64*f*
Goiter, 342–343, 343*f*
Goodpasture syndrome, 221, 294
Gout, 373*t*, 375–377, 376*f*
   saturnine, 377
Grade of tumor, 46
Graft-versus-host disease (GVHD), 27
Granulation tissue, 20
Granuloma, 19, 20*f*
Granuloma annulare, 388
Granulomatous inflammation, 19
Granulosa cell tumor, 326

Graves disease, 24, 344, 344*f*
Gray hepatization, 223
Growth hormone-secreting adenoma, 339
G6PD deficiency (glucose-6–phosphate dehydrogenase deficiency), 187
Guillain-Barré syndrome, 169
Gunshot wound, 50, 51*f*
GVHD (graft-versus-host disease), 27

Hairy cell leukemia, 202, 202*f*
Hairy leukoplakia, 44*t*, 234
Hamartoma, 36
HbH disease, 177
HBV. *See* Hepatitis B virus
HCC. *See* Hepatocellular carcinoma
Headache, 136
Healing, regeneration, 19
    first intention, 20
    general wound, 21
    mediators, 20
    scar replacement, 20
    second intention, 21
Heart. *See* Cardiac disorders
Heart failure cells, 83
Heat cramps, 50
Heat exhaustion, 51
Heat stroke, 51
Heavy chain disease, 205
Heberden nodes, 374
Heinz bodies, 187
Helicobacter pylori, 241–242
HELLP syndrome, 97, 331
Hemangioma, 106, 277, 278*f*
Hematemesis, 231
Hematocele, 313
Hematochezia, 231, 254
Hematoma, 85
Hematopathology
    anemia, 173–187, 174*t*, 176*f*, 176*t*, 178*f*, 180*t*,180*f*–181*f*, 184*t*, 185*f*-186*f*
    hemolytic anemia, 181–182, 185
    Hodgkin lymphoma, 196–198, 197*f*–198*f*, 197*t*
    immune-mediated platelet destruction, 205–206
    leukemia, 190–195, 190*f*, 191*t*, 192*f*–195*f*, 193*t*
    lymphoma, 190
    macrocytic anemia, 179–180, 180*f*, 180*t*
    myelodysplastic syndromes (MDS), 189
    microcytic anemia, 176–178, 176*f*, 176*t*, 178*f*
    myeloproliferative disorders, chronic, 195–196, 196*f*
    non-Hodgkin lymphoma, 197*t*, 199–202, 199*f*–202*f*
    nonimmune-mediated platelet destruction, 206–207, 206*f*, 207*f*
    plasma cell dyscrasias, 203–205, 203*f*
    platelet disorders, 207
    polycythemia, 188
    primary hemostasis disorders, 205
    red blood cell (RBC) destruction
        antibody-mediated, 182–185, 184*t*

        hereditary causes, 185–187, 186*f*
        infectious causes, 185, 185*f*
    secondary hemostasis disorders, 208
Hematopoietic transplantations, 27
Hemochromatosis, 9. *See also* Hereditary hemochromatosis
Hemodynamics
    edema, 82–83, 82*f*–83*f*
    embolus, 86–87, 86*f*–87*f*
    hemorrhage, 84–85, 84*f*–85*f*
    hemostasis, thrombosis, 85–86
    hyperemia, congestion, 83–84, 83*f*–84*f*
    infarcts, 81, 87*f*–88*f*, 88–89
    shock, 89–91, 90*f*–91*f*
Hemolytic anemia, 181–187, 184*f*, 184*t*, 185*f*–186*f*
Hemolytic uremic syndrome (HUS), 206
Hemophilia A, 208
Hemophilia B, 208
Hemorrhage, 84
    corticomedullary, 91
    Duret, 139, 139*f*
    ecchymoses, 84
    epidural, 146, 148*f*
    extracerebral, 146–148, 148*f*–150*f*
    gastric petechial, acute, 91, 91*f*
    germinal matrix, 75, 75*f*
    intracerebral, 48, 98, 145–146, 147*f*
    petechiae, 77, 77*f*, 84, 84*f*
    pulmonary, 220–221
    purpura, 84
    subarachnoid, 148, 150*f*
    subdural, 146–147, 149*f*
    terminology, 85, 85*f*
Hemosiderosis, 9
Hemostasis
    primary, 205 secondary. *See* Secondary hemostasis
    thrombus formation, 85–86
Henoch-Schönlein purpura (HSP), 294, 296
Heparin-induced thrombocytopenia, 205–206
Hepatic disorders. *See also* Hepatitis
    alcoholic liver disease, 271–272, 271*f*–272*f*
    circulation, 274–275
    cirrhosis, 9, 58, 82, 262, 262*t*, 266–268, 266*t*, 266*f*–268*f*
    drugs affecting, 271
    encephalopathy, 266
    failure
        complications, 265
        hepatic encephalopathy, 266
        hepatorenal syndrome, 266
        massive hepatic necrosis, 265
    metabolic liver disease, 272–273, 272*f*–273*f*
    neoplasms, 275–277, 276*f*–278*f*
    obstructive biliary tract disorders, 273–274, 274*f*, 274*t*
Hepatitis
    acute, 268, 268*f*
    alcoholic, 271–272, 272*f*
    autoimmune, 270–271
    chronic, 268, 268*f*–269*f*
    viral, 269–270, 269*t*

Hepatitis B virus (HBV), 38, 104, 269–270, 269t, 276, 291, 293
Hepatoblastoma, 277
Hepatocellular carcinoma (HCC), 38, 41t, 276, 276f
Hepatocellular dysfunction, 267–268
Hepatojugular reflux, 122
Hepatolenticular degeneration. *See* Wilson disease
Hepatorenal syndrome, 266
Hepcidin, 178
Hereditary hemochromatosis, 9, 9f, 59t, 60, 129–130, 266t, 267, 272–273, 273f
Hereditary immunodeficiency states, 31–33
    common variable immunodeficiency, 32
    hyper-IgM syndrome, 32
    isolated IgA deficiency, 32
    severe combined immunodeficiency disease (SCID), 32–33
    Wiskott-Aldrich syndrome, 33
    X-linked agammaglobulinemia of Bruton, 31–32
Hereditary nonpolyposis colon cancer, 257
Hereditary spherocytosis, 56, 56t, 186, 398, 416
Herniation
    cerebellar tonsillar, 82, 138, 138f
    cerebral edema, 82, 138–139, 138f–139f
    cingulate (subfalcine), 82, 139
    transcalvarial, 139
    uncal (transtentorial), 82, 139, 139f
Herpes simplex virus (HSV), 75, 154–155, 238, 238f, 317
Her-2–Neu, 335
HHV-8. *See* Human herpesvirus 8
Hiatal hernia, 235–236
Hill sign, 127
Hirschsprung disease, 233
HIV. *See* Human immunodeficiency virus
Hives (urticaria), 24, 384
HLA-B27, 27, 375, 385
Hodgkin lymphoma, 196–197, 197f, 197t
    lymphocyte predominant, 198
    mixed cellularity, 198, 198f
    nodular sclerosis type, 198, 198f
Holoprosencephaly
    alobar, 140
    lobar, 141
    semilobar, 141
Homer-Wright rosettes, 78, 160, 372
Horner syndrome, 228
Horseshoe kidney, 67, 67f, 73
HPV. *See* Human papillomavirus
HSP (Henoch-schönlein purpura), 294, 296
HSV. *See* Herpes simplex virus
HTLV-1 (human T-cell leukemia virus type 1), 38, 202
Human herpesvirus 8 (HHV-8), 39, 106, 201
Human immunodeficiency virus (HIV), 33–34, 234, 388
Human papillomavirus (HPV), 38, 42f, 313, 316–317, 317f, 388
Human T-cell leukemia virus type 1 (HTLV-1), 38, 202
Humoral rejection, 26
Huntington chorea, 164
HUS (hemolytic uremic syndrome), 206
Hutchison teeth, 76
Hyaline arteriolosclerosis, 98, 98f, 292f

Hyaline membrane disease, 74, 74f
    bronchopulmonary dysplasia, 75
    retrolental fibroplasia, 74
Hyaline membranes, 74, 74f, 90, 216, 216f
Hydatidiform mole, 327–329, 328f, 328t, 344
Hydrocele, 313
Hydrocephalus
    communicating, 137, 137f
    noncommunicating, 138
    normal pressure, 138, 164
    pseudotumor cerebri, 138
Hydrocephalus ex vacuo, 138
Hyperadrenalism. *See* Cushing syndrome
Hyperaldosteronism, 286, 358
Hyperemia, congestion, 83
    passive liver chronic, 84, 84f
    passive lung chronic, 83, 83f
Hyper-IgM syndrome, 32
Hyperkalemia, 284, 307, 356
Hypernatremia, 286, 307
Hyperparathyroidism, 349, 349t, 350f
    primary, 350, 350f
    secondary, 350
    tertiary, 350
Hyperpituitarism, 337–339
    pituitary adenomas, 338f, 338–339
Hyperplasia, 1
    adrenal, 355f, 355t
    benign prostatic, 314, 314f
    endometrial, 320–321, 321f
    focal nodular, 276, 277f
Hyperplastic arteriolosclerosis, 98, 98f
Hypersensitivity pneumonitis, 220
Hypersensitivity reactions
    Type I, 23–24
    Type II, 24–25
    Type III, 25
    Type IV, 25
Hypertension, 2f, 96–98, 354
    benign (idiopathic), 97
    chronic, 97
    gestational, 97
    malignant, 97
    preeclampsia, 97
    pulmonary, 86, 99–100, 219, 221, 221f
    secondary. *See* secondary hypertension
    systemic. *See* Systemic hypertension
Hypertensive cardiovascular disease, 2f, 120
Hyperthermia, malignant, 51
Hyperthyroidism, 245t, 343–344, 343t
Hypertrophic cardiomyopathy, 129, 129f
Hypertrophy
    concentric, 120
    pathologic/physiologic, 2, 2f, 98
Hypoadrenalism, 356–357, 356f–357f
Hypokalemia, 51, 308
Hyponatremia, 284, 286, 307, 342, 356
Hypoparathyroidism, 350

Hypopituitarism, 340, 340f
Hypoplasia, 2
Hypospadias, 73
Hypothyroidism, 343t, 345–346
    cretinism, 345
    myxedema, 345–346
Hypovolemic shock, 89
Hypoxia, 3–4

Icterus, 262, 262f
Idiopathic (benign) hypertension, 97
Idiopathic Parkinson disease, 165, 165f
Idiopathic pulmonary fibrosis, 219–220
Idiopathic thrombocytopenic purpura, 185, 205
IgA nephropathy, 295–296
Ileus, 245
Immune complex deposition-mediated vasculitis, 102
Immune-mediated platelet destruction, 205
Immune system disorders
    AIDS, 33–34, 33f, 34f
    amyloidosis, 31, 31t, 32f
    antibody-mediated red blood cell (RBC) destruction, 182–185
    autoimmune diseases, 27t, 27–30
    fetal hydrops, 77
    hematopoietic transplantations, 27
    hereditary immunodeficiency states, 31–33
    immune cytopenic purpura (ITP), 205
    neuropathy, 169
    transplantation pathology, 25–26, 26f
    Type I hypersensitivity reaction, 23
        early phase, 23–24
        late phase, 24
    Type II hypersensitivity reaction, 24
        antibody-dependent cell-mediated cytotoxicity, 24
        antibody-dependent cellular dysfunction, 24–25
        complement-dependent reactions, 24
    Type III hypersensitivity reaction, 25
    Type IV hypersensitivity reaction, 25
        cell-mediated cytotoxicity, 25
    vasculitis, 102
Immune thrombocytopenic purpura (ITP), 185, 205
Impetigo, 388
Incised wound, 50
Inclusion body myositis, 171
Ineffective erythropoiesis, 180
Infarcts, 81, 88–89, 88f
    cerebral, 143–145, 143f–146f, 143t
    lacunar, 145, 146f
    myocardial, 113, 116–120, 116f, 117t, 119t, 118f–121f
    red (hemorrhagic), 87f, 88
    white (anemic), 88, 88f
Infective endocarditis, 122f–123f, 123–124
    Janeway lesions, 123
    Osler nodes, 123
    Roth spots, 123
Inflammation
    acute 14–18
        mediators of, 14–16, 14t

morphology of
    fibrinous, 17
    purulent, 17, 17f
    serous, 17
outcomes of
    abscess, 18, 18f
    fistula, 18, 19f
    resolution, 17–18
    ulcer, 18, 18f
    signs of 14, 14t
chemotaxis, 16
chronic, 19
healing versus regeneration, 19–20
impaired inflammatory response diseases
    Chédiak-Higashi syndrome, 17
    chronic granulomatous disease, 16–17
increased vascular permeability, 14–15
    delayed prolonged response, 15
    endothelial cell retraction, 15
    endothelial contraction, 15
scar formation, 18
vasodilation, 14
white blood cell movement
    pavementing, 15
    rolling, 15
    transmigration, 15
Inflammatory carcinoma of the breast, 335
Inherited bone diseases
    achondroplasia, 361–362
    osteogenesis imperfecta, 362
    osteopetrosis, 362–363
Inherited skin neoplasia syndromes
    basal cell nevus, 383
    dysplastic nevus, 383
INK4a/ARF, 44
Interstitial nephritis
    acute, 297, 297f
    chronic, 297–298
Intestinal metaplasia, 242, 242f
Intestinal tumors
    adenomas, 256–257, 256f–257f
    carcinoid tumor, 258–259, 258f–259f
    colonic adenocarcinoma, 257–258, 257f–258f
    nonneoplastic polyps, 256
Intracerebral hemorrhage, 48, 98, 145–146, 147f
Intraductal papilloma, 333, 333f
Intratubular germ cell neoplasia, 311
Intrinsic azotemia, 284
Intussusception, 233
Involucrum, 365
Inv16, 193t, 194
Iron deficiency anemia, 176, 176f, 176t
Ischemia, 3
Ischemic bowel disease, 253–254, 253f
Ischemic heart disease
    clinical syndromes, 113–115, 114f–115f
    myocardial infarction, 113, 116–120, 116f, 118f–121f, 117t, 119t

non-ST segment elevation (NSTEMI), 113, 116–117, 116*f*
ST segment elevation STEMI, 113, 116–117
stable angina, 114, 114*f*
unstable angina, 113–117
variant angina, 115
Islet cell tumor, 281
Isohemagglutinin reaction, 182
Isolated IgA deficiency, 32
ITP (immune thrombocytopenic purpura), 185, 205

Janeway lesions, 123
Jaundice, cholestasis, 11, 262–265, 262*f*, 263*t*, 264*f*
Crigler-Najjar syndrome, 264
Dubin-Johnson syndrome, 264
Gilbert syndrome, 263–264, 263*t*
neonatal cholestasis, 264
physiologic jaundice of newborn, 263

Kaposi sarcoma, 34, 34*f*, 39, 106–107
Kartagener syndrome, 214–215
Karyolysis, 5
Kasabach-Merritt syndrome, 106
Kawasaki disease, 103*t*, 105
Kayser-Fleischer rings, 61
Keloid scar, 21, 21*f*
Kernicterus, 183
Kernig sign, 153
Kidney disorders. *See also* Renal disorders
asymptomatic hematuria, 295–296
congenital anomalies, 73
cystic diseases, 301–303, 302*f*
glomerular disorders, 82, 287–288
glomerulonephritis, chronic, 295, 295*f*
infections, 298–300, 299*f*–300*f*
neoplasms, 303–304, 303*f*–304*f*
nephritic syndrome, 289*t*, 292*t*, 292–295, 293*f*–294*f*
nephrolithiasis, 301, 301*f*, 301*t*
nephrotic syndrome, 288–292, 288*f*, 289*t*, 290*f*–292*f*, 292*t*
renal failure
acute 283–285, 284*t*
chronic renal failure, 285–286
tubulointerstitial disease, 296–298, 297*f*–298*f*
volume disorders, 286
Kidney stones. *See* Nephrolithiasis
Kimmelstiel-Wilson lesion, 292, 292*f*, 353
Klinefelter syndrome, 67
Koilocytes, 317, 317*f*
Korsakoff syndrome, 48, 52, 136
Krukenberg tumor, 326
Kussmaul sign, 122, 131
Kwashiorkor, 51

Laceration, 50, 50*f*
Lactose intolerance. *See* Disaccharidase deficiency
Lacunar infarcts, 145, 146*f*
Lambert-Eaton syndrome, 40, 171–172, 227
Laminar cortical necrosis, 142–143

Large cell carcinoma, 227, 228*f*
Laron dwarfism, 362
LCIS (lobular carcinoma in situ), 334
Left-sided heart failure, 83, 83*f*, 121–122
Leiomyoma, 36, 322–323, 323*f*
Leiomyosarcoma, 36, 323
Leipidic growth, 227
Lentigo, 380
Lesch-Nyhan syndrome, 376
Leser-Trélat, sign of, 381
Leukemia, 191, 191*t*
acute lymphoid (ALL), 191–192 191*t*, 192*f*
acute myeloid (AML), 191*t*, 193–194, 193*t*, 194*f*
adult T-cell leukemia, 38, 202
chronic lymphoid (CLL), 192–193 191*t*, 193*f*
chronic mycloid (CML), 191*t*, 194–195, 195*f*
cytogenetic abnormalities of acute lymphoid, 194
hairy cell, 202, 202*f*
T-cell lymphoblastic, 201
Leukoplakia, 234
Leukotrienes, 14, 14*t*, 16
Lewy body, 165, 165*f*
Lewy body disease, diffuse, 163
LFA-1, 14*t*, 15
Libman-Sacks endocarditis, 28
Li-Fraumeni, 41*t*
Lines of Zahn, 86, 86*f*
Linitis plastica, 245
Lipofuscin, 7–8, 8*f*
Lipoprotein A (Lpa), 94
Lisch nodules, 57
Lissencephaly, 141
Liver disorders. *See* Hepatic disorders
Liver neoplasms
angiosarcoma, 277
cholangiocarcinoma, 276, 277*f*
focal nodular hyperplasia, 276, 277*f*
hemangioma, 277, 278*f*
hepatic adenoma, 277
hepatoblastoma, 277
hepatocellular carcinoma (HCC), 38, 41*t*, 276, 276*f*
Lobar holoprosencephaly, 141
Lobar pneumonia, 222, 223, 223*f*
Lobular carcinoma in situ (LCIS), 334
Lou Gehrig disease [amyotrophic lateral sclerosis (ALS)], 166
LPL (lymphoplasmacytic lymphoma), 204
Luetic aortic aneurysm. *See* Syphilitic aortitis
Lymphocyte predominant Hodgkin lymphoma, 197*t*, 198
Lymphocytic (aseptic) meningitis, 151–152
Lymphocytic myocarditis, 130, 130*f*
Lymphoma, 190
cell markers, 197*t*
central nervous system (CNS), 160, 161*f*
Hodgkin, 196–198, 197*f*–198*f*, 197*t*
non-Hodgkin, 197*t*, 199–202, 199*f*–202*f*
testicular, 313
translocations, 197*t*

Lymphomatoid polyposis, 202
Lymphoplasmacytic lymphoma (LPL), 204
Lysosomal storage disorders, 62–63

Mac-1, 14t, 15
Macrocytic anemia
    B$_{12}$ deficiency, 179–180, 180f, 180t
    folate deficiency, 180, 180f, 180t
Macrovesicular steatosis, 262
Malabsorption, 248, 248t
    celiac sprue, 249
    Crohn disease, 250t, 251–252, 251f
    disaccharidase deficiency, 249–250
    inflammatory bowel disease, 250, 250t
    steatorrhea, 248–249
    ulcerative colitis, 252–253, 252f
    Whipple disease, 253
Male pseudohermaphrodite
    5α-reductase deficiency, 69
    testicular feminization, 69
Male reproductive tract disorders. See also Testicular
        neoplasms
    congenital anomalies, 73
    prostate pathology, 314–316, 314f–315f
    squamous cell carcinoma of penis, 313
    testicular neoplasms, 309–313, 310t, 310f–312f
Malignant hypertension, 97
Malignant hyperthermia, 51
Malignant melanoma, 44t, 380–381, 381f
Malignant peripheral nerve sheath tumor, 57, 57f
Mallory hyaline, 9, 9f, 271f, 272
Mallory-Weiss laceration, 236, 236f
Maltese cross, 288
MALToma, 30, 202
Mantle cell lymphoma, 202
Maple syrup urine disease, 61
Marasmus, 51
Marfan syndrome, 56–57, 56t, 98–99, 100f
Marginal zone lymphoma. See MAL Toma
Marjolin ulcer, 382
Mass effect, endocrine disorders, 339–341
Massive hepatic necrosis, 265
Mast cell tryptase, 213
Mastitis, acute, 331
McArdle syndrome, 10
McCune-Albright syndrome, 371
MDS (myelodysplastic syndrome), 189
Meckel diverticulum, 233, 254, 254f
Meconium ileus, 59
Medullary thyroid carcinoma, 348–349, 349f, 359–360
Medulloblastoma, 78, 78t, 160, 161f
Megaloblastic anemia. See Macrocytic anemia
Meigs syndrome, 326
Meiosis, 228
Melanocytic nevus, 380, 380f
Melanocytic proliferations
    acanthosis nigricans, 382, 382f
    basal cell carcinoma, 383, 383f

    cutaneous squamous cell carcinoma, 382–383
    dysplastic nevus, 380
    malignant melanoma, 380–381, 381f
    melanocytic nevus, 380, 380f
    seborrheic keratosis, 381, 382f
Melanoma, malignant, 44t, 380–381, 381f
Melena, 231, 237, 243
Membranoproliferative glomerulonephritis (MPGN), 289t,
        294–295, 294f
Membranous glomerulonephropathy, 289t, 291, 291f
MEN (multiple endocrine neoplasia), 359–360
Meningioma, 57, 161, 162f
Meningitis, 151t, 154t
    bacterial, 151–153, 151t, 152f
    brain abscess, 153–154, 154f
    Brudzinski sign, 153
    chemical, 151
    chronic, 151
    cryptococcal, 152, 153f
    fungal, 153
    Kernig sign, 153
    lymphocytic (aseptic), 151–152
    purulent (pyogenic), 151, 152t
    tuberculous, 152–153, 153f
    viral, 151–152
    Waterhouse-Friderichsen syndrome, 152, 357, 357f
Mesocapillary glomerulonephritis, 294
Mesothelioma, 230
Metabolic acidosis, 306
Metabolic alkalosis, 306
Metabolic syndrome, 94
Metaplasia, 3, 3f
    glandular, 238, 239f
    intestinal, 242, 242f
Metastic calcification, 8
MGUS (monoclonal gammopathy of undetermined
        significance), 204
Microalbuminuria, 291
Microatelectasis, 210
Microcytic anemia, 176t, 176–178, 176f, 178f
Microglial reactions, 137, 155, 155f
Microscopic polyarteritis, 102, 105
Microvesicular steatosis, 262
Miliary TB, 225
Minimal change disease, 289–290, 289t
Mismatched ventilation-perfusion, 211
Mitochondrial cytosolic calcium, 4
Mitral regurgitation
    mitral annular calcification, 128
    myxomatous mitral valve, 127–128, 128f
Mitral stenosis, 124, 124f, 127
Mitral valve prolapse, 128
Mixed acid-base disorders, 306
Mixed cellularity Hodgkin lymphoma, 198, 198f
Mixed connective tissue disorder, 30
Mönckeberg medial calcification, 93
Monoclonal gammopathy of undetermined significance
        (MGUS), 204

MPGN. *See* Membranoproliferative glomerulonephritis

MPS. *See* Mucopolysaccharidosis

MS. *See* Multiple sclerosis

M-spike, 203

Mucinous ovarian tumors, 325, 326*f*

Mucocutaneous lymph node syndrome. *See* Kawasaki disease

Mucoepidermoid carcinoma, 235

Mucopolysaccharidosis (MPS)
    Hunter disease (type II), 59*t*, 62
    Hurler disease (type I), 59*t*, 62

Multiple endocrine neoplasia 1, 359. *See also* Wermer syndrome

Multiple endocrine neoplasia 2A, 359. *See also* Sipple syndrome

Multiple endocrine neoplasia 2B, 358, 360

Multiple myeloma, 203–204, 203*f*

Multiple sclerosis (MS), 167–168
    acute (Marburg), 167
    Baló disease, 167
    clinical presentation, lab studies, 167–168
    Devic disease, 167
    morphology, 167, 167*f*

Munro microabscesses, 385

Mural thrombi, 119, 119*t*, 119*f*–120*f*

Myasthenia gravis, 25, 171

MYC, 42–43, 79, 201, 257

Mycosis fungoides/Sézary syndrome, 202

Mycotic aneurysm, 100

Myelin ovoids, 169

Myelodysplastic syndromes (MDS), 189

Myelofibrosis with myeloid metaplasia, 196, 196*f*

Myeloperoxidase, 16

Myelophthisic anemia, 181, 181*f*

Myeloproliferative disorders, chronic
    chronic myeloid (myelogenous) leukemia, 191*t*, 194–195, 195*f*
    essential thrombocytosis, 195–196
    myelofibrosis with myeloid metaplasia, 196, 196*f*
    polycythemia rubra vera, 196

Myocardial infarcts
    complications of, 119*t*
        aneurysm, 119, 121*f*
        arrhythmia, 119
        cardiogenic shock, 118, 118*f*
        conduction abnormalities, 119
        electrical, 119
        infarct expansion, 120, 120*f*
        infarct extension, 120
        mural thrombi, 119, 119*f*–120*f*
        pericarditis, 119, 119*t*, 131, 131*t*
        pseudoaneurysm, 119
        right ventricular infarct, 120
        rupture, 118–119, 119*f*–120*f*
    morphology of, 117–118, 117*t*, 116*f*–118*f*
    non-ST segment elevation (NSTEMI), 113, 116–117, 116*f*
    reperfusion of, 116*f*, 118
    ST segment elevation (STEMI), 113, 116–117, 116*f*

Myocardial rupture, 118–119, 120*f*

Myocarditis, lymphocytic, 130, 130*f*

Myocyte disarray, 129, 129*f*

Myopathies, 170–171
    congenital, 171
    mitochondrial, 171

Myotonic dystrophy type 1, 58

Myxedema, 345–346, 346*f*

Myxomatous mitral valve, 57, 127–128, 128*f*

NAFLD (nonalcoholic fatty liver disease), 272, 272*f*

Nasopharyngeal carcinoma, 38

Necrobiosis lipoidica, 389

Necrosis, 6–7
    caseous, 7, 7*f*
    centrilobular, 90, 90*f*
    coagulative, 6, 6*f*, 117, 117*t*, 118*f*
    fat, 7
    laminar cortical, 142–143
    liquefactive, 6–7, 6*f*
    massive hepatic, 265
    osteo-, 364
    subendocardial contraction band, 90
    tubular, acute, 90–91

Necrotizing enterocolitis, 75, 75*f*

Necrotizing pneumonia, 224

Negri bodies, 155

Nelson syndrome, 339

Neonatal cholestasis, 264

Neonates, acquired CNS abnormalities, 141, 141*f*

Neoplasm/neoplasia, 34, 34*f*, 35. *See also specific types of* Tumors
    adrenal, 358–360, 359*f*
    benign *versus* malignant
        growth rates, 37
        histologic features, 36–37, 38*f*–39*f*
        invasion, metastases, 37, 39*f*–40*f*
    cancer epidemiology, etiology, 37–39
    cancer morphology, 45
    cancer stem cells, 37
    carcinogenesis, 40, 42–45
    carcinogens, 42*t*
    central nervous system (CNS), 156–161, 156*t*, 158*f*–162*f*
    diagnosis of, 44*t*–45*t*, 46
    effects of, 39–40
    endometrial, 321–323, 322*f*
    gastric, 244–245, 244*f*–245*f*
    germ cell, 35, 310, 310*t*
        intratubular, 311
    grade and stage, 46
    liver. *See also* Liver neoplasms
    microscopic appearance of
        anaplasia, 36, 38*f*
        carcinoma in situ, 36
        differentiation, 36, 37*f*
        dysplasia, 36, 38*f*
    nomenclature, general, 35, 36*f*
    pediatric, 77–80, 78*f*–79*f*, 78*t*
    pulmonary, 226–228, 227*f*–229*f*

Neoplasm/neoplasia (*continued*)
　renal, 303–304, 303*f*–304*f*
　testicular. *See also* Testicular neoplasms
　thyroid, 347–349, 347*f*–349*f*
　tumor antigens, 45
　urothelial, 304–305, 304*f*–305*f*
　viruses associated with, 38
Nephritic syndrome, 289*t*, 292, 292*t*
　membranoproliferative glomerulonephritis (MPGN), 289*t*,
　　294–295, 294*f*
　postinfectious glomerulonephritis, 289*t*, 293, 293*f*
　rapidly progressive glomerulonephritis (RPGN), 289*t*,
　　293–294, 293*f*
Nephrolithiasis, 301, 301*f*, 301*t*
Nephrotic syndrome, 292*t*, 288–289
　components, complications, 288–289, 289*t*
　diabetic nephropathy, 291–292, 292*f*
　focal sigmental glomerulosclerosis (FSGS), 289*t*,
　　290, 290*f*
　membranous glomerulonephropathy, 289*t*, 291, 291*f*
　minimal change disease, 289–290, 289*t*
Neural tube defects, 139–140, 140*f*
Neuroblastoma, 78–79, 78*f*, 78*t*
　opsoclonus-myoclonus syndrome, 79
　prognostic factors, 79
Neurodegenerative diseases
　primarily with dementia
　　Alzheimer disease, 9, 9*f*, 162–163, 163*f*–164*f*
　　frontotemporal dementia, 163
　　Lewy body disease, diffuse, 163
　　normal pressure hydrocephalus, 164
　　vascular dementia, 164
　primarily without dementia
　　amyotrophic lateral sclerosis, 166
　　Huntington chorea, 164
　　idiopathic Parkinson disease, 165, 165*f*
　　Lou Gehrig disease, 166
　　progressive supranuclear palsy, 165–166
　　secondary Parkinsonism, 165
　　spinal muscular atrophy, 166
Neurofibrillary tangles, 162, 164*f*
Neurofibromatosis (NF)
　NF-1, 44, 57, 57*f*, 159
　NF-2, 57, 159
Neurofibromin, 44, 57
Neurogenic shock, 90
Neuroleptic malignant syndrome, 51
Neuromyelitis optica. *See* Devic disease
Neuronal migration disorders, 141
Neuropathology
　cerebral edema, herniation, 138–139, 138*f*–139*f*
　CNS infections, 150–155, 152*f*–154*f*, 151*t*, 154*t*, 155*f*
　CNS tumors, 156–161, 156*t*, 158*f*–162*f*
　consciousness disorders, 133–135
　cortical defects, localized, 135–136
　demyelinating diseases, 166–168, 167*f*
　dizziness, 136
　extracerebral hemorrhage, 146–148, 148*f*–150*f*

　general morphologic changes, 137, 137*f*
　headache, 136
　hydrocephalus, 137–138, 137*f*
　malformations, 139–141, 140*f*
　neonates, acquired abnormalities, 141, 141*f*
　neurodegenerative diseases
　　primarily with dementia, 162–164, 163*f*–164*f*
　　primarily without dementia, 164–166, 165*f*
　peripheral nerve pathology, 169
　seizures, 136–137
　skeletal muscle pathology, 170–172
　spongiform encephalopathies, 155–156
　trauma of parenchyma, 149–150, 151*f*
　vascular disease, 142–146, 143*f*–147*f*, 143*t*
　vascular malformations, 141–142
Neuropathy
　axonal, 169
　demyelinating, 169
　immune, 169
　infectious, 169
NF. *See* Neurofibromatosis
Niemann-Pick disease, Types A, B, and C, 63
Nikolsky sign, 386, 387
Nodular sclerosis Hodgkin lymphoma, 198, 198*f*
Nonalcoholic fatty liver disease (NAFLD), 272, 272*f*
Nonallergic asthma, 212
Non-Hodgkin lymphoma, 197*t*, 199–200, 199*f*
　adult T-cell leukemia/lymphoma, 202
　Burkitt, 201, 201*f*
　diffuse large B-cell (DLBCL), 200–201, 201*f*
　follicular, 200, 200*f*
　hairy cell leukemia, 202, 202*f*
　MALToma, 202
　mantle cell, 202
　mycosis fungoides/Sézary syndrome, 202
　precursor T-cell lymphoblastic leukemia/lymphoma, 201
　small lymphocytic (SLL), 200
Nosocomial pneumonia, 224
NSTEMI (non-ST segment elevation myocardial infarct),
　　116–117, 116*f*
Null cell adenoma, 338
Nutmeg liver, 84, 84*f*
Nutritional disorders. *See also specific* Nutritional deficiencies
　anorexia, 51
　bulimia, 52
　kwashiorkor, 51
　marasmus, 51
Nystagmus, 136

Obliterative endarteritis, 101
Obstructive atelectasis, 210
Obstructive biliary tract disorders
　primary biliary cirrhosis, 273–274, 274*f*, 274*t*
　primary sclerosing cholangitis, 274, 274*t*
Obstructive lung disease, 210–211
　asthma, 212–213, 213*f*–214*f*
　bronchiectasis, 214–215, 215*f*
　bronchitis, chronic, 214

chronic obstructive pulmonary disease, 215
  emphysema, 58, 211–212, 211*f*–212*f*
Obstructive pulmonary disease, chronic, 215
Ochronosis, 61
Oligodendroglioma, 159, 160*f*
Omphalocele, 73
Opsoclonus-myoclonus syndrome, 79
Opsonin, 14*t*, 16
Oral cavity, salivary glands
  hairy leukoplakia, 234
  leukoplakia, 234
  mucoepidermoid carcinoma, 235
  pleomorphic adenoma, 234–235, 235*f*
  salivary gland tumors, 234
  squamous cell carcinoma, 234
"Orphan Annie eye" nuclei, 347, 347*f*
Orthopnea, 109, 121
Osler nodes, 123
Osteitis deformans. *See* Paget disease
Osteitis fibrosa cystica, 350
Osteoarthritis, 373*t*, 373–374, 374*f*
Osteochondroma, 368*t*, 370, 370*f*
Osteodystrophy, renal, 366–367
Osteogenesis imperfecta, 362
Osteoma, 368–369, 368*t*
Osteomyelitis
  pyogenic, 364–365, 365*f*
  tuberculous, 365
Osteonecrosis, 364
Osteopetrosis, 362–363
Osteoporosis, 363–364
Osteosarcoma, 41*t*, 368*t*, 369, 369*f*
Ovarian disease, nonneoplastic, polycystic, 323
Ovarian tumors
  Brenner tumor, 325, 326*f*
  cystic teratoma, mature, 325–326, 327*f*
  dysgerminoma, 326
  endometrioid, 325
  epithelial, 324, 324*t*
  fibrothecoma, 326
  granulosa cell, 326
  Krukenberg, 326
  mucinous, 325, 326*f*
  serous, 324, 324*t*, 324*f*–325*f*
  surface epithelial, 324, 324*t*

Paget disease
  of bone, 365–366, 366*f*
  of breast, 333–334, 334*f*
Panacinar emphysema, 211
p-ANCA, 102, 105, 274
Pancreas divisum, 73
Pancreatic adenocarcinoma, 44, 44*t*, 281
Pancreatic disorders
  cysts, 281
  islet cell tumor, 281
  pancreatic adenocarcinoma, 44, 44*t*, 281
  pancreatic cysts, 281

pancreatitis
  acute, 280, 280*f*
  chronic, 281, 281*f*
Pannus, 374
Papillary necrosis, 187, 300, 300*f*
Papillary renal cell carcinoma, 304, 304*f*
Papillary thyroid carcinoma, 347, 347*f*–348*f*
Paradoxical embolus, 110–112, 153
Paraneoplastic syndromes, 39–40, 304
  ACTH (adreno corticotropic hormone)-like protein,
    40, 227
  erythropoietin, 40
  nerve, muscle, 40, 227
  PTH (parathyroid)-like protein, 39, 227
  syndrome of inappropriate antidiuretic hormone (SIADH), 40
Paraphimosis, 73
Parathyroid gland disorders
  hyperparathyroidism, 349–350, 349*t*, 350*f*
  hypoparathyroidism, 350
Parathyroid hormone (PTH), 39, 227
Paroxysmal cold hemoglobinuria. *See* Cold hemolysin
    hemolytic anemia
Paroxysmal nocturnal dyspnea, 109, 121
Paroxysmal nocturnal hemoglobinuria (PNH), 175
Patau syndrome, 66
Patched gene (PTCH), 183
Patent ductus arteriosus (PDA), 112
Pautrier microabscess, 202
Pavementing, 15
PCOD (polycystic ovarian disease), 321, 323
PDA (patent ductus arteriosus), 112
Pearson disease, 178
Peau d'orange, 335
Pediatric disorders, 71
  congenital anomalies, 71–73, 73*f*
  fetal hydrops, 76–77, 76*f*
  gastrointestinal
    congenital pyloric stenosis, 232
    duodenal atresia, 232
    Hirschsprung disease, 233
    intussusception, 233
    Meckel diverticulum, 233
  neoplasms, 77, 78*t*
    Burkitt lymphoma, 78, 78*t*, 197*t*, 201, 201*f*
    Ewing sarcoma, 78, 78*t*, 368*t*, 372, 372*f*
    medulloblastoma, 78, 78*t*, 160, 161*f*
    neuroblastoma, 78–79, 78*f*, 78*t*
    osteosarcoma, 41*t*, 368*t*, 369, 369*f*
    primitive neuroectodermal tumor (PNET), 78, 78*t*, 368*t*,
      372, 372*f*
    retinoblastoma, 41*t*
    rhabdomyosarcoma, 78, 78*t*
    Wilms tumor, 79–80, 79*f*, 399, 416
  perinatal infections, 75–76
  prematurity, 73–75
  sudden infant death syndrome (SIDS), 77
Peliosis hepatitis, 275
Pellagra, 52

Pelvic inflammatory diseases (PID), 317–318, 318f
Pemphigus, 386, 387t
Peptic ulcer disease, 242–243, 243f
Pericardial disease, 131–132, 131f–132f, 131t
   cardiac tamponade, 132
   pericardial effusion, 132
   pericarditis, 119, 119t, 131, 131f–132f, 131t
Perinatal infections
   congenital rubella, 76
   congenital syphilis, 76
   cytomegalovirus (CMV) infection, 76
   herpes simplex virus (HSV) infection, 75
Peripheral vascular disease, 95
Periventricular leukomalacia, 141
Pernicious anemia, 179, 242
Petechiae, 77, 77f, 84, 84f
Peutz-Jeghers syndrome, 256
p53 gene, 41, 41t, 43–44, 153, 240, 382
Phenylketonuria (PKU), 60–61
Pheochromocytoma, 96, 96t, 358–360, 359f
Phimosis, 73
Phosphatase and tensin homologue (PTEN), 44,
       321–322
Phyllodes tumor, 332–333
Physical trauma, 50, 50f–51f
   hyperthermia
      heat cramps, 50
      heat exhaustion, 51
      heat stroke, 51
   hypothermia, 51
   thermal burns, 50
Physiologic jaundice of newborn, 263
PID (pelvic inflammatory disease), 317–318, 318f
Pigment disorders
   freckles, 379
   lentigo, 380
   vitiligo, 379
Pigments, exogenous, 10, 10f
Pilocytic astrocytomas, 159, 159f
Pitting edema, 83
Pituitary disorders
   adenomas, 338f, 338–339
   hyperpituitarism, 337–339
   hypopituitarism, 340
   posterior gland disorders
      diabetes insipidus, 342
      syndrome of inappropriate antidivretic hormone
          (SIADH), 341–342
PKU (phenylketonuria), 60–61
Placental, pregnancy-related disorders
   abortion, 326–327
   abruption, 329, 394, 414
   chorioamnionitis, 327
   eclampsia/preeclampsia, 97, 330–331
   ectopic pregnancy, 329–330
   hydatidiform mole, 327–329, 328f, 328t
   hypertension, 97, 330–331
   placental abruption, 47, 48, 329

placenta accreta, 330, 330f
placenta previa, 330, 330f
toxemia of pregnancy, 97, 330–331
Plasma cell dyscrasias
   heavy chain disease, 205
   lymphoplasmacytic lymphoma (LPL), 204
   monoclonal gammopathy of undetermined significance
          (MGUS), 204
   multiple myeloma, 203–204, 203f
   plasmacytoma, 204
   Russell bodies, 203
   Waldenström macroglobulinemia, 204
Plasmacytoma, 204
Platelet destruction
   immune-mediated
      heparin-induced thrombocytopenia, 205–206
      immune thrombocytopenic purpura (ITP),185, 205
   nonimmune-mediated
      disseminated intravascular coagulation (DIC), 185,
          206–207, 207f
      hemolytic uremic syndrome (HUS), 206
      thrombotic thrombocytopenic purpura, 185,
          206, 206f
Platelet disorders, 205–207, 206f–207f
Pleomorphic adenoma, 234–235, 235f
Pleomorphism, 37
Pleural conditions
   effusions, 223f, 229
   mesothelioma, 218, 230
   pneumothorax, 210, 226, 229–230
Plummer-Vinson syndrome, 239
PNET. See Primitive neuroectodermal tumor
Pneumatosis intestinalis, 75
Pneumoconioses, 217–218, 217f–218f
Pneumocystis pneumonia, 32, 33f, 34, 226
Pneumonia
   aspiration, 224, 224f–225f
   bronchopneumonia, 222, 222f
   chronic, 224–225, 226t
   community-acquired
      atypical, 223–224, 224f
      typical, 222–223, 222f–223f
   in immunocompromised, 226
   lobar, 222, 223, 223f
   necrotizing, 224
   nosocomial, 224
   usual interstitial, 219–220
Pneumothorax, 210, 226, 229–230
   tension, 229
PNH (paroxysmal nocturnal hemoglobinuria), 175
Polyarteritis nodosa (PAN), 96t, 103t, 104, 104f
Polycystic ovarian disease (PCOD), 321, 323
Polycythemia, 188
Polycythemia rubra vera, 108, 196
Polymicrogyria, 141
Polymyositis, dermatomyositis, 170
Polyps, 36
   gastric, 244

intestinal, 256
  Peutz-Jeghers syndrome, 256
Pompe disease, 64f
Porencephaly, 141, 141f
Porphyria cutanea tarda, 389
Portal hypertension, 267, 267f-268f
Postinfectious glomerulonephritis, 289t, 293, 293f
Postrenal azotemia, 284–285
Pott disease, 365
Potter sequence, 71
Prader-Willi syndrome, 68
Precursor T-cell lymphoblastic leukemia/lymphoma, 197t, 201
Preeclampsia. See Toxemia of pregnancy
Pregnancy. See Placental, pregnancy-related disorders
Prematurity
  complications of
    germinal matrix hemorrhage, 75, 75f
    hyaline membrane disease, 74–75, 74f
    necrotizing enterocolitis, 75, 75f
  fetal causes of, 74
  maternal causes of, 74
  placental causes of, 74
Prerenal azotemia, 284
Primary biliary cirrhosis, 266t, 273–274, 274f, 274t
Primary ciliary dyskinesia, 215
Primary effusion lymphoma, 201
Primary hemostasis disorders, 205
Primary (essential) hypertension, 96–97
Primary pulmonary hypertension, 99–100, 221, 221f
Primary Raynaud disease. See Raynaud phenomenon
Primary sclerosing cholangitis, 274, 274t
Primitive neuroectodermal tumor (PNET), 78, 78t, 368t, 372, 372f
Prinzmetal angina. See Variant angina
Progressive massive fibrosis, 218
Progressive multifocal leukoencephalopathy, 168
Progressive supranuclear palsy, 165–166
Prolactinoma, 338, 359
Prolymphocytic leukemia, 192
Prostate disorders
  benign prostatic hyperplasia, 314, 314f
  prostatic adenocarcinoma, 315–316, 315f
  prostatitis, acute, 314, 314f
Prostate specific antigen (PSA), 44t, 315–316
Proteus vulgaris, 301
Prothrombin gene mutation, 85
PSA. See Prostate specific antigen
Psammoma bodies, 161, 324, 347, 348f
Pseudoaneurysm. See False aneurysm
Pseudogout, 377
Pseudohermaphrodite
  female, 68
  male, 69
Pseudomembranous colitis, 247, 247f
Pseudomonas, 59, 224, 301
Pseudomyxoma peritonei, 325

Pseudo Pelger-Huët anomaly, 189
Pseudopolyps in ulcerative colitis, 252, 252f
Psoriasis, 385, 385f
PTCH (patched gene), 183
PTEN. See Phosphatase and tensin homologue
PTH (parathyroid hormone), 39, 227
Ptosis, 228
Pulmonary disorders, 210t
  abscess, 226
  atelectasis, 210
  diffuse pulmonary hemorrhage, 220–221
  field effect, 230
  general categories, 210t
  Goodpasture syndrome, 221
  hypertension, 99–100, 211, 221, 221f
  infections
    aspiration pneumonia, 224, 224f–225f
    community-acquired
      atypical, 223–224, 224f
      typical, 222–223, 222f–223f
    dimorphic fungi, 225
    immunocompromised patient, 226
    lobar pneumonia, 392, 413
    necrotizing pneumonia, 224
    nosocomial pneumonia, 224
    pneumonia
      chronic, 224
    pulmonary tuberculosis, 225, 226f
  neoplasms
    adenocarcinoma, 227, 227f–228f
    large cell carcinoma, 227, 228f
    small cell carcinoma, 227–228, 229f
    squamous cell carcinoma, 226–227, 227f
  obstructive lung disease, 210–215, 211f–215f
  obstructive pulmonary disease, chronic, 215
  pleural conditions, 223f, 228–230
  respiratory failure, acute, 209–210
  restrictive lung disease
    acute, 215–216, 216f
    chronic, 216–220, 217f–220f, 216t
  sequestration, 72
  tuberculosis, 225, 226f
  upper respiratory tract pathology, 230
Pulmonary osteoarthropathy, 215
Pulmonary thromboembolus, 86–87, 86f, 221
Pulsus paradoxus, 131–132
Pure red cell aplasia, 181, 181f
Pure vasospastic angina, 115
Purpura, 84
Purulent inflammation, 17, 17f
Purulent (pyogenic) meningitis, acute, 151, 152t
Pyelonephritis
  acute, 299–300, 299f–300f
  chronic, 300, 300f
  xanthogranulomatous, 300, 301f
Pyknosis, 5
Pyoderma gangrenosum, 389
Pyogenic osteomyelitis, 364–365, 365f

QRS alternans, 132
Queen Anne sign, 345

Rabies, 154–155
Ranson criteria, 280
Rapidly progressive glomerulonephritis (RPGN), 289t, 293–294, 293f
RAS, 42, 44
Raynaud disease, 107
Raynaud phenomenon, 107
RB. *See* Retinoblastoma
RBC. *See* Red blood cell
Red blood cell (RBC), destruction of
    antibody-mediated, 182–185, 184t
        hereditary causes, 185–187, 186f
        infectious causes, 185, 185f
Red blood cell disorders. *See* Hematopathology
Red hepatization, 223
Red (hemorrhagic) infarct, 87f, 88
    reperfusion, 88
    venous infarcts, 88
Reed-Sternberg cell, 197, 197f, 198, 198f
Reflux esophagitis. *See* Gastroesophageal reflux disease
Regurgitation
    aortic, 126–127, 122f
    mitral, 127–128, 128f
Reid index, 214
Reiter syndrome, 375
REM (roentgen-equivalent-man), 49–50
Renal artery stenosis, 96t, 97
Renal disorders. *See also* Kidney disorders,
    congenital anomalies, 73
    cysts, 302
    hepatorenal syndrome, 266
    hypertension, 96, 96t
    neoplasms
        renal cell carcinoma
            chromophobe, 303
            clear cell, 303, 303f
            papillary, 304, 304f
    osteodystrophy, 366–367
Renal failure
    acute, 283–285, 284t
    azotemia
        intrinsic, 284, 284t
        postrenal, 284–285
        prerenal, 284, 284t
    chronic, 285–286
Respiratory acidosis, alkalosis, 305
Respiratory failure, acute, 209–210
Restrictive cardiomyopathy, 130, 130f
Restrictive lung disease
    acute, 215–216, 216f
    chronic, 216–220, 216t, 217f–220f
        asbestos, 217–218, 218f
        beryllium-induced, 218
        coal-induced, 218
        hypersensitivity pneumonitis, 220

idiopathic pulmonary fibrosis, 219–220
        pneumoconioses, 217–218
        sarcoidosis, 8, 18, 129–130, 130f, 219, 220f
        silica-induced, 218, 219f
RET proto-oncogene, 41t, 42, 359–360
Retinoblastoma (RB), 43
    familial, 41t
Retinopathy, 98
Retrolental fibroplasia, 74
Reye syndrome, 265
Rhabdomyoma, 132
Rhabdomyosarcoma, 78, 78t
Rheumatic fever
    acute, 124, 124t
    Aschoff nodules, 124
    rheumatic valvulitis, chronic, 124–125, 124f–125f
    stenotic, regurgitant valvular disease, 125
Rheumatic valvulitis, chronic, 124–125, 124f–125f
Rheumatoid arthritis, 29–30, 30f, 374–375, 375f, 375t
Richter transformation, 192
Right-sided heart failure, 121–122
Rodent ulcers, 383
Roentgen-equivalent-man (REM), 49–50
Rokitansky-Aschoff sinus, 279
Rolling, 15
Rosenthal fibers, 159, 159f
Rosettes, 78, 160
Roth spots, 123
Rouleaux, 175
RPGN. *See* Rapidly progressive glomerulonephritis
Rubella, 76
Russell bodies, 203

Saccular aneurysm, 100
Salivary gland tumors, 234
Salmonella osteomyelitis, 187
Sarcoidosis, 8, 18, 129–130, 130f, 219, 220f
Saturnine gout, 377
Schaumann bodies, 219
Schiller-Duval bodies, 311
Schistocytes, 175, 206
SCID (severe combined immunodeficiency disease), 32–33
Sclerosing adenosis, 331t, 332
Seborrheic dermatitis, 385–386
Seborrheic keratosis, 381, 382f
Secondary hemochromatosis, 273
Secondary hemostasis
    hemophilia A, 208
    hemophilia B, 208
    von Willebrand disease, 208
Secondary hypertension, 97
    cardiovascular causes, 96, 96t
    endocrine causes, 96, 96t
    neurologic causes, 96, 96t
    renal causes, 96, 96t
    stress-induced causes, 96
Secondary Parkinsonism, 165
Second intention, 21

Secondary Raynaud disease. *See* Raynaud phenomenon
Seizures, 136–137, 349
    absence, 137
    epilepsy, 136–137
Semilobar holoprosencephaly, 141
Seminoma, 311, 311*f*
Senile (neuritic) plaques, 162, 163*f*
Septic shock, 89–90
    superantigen, 90
Sequestration crises, 187
Sequestrum, 365
Serous inflammation, 17
Serous ovarian tumors, 324, 324*f*–325*f*
Severe combined immunodeficiency disease (SCID),
        32–33
Sex chromosome abnormalities, 67–68
Sexual differentiation disorders, 68–69
Sézary syndrome, 202
Shagreen patch, 58
Sheehan syndrome, 340
Shock
    anaphylactic, 90
    cardiogenic, 89, 118, 118*f*
    complications of
        corticomedullary hemorrhage, 91
        diffuse alveolar damage, 90
        gastric petechial hemorrhage, acute, 91, 91*f*
        global hypoxic-ischemic encephalopathy, 90, 90*f*
        necrosis
            acute tubular, 90–91
            centrilobular, 90, 90*f*
            subendocardial contraction band, 90
    hypovolemic, 89
    neurogenic, 90
    septic, 89–90
    stages of, 91
SIADH. *See* Syndrome of inappropriate antidiuretic hormone
Sickle cell anemia, 186–187, 186*f*, 300
Sideroblastic anemia, 178
SIDS (sudden infant death syndrome), 77
Signet-ring cell adenocarcinoma, 244, 245*f*
Simple renal cysts, 302
Sipple syndrome, 358–359
Sjögren syndrome, 30, 202
Skeletal muscle disorders
    inclusion body myositis, 171
    Lambert-Eaton syndrome, 171–172
    myasthenia gravis, 171
    polymyositis, dermatomyositis, 170
Skin. *See* Dermatopathology
SLE. *See* Systemic lupus erythematosus
SLL (small lymphocytic lymphoma), 192, 200
SMAD, 44
Small cell carcinoma, 227–228, 229*f*
Small lymphocytic lymphoma (SLL), 192, 200
Smudge cells, 193
Spermatocytic seminoma, 313
Spherocytes, 175, 186

Spina bifida, 139–140
Spina bifida occulta, 139
Spinal muscular atrophy, 166
Splenomegaly, 195, 267
Spongiform encephalopathies, 155–156
Squamous cell carcinoma
    cervix, 316–317
    cutaneous, 382–383
    esophageal, 239–240
    larynx, 230
    oral cavity, 234
    penis, 313
    pulmonary, 226, 227*f*
Squamous intraepithelial lesion, 316–317
Stable angina, 113–114, 114*f*
Stab wound, 50
Stage of tumor, 46
Staghorn calculi, 301, 301*f*
Staphylococcus, aureus, 59, 203, 222, 224, 293, 317, 388
Steatorrhea, 248–249
Steatosis, 9, 9*f*
    macrovesicular, 262
    microvesicular, 262
Stein-Leventhal syndrome, 323
STEMI (ST segment elevation myocardial infarct),
        116–117, 116*f*
Stenosis
    aortic, 112, 125–126
    mitral, 127
Stenotic, regurgitant valvular disease, 125
Stevens-Johnson syndrome, 384, 384*f*
Stillbirth, 326
Streptococcus pneumoniae, 151–152, 152f, 203, 222–223, 293,
        297, 317, 388
Stroke, 142
Struma ovarii, 344
Struvite stones, 301, 301*f*
Sturge-Weber syndrome, 358
Subacute combined degeneration, 179
Subacute thyroiditis, 346–347
Subarachnoid hemorrhage, 148, 150*f*
Subdural hemorrhage, 146–147, 149*f*
Subendocardial contraction band necrosis, 90
Subependymal giant cell astrocytoma, 58, 58*f*
Subpial sparing, 145*f*
Sudden infant death syndrome (SIDS), 77
Superior vena cava syndrome, 228
Superoxide dismutase, 4
Sydenham chorea, 124, 124*t*
Syndrome of inappropriate antidiuretic hormone (SIADH),
        40, 286, 341–342
Syphilis, 76
Syphilitic aortitis, 76, 100–101
Systemic disease, cutaneous manifestations
    ecthyma gangrenosum, 389
    necrobiosis lipoidica, 389
    porphyria cutanea tarda, 389
    pyoderma gangrenosum, 389

Systemic hypertension, 2f, 96
    complications of
        aortic dissection, 98–99, 99f–100f
        arteriolosclerosis, 98
            hyaline, 98, 98f
            hyperplastic, 98, 98f
        atherosclerosis, 97
        cardiac hypertrophy, 98
        intracerebral hemorrhage, 98
        retinopathy, 98
    chronic, 97
    eclampsia, 97, 330–331
    gestational, 97
    HELLP syndrome, 97, 331
    idiopathic, 97
    malignant, 97
    preeclampsia, 97, 330–331
    primary, 96
    secondary, 96, 96t
Systemic lupus erythematosus (SLE), 28–29, 131t, 132, 294
    antiphospholipid antibody syndrome, 29
    drug-induced lupus, 29
    Libman-Sacks endocarditis, 28
Systemic sclerosis, 30, 130

t(8;14), 197t, 201
t(8;21), 191t, 193t, 194
t(9;22), 191t, 192, 195
t(15;17), 191t, 193t, 194
Tabes dorsalis, 76
Takayasu arteritis, 103–104, 103t, 104f
Tamm-Horsfall protein, 298
Target cells, 175
Tay-Sachs disease, 63
TB. See Tuberculosis; Tuberculous entries
Telomerase, 11
Temporal arteritis. See Giant cell arteritis
Teratoma, 76f, 312
    immature, 312
    mature, 312
    mature cystic, 325–326, 327f
Testicular neoplasms, 309–310
    choriocarcinoma, 312, 312f
    embryonal carcinoma, 311
    germ cell tumors, 310, 310t
    intratubular germ cell neoplasia, 311
    lymphoma, 313
    seminoma, 311, 311f
    spermatocytic seminoma, 313
    teratoma, 312
    yolk sac tumor, 311, 311f
Tetralogy of Fallot, 110
TGF-β (transforming growth factor β), 44
Thalassemias, 176t, 177–178, 178f
    major, 177
    minor, 177
Thin basement membrane disease, 196
Thromboangiitis obliterans, 103t, 105

Thrombotic thrombocytopenic purpura (TTP), 185, 206
Thrombus 85–86, 86f
    fates of thrombi, 85
    hereditary conditions
        factor V Leiden mutation, 85
        prothrombin gene mutation, 85
    predispositions, 85
Thymoma, 181, 181f
Thyroid disorders
    Graves disease, 344, 344f, 400, 416
    hyperthyroidism, 343–344, 343t
    hypothyroidism, 343t, 345–346, 346f
    neoplasms, 347–349, 347f–349f
        anaplastic carcinoma, 349, 349f
        follicular adenoma/carcinoma, 347–348, 348f
        medullary thyroid carcinoma, 348–349, 349f, 359–360
        papillary thyroid carcinoma, 347, 347f
    thyroiditis, 346–347
    thyroid storm, 344
Tophi, 376, 376f
Torsion of testis, 313
Toxemia of pregnancy, 97, 330–331
Toxic epidermal necrolysis, 385, 385f
Toxic megacolon, 233
Toxic substances
    carbon monoxide, 49, 49f
    cigarette smoke, 47
    cocaine, 48
    cyanide, 49
    ethanol, 48, 271–272, 271f–272f
        Korsakoff syndrome, 48
        Wernicke encephalopathy, 48, 48f
    ionizing radiation, REM exposure, 49–50
    lead, 49
Tracheoesophageal fistula, 72
Tram-track, 294
Transcalvarial herniation, 139
Transforming growth factor-β (TGF-β), 44
Transient ischemic attack, 142
Transitional cell carcinoma. See Urothelial neoplasm
Transmigration, 15
Transplantation disorders, rejection of
    cellular, 26, 26f
    chronic, 26
    humoral, 26
    hyperacute, 26
Transudate, 83, 229
Tricuspid atresia, 110–111
Trisomy 13. See Patau syndrome
Trisomy 18. See Edward syndrome
Trisomy 21. See Down syndrome
Tropical sprue, 249
Troponin I, 117
Trousseau sign, 350
Trousseau syndrome, 281
True hermaphrodite, 68
Truncus arteriosus, 111
TTP (thrombotic thrombocytopenic purpura), 185, 206

Tuberculosis, pulmonary, 225, 226t
Tuberculous meningitis, 152–153, 153f
Tuberculous osteomyelitis, 365
Tuberous sclerosis, 58, 58f
Tubulointerstitial disease, 296–297
    acute, 297
    acute interstitial nephritis 297, 297f
    acute tubular necrosis, 90–91, 298, 298f
    chronic, 297–298
Tumor lysis syndrome, 201
Turner syndrome, 67, 67f, 318, 346
22q11.2 deletion, 66–67
    DiGeorge syndrome, 66
    velocardiofacial syndrome, 66
Two-hit hypothesis, 43

Ulcerative colitis, 250t, 252–253, 252f, 389
Uncal (transtentorial) herniation, 139, 139f
Unstable angina, 113–115, 115f
Upper respiratory tract disorders, 230
Uremia, 131, 131f, 131t, 285–286
Ureter obstruction, 305
Uric acid stones, 301
Urothelial neoplasm, 304–305, 304f–305f
Urticaria. See Hives
Usual interstitial pneumonia, 219–220
Uterine disorders
    bleeding, abnormal, 320
    fibroids, 322–323, 323f
    nonneoplastic, 319–321, 319f–321f
    tumors, 321–323, 322f, 323f
        endometrial adenocarcinoma, 321–322, 322f
        endometrial stromal sarcoma, 323
        leiomyoma, 322, 323f
        leiomyosarcoma, 323
        neoplasms, other, 323

Vacuolar myelopathy, 34
Vaginal adenosis, 316
Vaginal tumors, 316
Valvular disease
    aortic, 125–127, 125f–126f
    general, 122–125, 122f–125f
    mitral, 127–128, 128f
    stenotic, regurgitant, 125
Variant angina, 115
Varicocele, 313
Vascular disorders, 93
    aneurysms, 100–101, 100f–101f
    aortic dissection, 98–99, 99f–100f
    arteriosclerosis, 93
    arteriovenous fistula, 101
    atherosclerosis, 93–95, 94f–95f
    ischemic bowel disease, 253–254, 253f
    malformations
        arteriovenous malformation, 141
        capillary angioma, 142
        cavernous angioma, 142

pulmonary hypertension, 99–100
Raynaud phenomenon, 107
systemic hypertension, 96–99, 96t, 98f–100f
tumors
    angiosarcoma, 107
    hemangioma, 106
    Kaposi sarcoma, 106–107
vasculitis, 102–106, 103f–104f, 103t
Vasculitides, major, 102, 103t
    Buerger disease, 103t, 105
    Churg-Strauss syndrome, 106
    giant cell arteritis (temporal arteritis), 103, 103f–104f, 103t
    Kawasaki disease, 103t, 105
    microscopic polyarteritis, 105
    polyarteritis nodosa, 103t, 104, 104f
    Takayasu arteritis, 103–104, 103t, 104f
    Wegener granulomatosis, 103t, 104–105
Vasculitis
    ANCA-mediated, 102
    direct antibody interaction-mediated, 102
    immune complex deposition-mediated, 102
    major vasculitides. See Vasculitides, major
Velocardiofacial syndrome, 66
Veno-occlusive disease of the liver, 275
Venous infarct, 88
Ventricular septal defect (VSD), 110–111, 111f
Verrucae vulgaris, 388
Vertigo, 136
VHL syndrome. See von Hippel-Lindau syndrome
Viral hepatitis, 268f–269f, 269–270, 269t, 270f
Viral meningitis, 151–153
Virchow node, 228
Virchow triad, 85
Vitamin deficiencies, 52, 52t, 179–180, 180t
    B_1 (thiamine), 52
    B_2 (riboflavin), 52
    B_3 (niacin), 52
    B_6 (pyridoxine), 52
    B_{12}, 52, 179–180, 180f, 180t
    folate, 52, 180, 180f, 180t
    vitamin A, 52, 52t
    vitamin C, 52t, 53
    vitamin D, 52t, 53
    vitamin E, 52t, 53
    vitamin K, 52t, 53, 53f
Vitiligo, 379
Volume disorders, 286
Volvulus, 253, 253f
von Gierke disease, 63
von Hippel-Lindau (VHL syndrome), 41t, 44, 57, 304
von Willebrand disease, 208
VSD (ventricular septal defect), 110–111, 111f

WAGR syndrome, 79
Waldenström macroglobulinemia, 204
Wallerian degeneration, 169
Waterhouse-Friderichsen syndrome, 152, 357, 357f
Wegener granulomatosis, 102, 103t, 104–105

Wermer syndrome, 359
Werner syndrome, 11
Wernicke aphasia, 135
Wernicke encephalopathy, 48, 48f, 52
Werdnig-Hoffmann disease, 166
Wet beriberi, 52, 52t, 121
Whipple disease, 253
White (anemic) infarct, 88, 88f
White blood cell disorders. *See* Hematopathology
Wilms tumor, 79, 79f
    Beckwith-Wiedemann syndrome, 80
    Denys-Drash syndrome, 80
    WAGR syndrome, 79
Wilson disease, 61, 273, 276
    Kayser-Fleischer rings, 61

Wiskott-Aldrich syndrome, 33
Woltman sign, 345
Wound, incised, 50

Xanthogranulomatous pyelonephritis, 300,
    301f
Xeroderma pigmentosa, 41t
X-linked agammaglobulinemia of Bruton, 31–32
X-linked inheritance patterns, 64–65

Yolk sac tumor, 311, 311f

Zellballen pattern, 359
Zenker diverticulum, 239
Zollinger-Ellison syndrome, 243